PSYCHOSOCIAL CARE OF THE PHYSICALLY ILL

SECOND EDITION

PSYCHOSOCIAL CARE OF THE PHYSICALLY ILL

what every nurse should know

Vickie A. Lambert, R.N., D.N.Sc.
Medical College of Georgia

Clinton E. Lambert, Jr., R.N., M.S.N., C.S.
Dwight David Eisenhower Army Medical Center

Prentice-Hall, Inc., Englewood Cliffs, N.J. 07632

Library of Congress Cataloging in Publication Data

LAMBERT, VICKIE A.
   Psychosocial care of the physically ill.

   Includes bibliographies and index.
   1. Nurse and patient. 2. Sick—Psychology.
I. Lambert, Clinton E. II. Title. [DNLM:
   1. Nursing Care. 2. Patients—psychology—
nurses' instruction. WY 100 L222p]
RT86.3.L36 1985   610.73   84-16019
ISBN 0-13-736869-0

Editorial/production supervision
  and interior design: Fay Ahuja
Cover design: Wanda Lubelska
Manufacturing buyer: John B. Hall

Previously published under the title *The Impact of Physical Illness*.

Printed in the United States of America

10 9 8 7 6 5 4 3 2 1

ISBN 0-13-736869-0   01

Prentice-Hall International, Inc., *London*
Prentice-Hall of Australia Pty. Limited, *Sydney*
Editora Prentice-Hall do Brasil, Ltda., *Rio de Janeiro*
Prentice-Hall Canada Inc., *Toronto*
Prentice-Hall of India Private Limited, *New Delhi*
Prentice-Hall of Japan, Inc., *Tokyo*
Prentice-Hall of Southeast Asia Pte. Ltd., *Singapore*
Whitehall Books Limited, *Wellington, New Zealand*

To our daughter
ALEXANDRA KRISTINA
"Lexy"

CONTENTS

CHAPTER 10 MYOCARDIAL INFARCTION   176

CHAPTER 11 CHRONIC OBSTRUCTIVE PULMONARY DISEASE   206

PREFACE

The necessity of dealing with physically ill adults as holistic beings has become an increasingly important focus in comprehensive nursing care. Existing nursing literature has not adequately addressed the importance of psychosocial aspects as they relate to physical illness. Therefore, the purpose of this book is to demonstrate how the nurse and other health care providers can integrate, with ease, psychosocial concepts into the care of physically ill adults.

The book has been divided into two parts: Psychosocial Concepts and Coping with Specific Physical Illnesses. In Part I, three major concepts are discussed: the wellness/illness role, body image, and loss. An understanding of these concepts and their effects on the adult during the course of illness is vital to those who provide health care since the concepts are applied to material presented in later chapters.

In Part II of this book, specific physical illnesses are addressed and methods for the application of psychosocial concepts when caring for individuals with these illnesses are carefully delineated. The illnesses presented are those which we believe are encountered frequently by nurses and other health care providers.

The text demonstrates how each of the physical illnesses presented can impact upon the afflicted person in terms of the individual's psychological well-being, somatic identity, sexuality, occupational identity, and social role. Psychosocial problems incurred in conjunction with each of these areas of impact are presented and modalities for dealing with these problems are described in detail. To further aid in demonstrating how psychosocial concepts can be integrated into the care of the adult with a specific physical illness, we have provided, at the end of each chapter in Part II, a hypothetical patient situation with a corresponding nursing care plan and patient care cardex. Also at the end of each chapter is a list of references for further reading. It is our intent that this text, with its integrated approach to psychosocial care of the physically ill adult, will assist the student and the practitioner of nursing in diagnosing psychosocial problems incurred as a result of physical illness and in planning, developing, and initiating appropriate nursing care measures.

Vickie A. Lambert, R.N., D.N.Sc.
Clinton E. Lambert, Jr., R.N., M.S.N., C.S.

ACKNOWLEDGMENT

We wish to express our appreciation to Martha Temples for her loyal assistance in the preparation of the manuscript.

NOTE

The opinions or assertions contained herein are the private views of the authors and are not to be construed as official or as reflecting the views of the Department of the Army or the Department of Defense.

PSYCHOSOCIAL CARE OF THE PHYSICALLY ILL

part I: psychosocial concepts

1 ||||||||||||||||||||||||||||||||||||||||||||||||||||||||

WELLNESS/ILLNESS ROLE

INTRODUCTION

People are complex beings consisting of many parts. Each person is physiological, cultural, religious, and psychosocial. In order for people to be dealt with as holistic beings, nursing needs to become increasingly aware of how their many parts contribute to an optimal state of wellness. When individuals become ill or undergo diagnosis for altered states of health, their complex parts contribute to their reactions to illness. For example, how individuals react to illness may depend upon their self-perception and how they believe others view them and the existing illness. For some individuals, illness is more a way of life than wellness. The presence of illness often provides a vehicle for both primary and secondary gain. Recognition by the family that one is ill might represent a primary gain since the tension or conflict of thinking one is ill has been reduced (Freedman, Kaplan, and Sadock, 1980). The increased attention, flowers, and gifts might demonstrate secondary gains. Thus, illness often becomes a means toward an end for self-recognition.

In an attempt to achieve self-recognition in our complex and ever changing society, one is constantly expected to assume a variety of roles. Role assumptions are necessary for survival in today's demanding world. Commonly accepted societal roles include breadwinner, family member, community leader, and spiritual advisor. One is expected to take on a set role during both the state of wellness and the course of illness.

An individual assumes the state of wellness when an optimal level of physiological function and psychosocial integrity is attained in relationship to his or her particular stage of growth and development within the lifeline. By

1

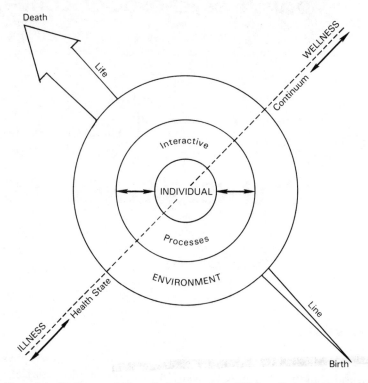

Figure 1.1   Wellness and Illness in Relation to the Lifeline. From Vickie A. Lambert, Clinton E. Lambert, The impact of physical illness and related mental health concepts, © 1979, p. 344. Reprinted by permission of Prentice-Hall, Inc., Englewood Cliffs, N.J.

KEY

INDIVIDUAL: A continuously emerging bio-psychosocial being who is constantly interacting with his or her environment.

ENVIRONMENT: The aggregate of things, conditions, and influences which impinge upon the individual's health.

INTERACTIVE
PROCESSES: All interchanges in which the individual engages.

HEALTH STATE
CONTINUUM: The varying and ever changing course of an individual's level of wellness and illness.

WELLNESS: The optimal level of an individual's physiological function and psychosocial integrity in relationship to his or her stage of growth and development within the life line.

ILLNESS: An alteration in physiological function and/or psychosocial integrity which impedes an individual's ability to achieve an optimal level of performance.

LIFELINE: An individual's growth and development trajectory.

BIRTH: An individual's emergence into the world.

DEATH: An individual's cessation of life.

comparison, the state of illness emerges when an alteration in physiological function and/or psychosocial integrity occurs and impedes the person's ability to achieve an optimal level of performance. As depicted in Figure 1.1, individuals (as they interact with the environment) progress unidirectionally from birth to death along the lifeline. At the same time, they move back and forth between the state of wellness and the state of illness on the health state continuum. In order for the professional nurse to provide in-depth care, he or she needs to be cognizant of the basic theories utilized in explaining and predicting the behaviors related to the wellness/illness role.

WELLNESS/ILLNESS ROLE

Guidelines for understanding the wellness/illness role have evolved from two major schools of thought: functionalism and interactionalism. Functionalism has dealt *exclusively* with the component of illness and has provided sets of rules and norms for guiding appropriate behavior. The emphasis of this approach has been on systems of interrelated roles (Nadel, 1957). By comparison, interactionalism has dealt with both wellness and illness and links these two components to a reciprocal interrelationship of roles that do not identify norms or rules for guiding or describing appropriate behavior (Mead, 1934; Turner, 1962).

Over the past three decades, nurses have tended to utilize functionalism as the major framework for guiding their understanding of the role of illness. Nurses now tend to rely more upon interactionalism as the theoretical basis for guiding their practice and research (Lambert & Lambert, 1981; Dracup & Meleis, 1982; Meleis & Swendson, 1978) since it provides a framework for describing both wellness and illness behavior. Since both functionalism and interactionalism continue to be used, each approach will be presented in conjunction with the contributions it makes for explaining behavior as it relates to the state of illness.

Functional Approach to the Illness Component of the Wellness/Illness Role

The major functionalist cited in describing illness behavior has been Parsons (1951). Parsons has identified four components to his "sick role theory": (1) exemption from social responsibility; (2) inability to achieve wellness simply by decision or will; (3) obligation to seek wellness; and (4) responsibility to seek and cooperate with technically competent assistance.

The first component characterizes the individual as being exempt from his or her usual social responsibilities. The degree of exemption, however, is related to the nature and severity of the illness. Examples of this might include the decrease or total release of accountability in carrying out family or job requirements. Illnesses that are familiar to the general public are more likely to be accepted as an exemption from responsibilities than are illnesses that are unfamiliar. This may be seen in the comparison of society's understanding of coronary disease versus diseases of the integumentary system. The advertising media has stressed the do's and don'ts of heart disease to such a degree that most individuals comprehend with little negative reaction some of the necessary restrictions of an individual who has coronary problems. An individual who has lesions on the skin, however, may not receive the same positive understanding about health care restrictions because society lacks knowledge about this particular problem. Before the exemption from social responsibility is complete, legitimization of the illness is necessary, and members of the health team serve as the major legitimatizing agents. Once a health team member has acknowledged the existence of a health problem, the existence of the illness is legitimatized for society. One of the most typical statements made concerning legitimization is, "Have you been to see a physician?"

The second component of the sick role is the individual's inability to achieve wellness by an act of decision or will. Illness then becomes a state of "no-fault" on the part of the individual. This second component of the sick role also implies an exemption from responsibility and the necessity of seeking assistance in order to alleviate or modify the condition. Identification of the fact that the individual has lost control of his or her situation is crucial in bridging the gap between the recognized illness and the acceptance of assistance (Parsons, 1951).

The third component of the sick role is the obligation of the individual to want to be well. The state of illness is a negatively acquired role, and one is obliged to set such a deviated role into a positive state, the state of wellness. Society tends to frown upon the individual who walks about in a state of illness and does not try to attain wellness. This is particularly true in the case of a communicable disease such as the common cold. The individual is obligated not to disseminate the illness to others and to seek a state of wellness.

The fourth and final component of the sick role is closely related to the element of obligation to achieve wellness. This fourth component of the sick role requires the individual to obtain technically competent assistance and to cooperate with the administrator of that assistance in the process of achieving a state of wellness. It is at this point that the ill individual becomes a complementary component in the health team structure.

The definition of what constitutes a technically competent health care provider varies among cultures and subcultures within our society. Judgment of proper selection of assistance should be based upon these cultural definitions (Bullough & Bullough, 1982). For example, the black patient may resort to using the special herbs, oils, and ointments of the root doctor while the Latin patient may seek the prayers, rituals, and the laying on of hands of the curandero (folk healer). The nurse must be competent in identifying these cultural differences in health care selection and make available to the individual appropriate avenues of assistance to insure meaningful health care.

In dealing with the individual in the state of illness, the seeking of assistance is simply one aspect of the fourth component of the sick role. In order for health care therapies to be successful, the patient must cooperate in the implementation of these therapies. It is most assuredly the role of the professional nurse to understand individual and cultural differences that may affect the patient's cooperation in the execution of optional health care (Spector, 1979). For example, a person of Italian ancestry has sought guidance in obtaining an appropriate diet for weight control. The person is given a diet that includes the necessary caloric restrictions. The patient notices that the diet generally decreases the amount of pasta that can be consumed and finds this restriction difficult to accept because of the importance placed on pasta. Unless the person truly understands and accepts the necessity for this restriction, the person may fail to carry out the necessary decrease in caloric intake. Thus, the execution of optimal health care therapy is rendered unsuccessful.

The four components of Parsons' sick role theory (exemption from social responsibility; inability to achieve wellness, simply be decision or will; obligation to seek wellness; and responsibility to seek technically competent assistance and cooperation with this assistance) provide a framework for understanding patterns of behavior during an individual's assimilation of the illness role.

However, Parson's theory has limitations in its applicability to certain physical illness situations. For example, it is not useful or appropriate for understanding patterns of behavior related to the physically ill individual with a chronic disease or a disability (Segall, 1976). Being a functional theory, Parsons' sick role theory mandates that the ill individual be exempt from social responsibility as a result of his or her condition and be obliged to seek wellness since illness is a negatively acquired role. The chronically ill and/or physically disabled person rarely is exempt from social responsibility or is obliged to seek a state of total wellness since both of these health care states are permanent and are caused by irreversible pathological processes (McKinley, 1972). The chronically ill and/or physically disabled individual generally is encouraged to meet as many of his or her social obligations as possible. Recommending that one not rely upon illness or disability as an exemption from responsibility is a primary focus of rehabilitative health care.

Seeking a state of total wellness is not feasible with the chronically ill and/or physically disabled person since *complete* removal or recovery from the illness or disability is impossible. Attempting to attain and maintain an *optimal* level of health within the context of the chronic illness and physical disability is more realistic. Thus Parsons' sick role theory serves best as a guideline for understanding illness behavior related to physical ailments which are acute rather than chronic in nature.

Interactional Approach to the Wellness/Illness Role

The interactional approach to the wellness/illness role stresses a reciprocal interrelationship of roles where each actor regulates his or her behavior and reactions dependent upon what is expected from other individuals (Turner, 1978). In other words, roles are perceived as relationships between what a person does and what others do.

According to two interactionalists, Lindesmith and Strauss (1968), in order for a person to enact a role (such as the wellness/illness role) the four following components must be present: (1) an identification of self; (2) behavior appropriate to the given situation; (3) a background of related acts by others (counter-roles) that serve as cues to guide specific performance; and (4) an evaluation by the individual, and by others, of the role enactment.

Enacting the wellness/illness role from the interactionalists' point of view does not involve a single, unvarying routine. The individual must identify "self" by going outside the self and viewing the self from the perspectives of significant others. Thus the individual assumes a set of organized attitudes about his or her state of health and responds to these attitudes. These attitudes evolve from the attitudes of the organized community of social groups that give the individual an identity of "self."

To enact the wellness/illness role one needs to name, categorize, and catalogue prior situations, scenes, and episodes. If this is not done, appropriate behavior for the health state cannot occur. Granted, no two situations are alike; however, adequate resemblance between the present state of health and one formerly encountered allows for the recognition and enactment of expected behavior.

No role can be enacted without an understanding of the "contrasting" or counter-role (Turner, 1962). For example, the patient role makes no sense without its counter-role, the health care provider, since both roles are formulated and evaluated by each other. The relationship that occurs between the patient role and the health care provider role is continually changing and emerging. An individual who misunderstands the counter-role is likely to enact his or her role in an invalid manner. If the ill individual incorrectly interprets the role of the professional nurse, then his or her illness behavior is likely to be enacted inappropriately.

Wellness/illness role enactment is incomplete unless ensuing behavior is evaluated both by the individual and by relevant others. Evaluation can lead to role maintenance or to a change in role behavior. Meleis (1975) states that a change in one's role behavior generally reflects a changed assessment or perception of the role by the individual or by relevant others. Thus the interactional approach to the wellness/illness role involves learning, reciprocal interaction, change, and growth.

The four components of the interactional approach to the illness role (identification of self; behavior appropriate to the given situation; counter-roles; and role enactment evaluation) provide a basis for understanding behavior during the enactment of the wellness/illness role. Unlike Parsons' sick role theory, the interactional approach to the wellness/illness role does not mandate a set of rules or norms for governing role behavior. Neither a sense of dictation nor a sense of conformity in role performance exists. The interactional approach to the wellness/illness role is flexible and non-constricting. It takes into account personal, cultural, and societal aspects which influence health behavior. Thus the interactional approach to the wellness/illness role can provide guidelines for understanding patterns of behavior related to wellness and/or acute or chronic physical illness.

COPING BEHAVIORS SEEN DURING DIAGNOSIS AND ILLNESS

During enactment and incorporation of the illness component of the wellness/illness role, individuals often demonstrate a variety of coping behaviors. These behaviors serve the important function of relieving stress, protecting self-esteem, and assisting the individual in dealing with problems connected with the stress of illness (Cohen & Lazarus, 1979). The manner and degree to which these behaviors are exercised may vary among individuals. Some individuals need few psychological mechanisms in dealing with illness, others require a host of mechanisms, and there are some who, even with the use of all of their adaptive mechanisms (Kolb, 1982), never come to accept the illness component of the wellness/illness role.

The nurse must assess where the individual stands in relation to his or her assimilation of the illness component of the wellness/illness role in order to appropriately plan and initiate nursing care. Important issues to incorporate in this assessment are the person's: 1) knowledge about the specific illness and its related therapies; 2) understanding of possible required alterations in usual activities of daily living; and 3) adherence and active participation in necessary health care therapies. Using this data, the nurse decides the appropriate intervention. If the individual is having difficulty accepting the fact that health assistance is needed, the nurse may have to intervene and, with the patient, attempt to identify this fact. An individual may seek assistance, faithfully carry out health care instructions, and then suddenly stop all necessary health care therapies. In this case, the nurse may have to assist the patient in identifying his or her reason for the sudden cessation of therapy. This assistance needs to be in the form of a supportive, non-judgmental approach whereby the rights of the individual to make decisions about his or her health care are recognized. However, the patient should be encouraged to identify the rationale for the prescribed therapy and to investigate alternative options if cessation of therapy is to continue. The lack of desirable behavior may suggest that ambiguities exist in the health care situation, and these ambiguities are restricting the individual's awareness of what is expected (Meleis, 1975). Thus, it can be seen that individuals vary both in their ability to assume and to maintain the illness component of the wellness/illness role.

The following discussion will deal with some of the human responses that might be seen in individuals who are attempting to cope with their newly defined state of illness.

Anxiety

The most commonly occurring human response to illness and diagnosis is anxiety. Anxiety can be described as the uneasiness, apprehension, or dread that is associated with an unrecognizable source of anticipated danger. It differs from fear in that with fear an identifiable source of danger can be designated (Freedman, Kaplan, and Sadock, 1980). One can be afraid of dogs, crowds, elevators, or lightning; however, one may not be aware of why he fears illness. Anxiety is essentially a human experience that is ever present and has always been a part of our human existence. It is the result of conflicts and frustrations in our daily lives, and it is a lifelong partner that one can either use constructively or succumb to its destructive forces.

When assuming the state of illness, individuals are not always capable of determining the source of danger in their lives; consequently, anxiety can occur. Illness is both physically and mentally taxing and unknowns are ever present. Questions that come to the mind of the ill individual may include: "Why do I feel this way?" "What is wrong with me?" "How do ill people act?" "Should I seek medical attention?"

The degree and duration of anxiety demonstrated by each individual vary. The nurse may identify the presence of an anxiety-provoking situation for the patient, such as an impending hospitalization, and notes that individuals of the same sex, age, and socioeconomic status will react entirely differently. Each individual's perception of the same anxiety-provoking situation produces entirely different individual responses. Each response depends upon past experiences, learning, and the degree of emotional maturation. The results of such unpleasant feelings can be manifested in a variety of both physical and mental states. The nurse may identify a quavering voice, increased perspiration, breathlessness, pacing, and hand wringing. The individual may note difficulty in concentrating and tend to lose track of the environment. These physiological and psychological manifestations are just a few of the human responses to anxiety.

The indvidual's level of anxiety must be identified before efficient and effective health care therapies can be successfully instituted. Mild to moderate degrees of anxiety can be an asset to successful adaptation in life. When one is moderately anxious, one is more aware of environmental surroundings and is more receptive to learning. Such an aroused state can be conducive to patient learning (Mischel, 1981). The individual who is mildly anxious about learning the procedure of insulin injection is more likely to be attentive to details in aseptic technique than the individual who is apathetic or extremely anxious.

As the level of anxiety increases, however, one loses the capability to function efficiently over a period of time (Mischel, 1981). In most instances, one is unable to tolerate feelings of high anxiety for sustained periods of time and attempts are made to terminate the anxiety in any way possible. As anxiety increases, one's perceptual field is reduced. The overly anxious individual loses track of time, space, and the meaning of environmental events. Situations become distorted and simple happenings may be blown out of proportion. For example, a patient may become verbally loud and abusive to the nurse because a drinking straw has been omitted from the dietary tray. Heightened anxiety may produce panic and the individual's attention is so scattered that goal-directed activity is impossible (Luckmann and Sorenson, 1980). When anxiety is recognized, the nurse must refocus the patient's coping behavior so that more therapeutic coping modes may be implemented. This can be accomplished by providing privacy, demonstrating competent care, and giving feedback regarding the individual's actions. Such interventions aid in facilitating the individual's progression toward a state of wellness on the health care continuum.

During high anxiety both verbal and nonverbal communication is imperative. Communications should be brief and simple since individuals experiencing anxiety often have difficulties comprehending details of their surroundings. When the nurse directs the spouse of the surgical patient to the family waiting room the morning of surgery, the nurse should give clear, concise, and uncomplicated directions. If the directions are too complex, most likely the spouse will not comprehend all of what is being said because of the level of anxiety caused by the fear of the unknown about the patient's surgery.

To summarize, anxiety is a universal reaction to illness that must be dealt with by both the patient and the nurse. The level of anxiety demonstrated is individualized and the manner in which it can be channelled varies from person to person. It should be realized that the existence of anxiety can be either an asset or a liability to the successful institution of health care therapies.

Denial

One of the ways in which an individual copes with a stress-producing situation, such as illness, is to deny the existence of the threat. Denial operates to allay anxiety by decreasing perception of the threat. The tendency of the individual to deny the existence or the seriousness of an illness is one example frequently seen by health care deliverers.

Denial is a coping behavior that indicates the failure to acknowledge either the existence of a known fact or its significance. Various steps are involved in the denying behavior. First, a reality situation exists and the individual either perceives or anticipates some component of the situation as a threat. Second, anxiety transpires in response to the perceived threat. Next, the individual either completely or partially disclaims the facts or their significance in the threat-producing situation. In the last step of the denying behavior, the individual ignores or rejects data connected with the threatening situation in an attempt to regain and maintain psychological equilibrium (Kiening, 1978a).

As one examines the response of denial, it can be seen that it merely minimizes the anxiety-producing components of reality that comprise the threat. The use of denial may act as a temporary protector of the ego by preventing the individual from becoming totally overcome by anxiety (Kiening, 1978). However, an adult's frank denial of obvious reality over a long period of time may indicate a more serious mental health disturbance.

In order to therapeutically intervene when denial occurs, the nurse must first be capable of recognizing manifestations of this coping behavior. These manifestations may be either subtle or explicit. The individual may be the quiet, "model" patient who never expresses doubt that his or her life-style has contributed to the recurrence of the ulcer. The individual may, on the other hand, be obnoxiously verbal and refuse medications stating that there is nothing wrong.

After identifying the patient's usage of denial, the nurse needs to determine the degree to which the denial hinders the individual's progress toward wellness. Is denial preventing the individual from seeking much needed health assistance or is it allowing the individual time to regain his or her composure in dealing with the shocking emotional experience? It is essential for the nurse to be aware that total realization and acceptance of an emotionally charged experience are never accomplished at once.

After the degree of denial is determined, the nurse should attempt to understand the need that this coping behavior serves for the specific individual. Why is this individual using denial? Possibly the existence of the state of illness is threatening the feeling of security, or the presence of illness may carry with it the anxiety of possible loss. (The reader is advised to consult Chapter 3.)

The nurse needs to make a professional decision on how to deal with an individual's behavior based upon the manifestations of denial, the degree to which denial is utilized, and the need that denial serves. It is essential for the nurse to keep in mind that psychosocial support of the individual demands a high priority in nursing intervention so that ego integrity can be maintained. The mechanism of denial should not be attacked directly while it is providing ego support. The nurse needs to explore the means available to the individual that would serve to decrease the anxiety at this time and hence to decrease the need for denial. This may be typified by a new postoperative patient who blatantly refuses pain medication and verbally denies being in pain. However, the patient has just experienced very extensive surgery, has a markedly increased pulse rate, and is extremely restless. The nurse should avoid directly attacking the patient's denial by abruptly saying, "Don't kid me, I know you are having pain!" Such a statement can be a threat to one's ego integrity. An approach that may serve the patient in a more therapeutic manner is to point out that the patient appears restless and uncomfortable and the pain medication will relieve some of the discomfort. The nurse at this point has not supported the patient's denial of pain yet the denial has not been directly attacked. Instead the individual has been given the opportunity to maintain ego integrity while being provided with the option of either admitting or denying his or her pain. In addition, the nurse needs to clarify further the situation by pointing out that discomfort after this type of surgery is common and that it is appropriate to request relief from discomfort. In most situations, additional data about health care therapies tend to alleviate anxiety because the data clarify the unknown. With a decrease in anxiety the need for the use of denial also is decreased.

Questioning

When illness occurs, individuals often review their lives in an attempt to find an answer to the reason or purpose for the illness. "Why me?" "What did I do to deserve this?" "Why am I so sick and you are so well?" Some individuals fail to find answers to these questions, while others find a variety of explanations. The individual may view the illness as punishment for a sin, the result of unhealthy living, or simply as part of life. Regardless of whether or not the individual finds answers to his or her questions, the occurrence of illness evokes anxiety. Since the individual has temporarily lost control of life, feelings of uneasiness and apprehension develop. These anxious feelings are often manifested by repeated questioning.

The nurse's responsibility is to supply reliable data to the patient about the illness and to provide support during periods of anxiety. Support can be furnished by allowing and encouraging the patient to do as much as possible. This demonstrates to the patient that he or she still has some control over life. In the hospital setting, if possible, the patient needs to be permitted to carry out personal hygiene and to take an active part in arranging the daily schedule. If the nurse works with the patient on the patient's daily plan of care, he or she identifies the nurse as an available means of support and an avenue by which to relieve anxiety. As such, the nurse serves as a sounding board and an information supplier. Although the nurse may be unable to supply answers to all questions, the fact that the patient is allowed to ask questions and seek answers allays some of the apprehension about the unknown. The patient feels that he or she has greater control of the surroundings and hence anxiety is decreased. In turn, the need for constant questioning usually diminishes.

Ambivalence

Another coping behavior that may occur during the course of an illness is ambivalence. Ambivalence can be described as the coexistence of opposing emotions, attitudes, and desires toward the same object or situation (Freedman, Kaplan, and Sadock, 1980). The individual often has opposing emotions and desires about whether seeking medical attention for the illness is in his or her best interest. Once health care assistance is sought, the individual may be ambivalent about whether medical advice should be followed. Both of these examples demonstrate that ambivalence can result from the frustration of making decisions about the newly imposed state of illness.

The expression by the individual of both negative and positive feelings can prove beneficial. With the expression of such feelings, the individual may need to be informed that the existence of ambivalent feelings about illness are not unusual. Verbalizing opposing feelings often enables the individual to identify more realistic approaches to problems. Although the individual may harbor ambivalent feelings about a health care situation, he or she may remain able to take appropriate action. The woman who after surgery feels reassured that her mastectomy may control her cancer but remains appalled by its mutilating effects demonstrates ambivalence. Thus, therapeutic nursing practice requires the realization that human existence takes into account the likelihood that where there is love there may also be some hate.

Suspicion

Some individuals look upon their illness with suspicion and do not completely accept the possibility that their diagnosis may be true. Such individuals may be suspicious if their diagnosis is serious or if their diagnosis does not appear to be serious. Suspicion is imagining the existence of guilt, fault, or defect on the part of another with little or no evidence. Individuals demonstrating suspicion attempt to find possible reasons for mistrusting their diagnosis and question the motives of others over minute matters. The suspicious individual thinks that the health team members are incorrect or defective in their judgments about the illness. The nurse can detect the suspicious individual by such statements as: "What are you trying to do, kill me? This food isn't mine!" "You are lying to me. I'm not well. I'm a very sick man!" Some doubt concerning illness is reasonable, but suspicion can be blown out of proportion so that the individual mistrusts everything. When carried to extremes, suspicious behavior can develop into a neurotic or psychotic disorder (Arieti, 1979).

An individual who is suspicious is frightened and often feels the need to be constantly on guard or feels that he or she may be taken advantage of. Such an individual lacks a sense of trust in others. In some cases, the absence of trust makes the successful institution of health care therapies difficult, if not impossible. When interacting with the suspicious individual, the nurse must be consistent in his or her approach, and must respond to questions in an open and truthful manner, since any demonstration of inconsistent behavior and/or false information increases the degree and usage of suspicion in an attempt to alleviate anxiety.

Hostility

Perhaps one of the most difficult barriers for the nurse to deal with when working with others is hostility. All humans experience hostility at some time or another. This coping behavior may be but one way a patient reacts to the threatening and frustrating situation of illness. Hostility can be delineated as the feeling of antagonism accompanied by the desire to harm or disgrace others. These desires subsequently may produce feelings of inadequacy and self-rejection on the part of the individual and lead to the loss of self-esteem (Kiening, 1978b).

Hostility is exemplified in a variety of ways in which each individual's display of such behavior is affected by each one's unique background and the situation itself. The manifestations can range from *extreme* polite behavior to external forms of rage or homicide or internal forms of depression or suicide (Freedman, Kaplan, and Sadock, 1980). What is important is that the individual may be unaware of these hostile feelings and wants control of his or her actions. The world may be perceived as unfriendly, dangerous, and hostile. Terms that may be used to describe the behavior of hostile individuals are picky, argumentative, irritable, sarcastic, demanding, critical, and uncooperative. However, nurses must be careful not to hastily label an uncooperative patient as hostile since ill-founded labels can create detriments to future therapeutic interactions. Some individuals may demonstrate uncooperative behavior because of healthy self-assertion which is part of the human process of experiencing individual rights. Individuals who assert themselves with justifiable reason may not conform to what the health team sees as expected patient behavior (Ramsden, 1980). These individuals are not necessarily hostile. Such an incident is demonstrated by the female patient who refuses to wear an open-back gown to X-ray because she feels that it overly exposes her body. She has not conformed to hospital regulation, but is not her noncompliance justifiable?

A patient who demonstrates hostility represents a barrier to the nurse's goal of assisting the patient. The patient poses a threat to the nurse's self-image as an authority figure since the nurse is unable to control the hostile behavior (Ujhely, 1976). Even though the patient's hostile behavior may be directed toward the nurse, such behavior ought not be taken as a personal threat. Immediate reactions of counterhostility toward the patient by the nurse may represent the nurse's own fear of impending threat. When the nurse is counterhostile, a vicious attack and counterattack cycle of hostility can develop between patient and nurse.

Awareness of personal hostile impulses and thoughts (and the mechanisms used in dealing with them) is essential for the nurse. This awareness is necessary before the nurse can effectively intervene with the patient. When the nurse perceives behavior that appears to indicate impending hostility (e.g., increased motor activity, angry facial expressions, increased verbal abuse), it is essential to validate these observations with the patient. Leading validating statements may include: "You appear upset." "Something seems to be bothering you." These leading statements can guide the patient toward describing what is being experienced and the possible reasons for these feelings. Approval or disapproval of the patient's comments should not be shown by the nurse's personal reaction during the interview. It is imperative that the nurse avoid conveying value judgments while demonstrating concern about the patient's well-being. One of the major aspects of nursing intervention is to identify and possibly to alter the condition leading to the hostility while ensuring the maintenance of the patient's self-respect. The patient has to express anger, but limits have to be provided so that the patient realizes that destructive aggression, such as striking someone or throwing a drinking glass, is not acceptable. Socially acceptable outlets for feelings of hostility may have to be suggested or provided. Possible suggestions may include running, pounding a table with the fist, stomping the floor with the foot, hitting a punching bag, squeezing a rubber ball, playing the piano, or typing. If the patient is unable to carry out any of the above activities, vicarious participation in much-loved television sports such as boxing or wrestling may provide an alternate, yet effective, outlet.

To recapitulate, when dealing with the hostile individual the therapeutic tasks of the nurse include the following: validating the existence of the behavior; allowing verbalization of feelings; providing firm but supportive direction; supplying alternate means of hostile expression and, above all, assisting the patient in regaining and maintaining self-esteem.

Regression

It is anticipated that during illness individuals may regress and demonstrate behavior that is not so mature as that which they assume during times of wellness. Regression can be defined as a protective reaction involving a retreat to the use of behavioral patterns that were appropriate during earlier stages of development. During stressful situations, such as illness, behavior from earlier developmental stages may be reassuring. Such behavior is less complicated than the behavior developed to maintain security and self-esteem in adult living (Freedman, Kaplan, and Sadock, 1980). Regression is seen in a variety of forms, such as helplessness, nail biting, inability to wash or feed oneself, crying, withdrawal from responsibility, preoccupation with self, untidyness, total dependence, giddiness, stubbornness, and an altered capacity for human relationships. When it is not extreme, regression during illness is a natural reaction and can facilitate recovery because it permits the patient to be more dependent than usual (Jack, 1980). For example, dependence in the form of bed rest can restore strength and hence assist in progress toward wellness. Therefore, patients must be allowed sufficient and appropriate regression and dependency upon others so that they may work toward recovery. Forms of regression and dependency that are encouraged by health personnel to facilitate the achievement of wellness are deemed legitimate. Legitimate forms of patient regression and dependency could include being fed during the acute phase following a myocardial infarction, requiring assistance on the first day of ambulation after surgery, and requesting help in splinting an abdominal wound during coughing and deep breathing.

However, individuals demonstrating inappropriate degrees of regression, such as demanding assistance with hygiene and elimination needs when they are unnecessary, may need encouragement to achieve adaptation to stress by other means. Alternate means can include the use of: 1) stress/coping group therapy sessions, 2) diversional activities such as craft work, and/or 3) biofeedback. Extreme degrees of regression are not conducive to the patient's achievement of optimal wellness and it is undesirable to foster such behavior.

Nurses have to recognize that regression is a function of the individual's relationship with his or her environment (Freedman, Kaplan, and Sadock, 1980). In other words, the nurse, to effectively intervene, has to understand the purpose or use that the behavior serves the individual in dealing with the environment. Does the individual cause family members or members of the health team to respond to what he or she wants? Is the individual capable of controlling and manipulating others? Is the individual's behavior a means of obtaining "mothering" or "fathering" from family members or from the nurse?

Regardless of what nursing intervention is used, nursing actions are to be developed around the individual patient and the patient's need for the use of regression. For successful institution of health care therapy, it is imperative that a therapeutic nurse-patient relationship be established. Therefore, the patient is provided with the opportunity to contribute his or her thoughts, feelings, and desires into the planning of the treatment. To illustrate: Does Mr. Jones prefer IPPB (intermittent positive pressure breathing) before or after his morning hygiene needs are carried out? Does Miss Kay prefer her morning bath before breakfast or after physical therapy? The decision process involved in the above examples is assumed easily by the nurse, but the decision should *include* the individual patient. By the nurse's not "taking over" for the patient an atmosphere of custodial care is avoided; hence, the individual is encouraged to be more independent.

In the process of assisting the patient in developing a plan of care, the nurse should always begin at the patient's level of ability. The nurse should avoid loading the patient with responsibilities he or she is unable to accomplish, since this can increase frustration and lead to further regression. Such a case might involve expecting the patient to carry out the change of a colostomy bag after only one demonstration by the nurse. Once the patient has assumed more responsibility or has done something unusually well, the nurse should compliment the patient's achievements. Positive reinforcement for a job well done does a great deal of good for anyone's self-esteem.

It can be seen that some form of regression during illness is expected. But if the degree of regression hinders the achievement of optimal wellness, the nurse must intervene to assist the individual in coping with the stress of illness and to limit regression throughout the various phases of health therapy. Otherwise, successful achievement of wellness will be deterred.

Loneliness and Rejection

The presence of illness can bring with it the feelings of loneliness and rejection. Patients often feel entrapped by the illness and feel isolated in dealing with its problems. Individuals who have a communicable disease may sense that others reject them because of the nature of the illness, such as in the case of a socially unacceptable disease like genital herpes. In the case of a long-term chronic illness, such as emphysema, friends and relatives may begin to take the illness for granted and proceed with their own lives. This state of affairs may be interpreted by the chronically ill individual as rejection by significant others. Once loneliness or rejection is felt, it is not uncommon to hear the patient say, ''I know what will become of me and there is nothing I can do to change it!'' Despondency sets in and the patient has a real need for attention and companionship during the illness.

If asked to describe inward feelings, the lonely and rejected individual may allude to a sensation of being cut off from others; a feeling that no one understands or cares; a feeling of being unloved; a feeling of being forgotten with no one to turn to; or a perception of being deserted by friends and relatives.

Feelings of loneliness and rejection are intensified at various times of the day. Patients often comment that night is the most lonely and unfriendly time. The nurse may note that complaints of pain are more frequent at night than during the day. This may be an unconscious attempt by the lonely individual to seek human contact. Darkness automatically decreases human interaction because it is the expected time for the privacy of rest. Night also is the end of the day for everyone, except possibly for the ill individual who views it as a continuation of both the illness and the separation from family and friends. Hence, feelings of loneliness and rejection tend to increase. If feelings of loneliness and rejection are severe, alterations in sensory experiences may occur. (Further discussion on alterations in sensory experiences are covered in Chapter 15.)

Avoiding pretense is important when dealing with the patient's feelings of loneliness and rejection. If approached, the nurse need not hide the fact that he or she also has experienced fear, loneliness, pain, or feelings of rejection since these are all human emotions which everyone experiences at one time or another. However, this does not mean that the nurse should proceed to unfold personal problems and life experiences to the patient. Instead, it is advisable to provide the patient with acknowledgment of the reality of these feelings. In other words, when the patient says that he or she feels lonely and rejected, these emotions need recognition. The nurse can achieve this by investigating with the patient how these feelings have been dealt with in the past. Prior measures which have proven beneficial in alleviating feelings of loneliness and rejection should be instituted. Such measures may include involvement with others in the form of visiting face to face or on the telephone. Fellow patients often are excellent resources for such involvement. As the patient utilizes effective measures for dealing with his or her feelings, positive feedback needs to be given to provide validation of appropriate coping behaviors and to support his or her ego.

Accepting the patient as he or she is becomes necessary if the nurse wishes to avoid a display of rejection. The behavior manifested by the nurse can demonstrate acceptance or rejection of the patient. Facial expressions, voice intonations, and body language are means of conveying these feelings toward another individual (Fast, 1977). Facial expressions and loud voice intonations displaying disgust while standing at a distance of 2½ feet to 4 feet from the patient during a personal conversation can be interpreted as non-acceptance. Touch also plays an important part in displaying acceptance. A light touch on the arm, shoulder, or hand indicates the presence and the existence of actual human contact (Hein and Leavitt, 1977). To illustrate, human contact made during the patient's evening back rub provides a message of "caring" on the part of the nurse. Since patients verbalize that increased loneliness occurs at night, the human contact during the back rub prior to sleep may increase the patient's awareness of someone to turn to in time of need. The importance of touch should not be minimized. Nursing research has demonstrated that even certain physiological changes can be related to the act of therapeutic touch (Krieger, 1975).

In the hospital setting, frequent superficial trips past or into the patient's room should be avoided. Simply walking by the patient's room or stepping into the doorway does not necessarily display acceptance. The extended distance between patient and nurse and the brief superficial encounter do not lend themselves to increasing the patient's self-worth. It would be more therapeutic to spend three to five minutes twice a day at the bedside conversing with the patient about how the patient feels about the illness instead of checking on the patient from the doorway every hour. Until the patient can adapt to the stress of illness, the patient may continue to feel lonely and rejected. With personalized human contact on the part of the nurse, loneliness and rejection can be minimized.

Depression and Withdrawal

One commonly occurring human response to illness is depression, a feeling of sadness and self-depreciation accompanied by difficulty in thinking, reduced vitality, and lowered functional activity. In depression there can be failure in the ability to carry out household tasks and job responsibilities. The individual's general mood is one of sorrow, and crying spells may occur without warning. Physically, the entire body appears to be slowed down or working improperly. Appetite is poor; sleep disturbances occur; constipation is not uncommon; libido decreases; and personal appearance fails to be maintained. A frequently occurring response by the depressed individual is preoccupation with his or her body. It is not unusual for the patient to be seen in the physician's office or at an outpatient clinic with the complaint that his or her body is malfunctioning in one way or another. Such preoccupations with body malfunction may be reflected in such a statement as, "I have these pains in my stomach. Lately my joints have been killing me and my bowels just aren't working right!" Our society has deemed social acceptability for one's concern of proper body function but little understanding to emotional instability. Thus, the feelings of depression are often vented through the physical functioning of the body.

In order to cope with depression, some individuals resort to withdrawal, the act of retreating or retiring away from someone or something. Manifestations of withdrawal might include sleeping a great deal, staying in one's room, avoiding people, sitting alone, and daydreaming. In the hospital setting, feigning sleep is an excellent way to withdraw in an attempt to avoid human contacts that may be stress producing.

In dealing with depression and withdrawal, the nurse's first task is to recognize their existence. Since nurses spend more time with patients and family members than any other individual on the health care team, they are in an opportune position to note the presence of depression. The existence of depression is not always clear-cut, and sometimes professionals may mistake depression in older individuals for organic conditions, such as cerebral arteriosclerosis, since some manifestations are common to both conditions (Diebel, 1976). To facilitate recognizing depression and withdrawal, the nurse should note changes in the individual's usual behavior, for example, refusal to eat, neglecting body hygiene, and sudden cessation of normal daily activities. The depressed and withdrawn individual may need assistance in mobilization. Setting up a schedule with the patient for personal hygiene, grooming, and eating may be helpful in mobilizing the patient's energies.

Since body functions are generally decreased in depression, constipation can occur. To assist in the prevention of constipation, the individual should be offered foods, such as fruits and bran, which facilitate elimination. In addition, fluids between meals and a regular schedule of exercise are helpful. Exercise is also therapeutic for the depressed and withdrawn individual because it allows for the release of internalized hostility in a socially acceptable manner. Playing table tennis, hitting a punching bag, working on leather tooling, or simply taking a brisk walk are other ways of releasing internalized feelings.

The nurse's presence also plays a vital role in working with the depressed and withdrawn person. It is important for the nurse to encourage the individual to express verbally feelings both of anger and sadness so that resolution of these feelings can occur. Since the depressed and withdrawn individual may not be extremely verbal, various techniques of interviewing may be required. To encourage the individual to start talking about these feelings, the use of open-ended statements may be necessary. The following statements may provide an opening for the depressed and withdrawn person to express his or her feelings: "You seem down today." "The day doesn't seem to be going well for you." "It must be upsetting to be here in the hospital with your family at home." The use of such open-ended statements also demonstrates that the nurse is sensitive to the individual's existing feelings.

Reflection is another interviewing technique that may be used. In reflection, the nurse restates part of the patient's statement in question form. The purpose of reflection is to clarify and initiate additional communication on the part of the patient. An example of reflection may be, *Patient:* "I'm really no good to the world." *Nurse:* "No good to the world?" Here the patient is provided with the cue to develop what he means by "no good." Additional feelings that the patient is experiencing may then be explored by both the patient and the nurse.

Summation, a third interviewing technique, may be used at the close of the nurse-patient interview. The nurse outlines or reiterates the basic issues that the patient has presented during the conversation. The nurse clarifies what has been said and seeks confirmation of what the patient believes has been expressed. Summation is important because it provides an opportunity to make sure that the patient and nurse are in agreement with what has occurred during their conversation. In addition, summation leaves the patient with the key points that have been verbalized and it plants a "seed" for further thought of what the patient is feeling.

The success of nursing interventions used in dealing with depressed and withdrawn individuals is best measured by the individual's ability to function in his or her usual manner in carrying out daily activities. Examples of improvement may be a good night's sleep for the first time in months, carrying out some aspect of personal hygiene, or an increase in appetite. The nurse, however, must keep in mind that a patient going into or coming out of depression is more prone to attempt suicide (Hendin, 1982). Sudden changes in mood should be noted and the patient should be closely observed. This is not to say that all depressed patients attempt suicide, but the nurse must be aware of the possibility with severely depressed and withdrawn individuals. In some cases, psychotherapy may be advisable.

In summary, depression and withdrawal are not uncommon behavioral reactions to illness. The body's response to depression is one of general slowing down of all body processes with possible withdrawal from surroundings. The nurse's goal entails assisting the individual in examining his or her feelings and modifying how the individual perceives his or her relation to others.

SUMMARY

Enactment and assimilation of the illness component of the wellness/illness role is not a simple task. Often it requires changes in one's usual patterns of behavior. To assist in understanding patterns of behavior related to illness, nurses have relied upon two theoretical frameworks: functionalism and interactionalism. Functionalism has associated the state of illness with a set of norms for guiding appropriate behavior. These norms include: (1) exemption from social responsibility; (2) inability to achieve wellness simply by decision or will; (3) obligation to seek wellness; and (4) responsibility to seek and cooperate with technically competent assistance (Parsons, 1951). By comparison interactionalism has linked both the state of wellness and the state of illness with a reciprocal interrelationship of roles where each actor regulates his or her responses based upon what is expected from other individuals. In order to enact the wellness/illness role from the interactional point of view the following components must be present: (1) an identification of self; (2) behavior appropriate to the given situation; (3) a background of appropriate acts related to the specific situation; and (4) an evaluation by the individual, and by others, of the role enactment (Lindesmith & Strauss, 1968).

Regardless of which theoretical framework is used to explain illness behavior, it must be remembered that incorporation of illness into one's life is not always easy. Often various behavioral reactions occur during the course of illness assimilation. Some of the more common behavioral reactions occurring during diagnosis and illness include: anxiety, denial, questioning, ambivalence, suspicion, hostility, regression, loneliness and rejection, and depression and withdrawal.

The nurse's role centers around identifying the existence of each behavioral reaction, assisting the individual in dealing with each behavior and facilitating the individual's assimilation of the illness component of the wellness/illness role. Without adequate role assimilation, successful health care therapies cannot be instituted and the individual will be unable to achieve an optimal state of wellness.

REFERENCES

ARIETI, S. *Understanding and helping the schizophrenic: a guide for family and friends.* New York: Basic Books, 1979.

BULLOUGH, V. & BULLOUGH, B. *Health care for the other Americans.* Englewood Cliffs, NJ: Prentice-Hall, 1982.

COHEN, F. & LAZARUS, R. Coping with the stresses of illness. In G. Stone, F. Cohen, & N. Adler (Eds.), *Health psychology: a handbook.* San Francisco: Jossey-Bass, 1979.

DIEBEL, A. Brief notes on brain syndrome in aging persons, *Journal of Psychiatric Nursing and Mental Health Services,* 1976, *14* (8), 51–52.

DRACUP, K. & MELEIS, A. Compliance: an interactionist approach, *Nursing Research,* 1982, *31* (1), 31–36.

FAST, J. *The body language of sex, power, and aggression.* New York: M. Evans & Co., Inc., 1977.

FREEDMAN, A., KAPLAN, H., & SADOCK, B. *Comprehensive textbook of psychiatry-III.* Baltimore: Williams & Wilkins, 1980.

HEIN, E., & LEAVITT, M. Providing emotional support to patients, *Nursing '77,* 1977, *7* (5), 38–41.

HENDIN, H. *Suicide in America.* New York: W.W. Norton & Co., Inc., 1982.

JACK, S. When regression becomes a problem, *The Canadian Nurse,* 1981, *77* (4), 31–34, 37.

KIENING, SISTER M. M. Denial of Illness. In C. Carlson & B. Blackwell (Eds.), *Behavioral concepts and nursing interventions.* Philadelphia: Lippincott, 1978a.

KIENING, SISTER M. M. Hostility. In C. Carlson & B. Blackwell (Eds.), *Behavioral concepts and nursing interventions.* Philadelphia: Lippincott, 1978a.

KOLB, L. *Modern clinical psychiatry.* Philadelphia: Saunders, 1982.

KRIEGER, D. Therapeutic touch: the imprimatur of nursing, *American Journal of Nursing,* 1975, *75* (5), 784–787.

LAMBERT, V. & LAMBERT, C. Role theory and the concept of powerlessness, *Journal of Psychosocial Nursing and Mental Health Services,* 1981, *19* (9), 11–14.

LINDESMITH, A. & STRAUSS, A. *Social Psychology.* New York: Holt, Rinehart & Winston, 1968.

LUCKMAN, J. & SORENSEN, R. *Medical-surgical nursing: a psychophysiologic approach.* Philadelphia: Saunders, 1980.

MCKINLAY, J. The sick role: illness and pregnancy, *Social Science and Medicine,* 1972, *6* (5), 561–572.

Mead, G. *Mind, self, and society.* Chicago: University of Chicago Press, 1934 (paperback, 1967).

MELEIS, A. Role insufficiency and role supplementation: a conceptual framework, *Nursing Research,* 1975, *24* (4), 264–271.

MELEIS, A. & SWENDSON, L. Role supplementation-an empirical test of a nursing intervention, *Nursing Research,* 1978, *27* (1), 11–18.

MISCHEL, W. *Introduction to personality.* New York: Holt, Rinehart, & Winston, Inc., 1981.

NADEL, S. *The theory of social structure.* London: Cohen & West, 1957.

PARSONS, T. *The social system.* New York: The Free Press, 1951.

RAMSDEN, R. Values in conflict: hospital culture shock, *Physical Therapy,* 1980, *60* (3), 289–292.

SEGALL, A. The sick role concept: understanding illness behavior, *Journal of Health and Social Behavior,* 1976, *17* (2), 162–170.

SPECTOR, R. *Cultural diversity in health and illness.* Englewood Cliffs, NJ: Prentice-Hall, 1979.

TURNER, R. Role taking: process versus conformity. In A. Rose (Ed.) *Human behavior and social processes.* Boston: Houghton Mifflin Co., 1962.

TURNER, R. The role and the person, *American Journal of Sociology,* 1978, *84* (1), 1–23.

UJHELY, G. Two types of problem patients and how to deal with them, *Nursing '76,* 1976, *6* (5), 64–67.

2

||||||||||||||||||||||||||||||||||||||||||||||||||||||||||

BODY IMAGE

INTRODUCTION

The concept of body image has its roots in history. Its historical basis, however, cannot be traced, for in reviewing the literature, one finds the concept of body image applied in many diverse disciplines. Some of the disciplines influenced by the body image concept include neurology, psychiatry, hypnology, and psychosomatology. Nursing now has been added to this list of disciplines since the concept of body image has relevance for comprehensive patient care (Marten, 1978; Williams, 1979).

Schilder (1958) describes body image as the picture or schema of one's own body formed in one's mind as a tridimensional unity involving interpersonal, environmental, and temporal factors. Body image, as delineated by Jourard and Landsman (1980), is the perceptions, beliefs, and knowledge an individual holds in regard to his or her body's structure, function, appearance, and limits. Fisher and Cleveland (1968) find the concept of body image too difficult to consolidate or methodize. Shontz (1974) tends to agree by stating that the body image concept has lost its abstraction and has become a "thing" because such diverse definitions exist.

For the purpose of simplicity in dealing with such a complex and incommensurable concept, the authors of this book have chosen to describe the body image concept as the conscious information, feelings and perceptions one uses to identify oneself as being unique and different from everyone else. The view of being unique and different from others includes not only one's concept of one's physical structure, but it also includes one's concept of personal space.

22

Space, the area around us, is where our physical body boundaries end and some other object or person begins. This personal territory has meaning to the individual and conveys a message to those around the individual. We tend to stand close to friends and keep our distance from strangers. For example, note the reshuffling of people in an elevator when someone gets off the elevator and makes more room for the continuing passengers. The automatic reaction is to back away.

Hall (1980) has identified four distinct zones of space in which most people operate. He classified these zones as (1) intimate distance, (2) personal distance, (3) social distance, and (4) public distance. As the terms imply, the zones are different areas in which we move, areas that either increase or decrease intimacy and consciously affect one's body image perception.

Intimate distance ranges from actual body contact up to 18 inches from the body. The close phase of intimate distance (body contact) is for making love, for very close friendships, and for children clinging to parents or to each other. A close intimate distance makes one overwhelmingly aware of the other individual. It is the most private zone of personal space. The far intimate phase ranges from 6 to 18 inches from the body. It is close enough for the clasping of hands, but the head, thighs, and pelvis are not easily placed in contact. The use of this distance in public is not considered appropriate by many adult, middle-class Americans (Hall, 1980).

Personal distance, the second zone of territory, ranges from a close distance of 1½ feet to 2½ feet to a far distance of 2½ feet to 4 feet. The close phase of personal distance allows one to hold or grasp the other individual's hand. This distance is frequently used between husband and wife. The far phase of personal distance lends a certain privacy to any encounter. The distance is close enough for personal discussion, yet one is unable to touch comfortably the other person. Hall (1980) refers to this distance as the limit of physical domination.

The third distinct zone, social distance, extends from a close distance of 4 feet to 7 feet to a far distance of 7 feet to 12 feet. Impersonal business is usually done at the close range. One usually assumes this distance at casual social gatherings. However, this distance also can be a manipulative distance, for it reminds the other individual of one's dominance (boss versus secretary). The far phase of social distance is more for formal social and business relationships. The husband and wife often assume this distance at home in the evenings while relaxing during conversation. This phase of social distance is almost a necessity in large families residing in the same household (Fast, 1977; Hall, 1980).

The fourth and final zone is public distance. Public distance is from 12 feet to 25 feet or more and is the farthest extension of our territorial bondage. The close phase of public distance ranges from 12 feet to 25 feet and is the most desirable range for informal gatherings, such as a teacher addressing a group of students. The far phase of public distance is any distance greater than 25 feet and is reserved for politicians and actors where space provides safety and security. This far distance makes it easier to hide the truth about motions of body language. It is a maneuver long used by stage actors.

In reviewing Hall's four distinct zones of space, one can see the relevance personal space plays in dealing with the body image of the adult patient. For example, the patient who requires any type of "hands on" treatment (i.e., breast examination or dressing change) may interpret the treatment as an assault to body image integrity since penetration of the intimate zone has occurred. As previously mentioned the intimate zone is reserved for very personal relationships and should not be invaded by "just anyone."

In order for the professional nurse to identify an appropriate role in dealing with patients who are experiencing alterations in physical structure and in personal space, the nurse must have a basic understanding of how an individual develops his or her body image. Erik Erikson's (1963) stages of personality development will be used as a framework for discussing an individual's body image development from infancy through senescence.

DEVELOPMENT OF ONE'S BODY IMAGE

Trust versus Mistrust (Oral-Sensory Stage)

The first stage of development, the oral-sensory stage, occurs during the first year of life. It is during this developmental stage that the infant acquires a basic sense of trust. As the name of the stage implies, oral-sensory, the mouth is the predominant zone. The infant meets basic needs by way of the mouth. For these basic needs the infant is totally dependent upon the mother. The quality of care that the mother transmits to the infant in meeting the infant's basic needs will determine the infant's feeling of trust. The infant will either develop a sense of trust that the basic needs will be met or will feel that most of what is needed will be lost. The development of a sense of trust becomes the foundation for a healthy personality (Erikson, 1963).

At birth no concept of physical body image exists except at the feeling level—for example, hunger, thirst, comfort, and rage. The infant has little knowledge about the body and relates to body parts as though they were strange environmental objects. Responses to bodily and environmental experiences solely are at the sensory level during the early months of life and the newborn controls those around him or her by screaming (O'Brien, 1980). Throughout the first year of life the infant progressively acquires some degree of visual, tactile, and motor coordination that allows exploration of the body to a greater extent and provides the infant with the opportunity to bring objects to the mouth more easily (Kolb, 1982). For example, the infant gazes at his or her clenched fist as though it were a toy, chews his or her fingers and toes, and bangs the head in rage. However, the center of the child's body image remains the oral zone (Erikson, 1963). It is during this developmental timeframe that the child must be allowed to examine with the mouth personal body parts, as well as non-hazardous play objects. Such activities assist in the rudimentary formulation of the child's "feeling" component of his or her body image.

As the infant reaches the end of the first year, the interest in observing the body has somewhat diminished. The child becomes aware of the fact that his or her body is separate from mother's body and from those of others. This nuclear body image structure forms the basis of the individual's later personality and, to a great extent, the ability to cope with the stresses of illness, trauma, and physical change (Kolb, 1982).

Autonomy versus Shame and Doubt (Muscular-Anal Stage)

The second developmental stage, the muscular-anal stage, occurs in the second and third years of life. It is during this developmental stage that muscular maturation evolves. The child learns to walk, to eat, to communicate verbally, and to control anal sphincter muscles. With this increased muscular maturation comes the choice of two social modes: that of holding on or letting go (Erikson, 1963).

It is during this second stage of development that parental figures become the most significant individuals to the child. The parents' approval or disapproval of the child's behavior and physical features impart an unforgettable impression on the child's body image perception. If the parents encourage the child to depend upon his or her own abilities and provide consistent and realistic support, the child will gain confidence in his or her own autonomy. Children who have been appropriately accepted by their parents usually do not underrate or overrate their body structures or functions. However, if the parental figures are not accepting of the child's behavior or physical features, the child, according to Erikson (1963), will feel that his or her actions and body do not measure up to the expectations of others. For example, if the child is made to believe that his or her feces are bad and if the child is overrestrained, the child feels enraged at his or her incapabilities and there is danger of the development of shame and doubt. It is at this stage that the child begins to expect defeat, in any venture, by those who are bigger and stronger.

The two- or three-year old child has a continuously changing body image because of rapidly changing motor activities. Frequently he or she has difficulties with definite body boundaries and may resist when the parental figure attempts to flush the feces away. The child also may be apprehensive when an adult attempts to cut the hair or nails since the feces, hair and nails are perceived as an extension of himself or herself. Reassurance that it is necessary to cut the nails or hair and to flush the feces away may be necessary.

During this stage of motor and environmental mastery the child learns to relate to the world. If environmental mastery is positively experienced, the child begins to attach significant value to autonomous will (Erikson, 1963).

Initiative versus Guilt
(Locomotor-Genital Stage)

The locomotor-genital stage, the third stage of development, begins at three years of age and ends at approximately the sixth year. The critical developments that take place during this period include: (1) start of sex typing and emergence of sexual curiosity, (2) identification with parental models, (3) rapid development of language and intellectual capacities, and (4) increased psychomotor skills.

Sex typing and gender identification are the two primary tasks of this developmental stage. It is during this period of development that the parents impose their attitudes upon the child about the appropriate behavior for femaleness and maleness. Historically it has been the general trend of our culture to deem muscular build, physical aggression, proficiency in athletics, and independence as desirable traits for males. Conversely, desirable female traits have been identified as neatness, politeness, social poise, inhibition of physical aggression, and dependency. It must be recognized that social trends are changing and one can observe a positive intermingling of these male and female traits. For example, it is not uncommon to see girls and boys playing on the same baseball teams or to see girls setting up their own hockey and football teams. Traditionally, parental expectations and stigmas have been attached to the biological appearance of their offspring. In today's society with the ever growing recognition of the rights of sexually liberated persons, the identification of various activities and physical appearance with a particular sex has diminished. It is speculated that in the future there will be even less significance attached to maleness and femaleness during this developmental stage.

Because of the rapid growth of the child's language skills, intellectual capacities, and psychomotor abilities, the child becomes avidly curious about himself or herself. The "I" component of the personality becomes stronger. The child's curiosity and increase in hand coordination direct attention to the pleasurable sensation of touching and manipulating the genital area. According to Kaplan (1974), boys demonstrate an interest in manipulating their genitals as soon as hand coordination permits. During this developmental stage most children take part in some form of modified masturbation. Parental attitudes toward the child's masturbation is an important determinant of later sexual attitudes. If the parent attaches punishment to sexual curiosity and masturbation, the child may feel anxiety and guilt. The child's genitals become the focus of conflict which may result in a body image distortion of the genital region (Erikson, 1963). Parental figures should be encouraged to obtain information about normal genital responses. In some circumstances, professional assistance may be required to aid the parents in exploring their personal feelings about sexual behavior, such as masturbation.

The locomotor-genital stage of development provides the child with the opportunity to begin learning an appropriate sex role. Sex role assimilation facilitates basic information, feelings, and perceptions about sexual identity as it relates to his or her body image.

Industry versus Inferiority (Stage of Latency)

From the ages of six to eleven years the child enters the fourth developmental stage, the stage of latency. It is during this developmental stage that basic technological skills are developed. There is a constant need to learn how to do things and how to make things for others. The child develops skills in the use of adult materials while he or she waits, learns, and practices to be a provider. It is at this time that new skills are experienced with the peer group.

The school becomes a way of life, whether the experience be in a formal classroom or on the playground. Since the school situation provides a less protective environment than home, the child may realize for the first time that he or she cannot perform as well as others. The presence of a physical alteration, such as defective vision or hearing, plays an important part in the formulation of the school age child's body image perception. Because of the presence of corrective lenses or hearing devices, the child may be led to feel inadequate or inferior to others. Inferiority and inadequacy are the greatest dangers during this stage of development and are more likely to occur if the child does not receive recognition for his or her efforts (Erikson, 1963). The presence of inferiority and inadequacy fails to provide a sound foundation upon which to build a healthy body image perception. Thus to deal with the issues of inferiority and inadequacy, parental figures may find it necessary to compliment the child frequently in the latency stage on physical and educational achievements.

During approximately the tenth and eleventh years the child undergoes sudden body changes as the result of rapid growth, with females physically outgrowing males. The child becomes more self-conscious and focuses on his or her body and the bodies of others. The child may be particularly aware of his or her height and is very concerned about how he or she looks to others. Positive feedback from significant adults and peers regarding appropriate behavior and appearance is essential and contributes to the development of a healthy body image perception.

Identity versus Role Confusion
(Stage of Puberty and Adolescence)

The fifth stage of development, adolescence, takes place during the eleventh to eighteenth years of life. It is during this period that childhood proper ends and youth begins. Erikson (1963) has referred to this developmental stage as a "moratorium, a psychosocial stage between childhood and adulthood, and between the morality learned by the child, and the ethics to be developed by the adult." The adolescent is faced with the task of opting for a career that receives parental consent or choosing one of his own. This indecision and perplexity in securing an occupational identity can lead to role confusion. In order for the youth to cope with such perplexities, he or she temporarily overidentifies with the leaders of cliques and crowds (Erikson, 1964). The youth in puberty also tends to be "chummy," often to the point of ostracizing those who are different in manner of dress, cultural background, and/or financial status. However, the adolescent generally fears a negative identity and attempts to become what his or her parents and community members desire. To assist the youth in developing a realistic identity, constructive feedback regarding his or her behavior and the effect it is having upon others is advisable.

Final physical growth occurs during this developmental stage with most males becoming taller than females. For those who do not experience this "last chance" for stature an incomplete sense of identity may result. It is not uncommon for youth to express concerns about being "too tall" or "too short" in relation to their peers. Exploring with adolescents their social and physical accomplishments which have occured in spite of their body size facilitates in establishing a meaningful sense of identity.

Body fat distribution, as well as height, plays a vital role in how adolescents view themselves. The location of the body fat is probably the more important aspect because females and males are becoming more conscious of their body contours. The adolescent female body takes on a rounded feminine form while the adolescent male body assumes a muscular, masculine appearance. The youth sees the body as something that is useful and allows him or her to engage in activities. The success with which adolescents can utilize their bodies is important since it contributes to the value they place upon themselves.

Another important aspect of physical maturation during the stage of adolescence is the development of sex organs and the appearance of secondary sex characteristics. Adolescent males often compare sex organ size with their peers since the scrotum and penis are external. Females, on the other hand, are unable to see their ovaries; consequently they pay more attention to the menstrual cycle than to the existence of the ovaries themselves. This significance can be seen by the various gynecological problems and complaints demonstrated during this developmental process. In addition, if negative social practices, such as calling the menstrual cycle "the curse" are used, the female's concept of womanhood may suffer further destruction (Brown, 1972). Dealing with the menstrual cycle as a normal physiological occurrence aids the adolescent female in contending appropriately with her new found mark of femininity.

Secondary sex characteristics play a vital role in the youth's concept of his or her body image since they are more observable to others than the development of sexual organs. Some of the more valued characteristics in the female are development of breasts and pubic hair. The adolescent female often attempts to draw attention to her increased breast size by wearing "accentuating" clothing. In the males the development of facial and body hair and voice changes are coveted signs of masculinity. The adolescent male frequently makes attempts to sport a mustache or beard as a sign of his achieved manhood. To assist the youth in dealing with their physical and sexual development, opportunities need to be provided to discuss, with responsible and knowledgeable adults, how they perceive their bodies. Appropriate incorporation of the rapid body growth and sexual maturity that occurs is necessary if the adolescent is to develop a healthy perception of his or her body image.

Intimacy versus Isolation
(Stage of Young Adulthood)

Young adulthood, the sixth stage of development, begins at the eighteenth year and terminates approximately at forty-five years of age. This period of development continues to be a time of change, even though the biological aspects of adolescence are completed and a sense of identity should have been formulated. The young adult is ready and willing to merge his or her identity with that of others. It is during this period that the individual either shares himself or herself with others, both in friendship and a mutually satisfying sexual relationship, or because of the fear of losing individual identity, develops a sense of isolation (Erikson, 1963). If successful negotiation has occurred in previous stages of development, the young adult is able to accept his or her body without unnecessary preoccupation with its functions. The acceptance of one's body image plays a major role in one's ability to relate to others. In summary, an individual who successfully integrates his or her body image is more capable of developing meaningful and satisfying interpersonal relationships.

In Western society a great deal of emphasis is placed upon the attractiveness of one's body (Woods, 1979). The attitudes one has about oneself are influenced by one's physical appearance and ability. Research has demonstrated that members of society equate certain behavior with specific body builds. A person of "stocky" build is described as being lazy, less strong, good-natured, and trusting; an individual of muscular build is characterized as being strong, adventuresome, mature, and self-reliant; and an individual of slender build is rated as being tense, stubborn, pessimistic, and quiet (Well and Siegel, 1961). Even a difference in body image exists between the sexes. According to Fisher (1964), the female develops a more clearly defined and articulate concept of her body image than does the male. Therefore, the female's body awareness involves more defined boundary regions (high-barrier person). In addition, the female tends to devote more attention to her body than does the male and her feminine role tends to be more specifically identified with her body and its functions. The male's role is more likely to be defined in terms of achievement rather than bodily attributes. Since the female has more clearly defined body boundaries, she has a greater tendency to show reaction to boundary regions, such as the skin and muscle. The male, on the other hand, with a less defined body boundary (low-barrier person), when under stress, will experience an internal physiologic response, such as problems of the cardiac and gastrointestinal systems (Fisher, 1964).

Fisher and Cleveland (1968) found that individuals who have a firm, well-defined body image are more likely to be independent, goal-oriented, and influential group members. Conversely, individuals who have a poorly integrated, ill-defined body image are more likely to be passive, less influential in groups, and less achievement oriented. Thus when planning health care for the adult, the nurse may need to consider the importance of providing an independent, self-care oriented regimen for the patient who manifests a firm, well-defined body image. By comparison a highly structured, clearly delineated treatment modality may prove more beneficial for the person with a poorly integrated, ill-defined body image.

In retrospect, we have seen that during the individual's life span large shifts in body image boundary occur. The infant has hazy boundaries and his or her more meaningful body experiences center around the mouth and stomach (Fisher & Cleveland, 1968). During childhood the boundaries approach the surface of the body wall; however, areas of intense contact with the world (mouth, anus) might reach the body wall earlier than the other body parts. Consequently, the child may perceive his or her contour to be highly irregular. As the individual approaches young adulthood, the maximum regular contour consistent with the body wall is realized. At this point the individual who successfully has integrated the conscious information, feelings, and perceptions of his or her body image is ready to move into the stage of adulthood.

Generativity versus Stagnation (Stage of Adulthood)

The seventh developmental stage, adulthood, occurs approximately between the forty-fifth and sixty-fifth year and spans the middle years of life. During this period in one's life a vital interest outside the home occurs. The major focus of one's interest is directed toward establishing and guiding future generations with an optimistic hope of bettering society. One must keep in mind that being a biological parent does not make one inherently generative. It is an individual accomplishment and the unmarried or childless person is capable of being generative in his or her own right.

The middle-aged adult who feels that he or she has failed to accomplish his or her life-long goals may undergo a middle-aged crisis (Peplau, 1975; Jaques, 1980) and feel incapable of being generative. As a result, the individual may become engulfed in satisfying personal needs and acquiring self-comforts because of the feeling that it is his or her last chance to succeed in life. The outcome is a sense of interpersonal impoverishment resulting from a state of self-absorption and stagnation (Erikson, 1963).

The fear of appearing old may be another concern of the middle-aged person. Difficulty accepting the existence of normal physiological changes due to aging can occur. This difficulty can lead to socially inappropriate dress and behavior. Such maneuvers by the middle-aged adult are attempts to present to others and to oneself a younger appearing body image.

Conversely, the middle-aged adult may resign himself or herself to old age. Every single physical change that occurs may be identified in an exaggerated manner. Chronic defeatism and depression may result and the person may isolate himself or herself in self-pity and retire to the "rocking chair" prematurely.

In dealing with the middle-aged adult, the nurse may have to involve the patient in a re-educative modality which emphasizes alternatives for dealing with body image changes and related psychosocial implications. The use of stylish eyeglasses, concealed hearing aids, appropriate supportive garments and shoes, and becoming facial makeup are just a few examples of realistic alternatives which might be offered. In addition, the involvement in physical activities (jazzercise, isometric exercises) which are specifically designed for the middle-aged adult are highly effective in dealing with chronic defeatism and depression. The middle-aged adult who has dealt successfully with his or her aging body image is more likely to manifest a sense of generativity and to be prepared to progress toward the final stage of development, the stage of maturity.

Ego Integrity versus Despair
(Stage of Maturity)

The eighth and final stage of development, the stage of maturity, occurs from sixty-five years of age and over. During this period the frequent thought of death and the concern about not being capable of caring for an ailing significant other become eminent. As a result, the mature adult may develop feelings of despair that are manifested by disgust. If the mature adult has developed a strong sense of self-worth and is able to place value on his or her past life experiences, feelings of despair will be overcome (Erikson, 1963).

Throughout life physiological changes are taking place, but when older individuals view themselves, they may find wrinkles and pigment changes in the skin, gray sparse hair, eyeglasses and hearing aids, dentures, enlarged knuckles, decreased taste sensations, body contour changes, and weight loss. With these internal and external changes mature adults may experience alterations in body-image boundaries and retreat their body boundaries to more internal sites (Fisher and Cleveland, 1968). An example of boundary retreat might be a constant fixation on bowel function, a manifestation often seen in the elderly. However, as with all the developmental stages, how mature adults view themselves is affected by how they feel others see them. The nurse's role in fostering a stable self-image in the mature adult involves reviewing with the individual his or her past accomplishments, as well as existing abilities to share both knowledge and experience with others. Being involved as a consultant to others for establishing small business operations, for learning gourmet cooking, or for making flies for trout fishing are examples of how the mature adult often shares skills with others. As a result the elderly individual is more likely to manifest a sense of self-worth and is better prepared to demonstrate ego integrity rather than feelings of despair.

SUMMARY

In reviewing the development of one's body image, in relationship to Erickson's developmental stages, it can be seen that the individual's self-perception undergoes many changes. During infancy the body boundaries are hazy and the focus of the body image is the mouth. The child progresses to an image of distorted contours with the focus of the body image being the genital region. It is during adolescence that final physical growth and sexual maturation occur resulting in a body image which incorporates one's role identity. A realistic contour consistent with the physical body wall is realized during adulthood, whereby one is able to accept his or her body without unnecessary preoccupation with its function. Finally, the elderly individual develops a body image that involves a retreat toward the interior of the body structure and a preoccupation with certain bodily functions.

Knowledge of these basic facts is important when developing individualized patient care since it assists the nurse in facilitating the individual's integration of the conscious information, feelings, and perception he or she has about his or her body image. The nurse should be cognizant of the normal developmental processes of the body image and be aware of what developmental state the patient is exemplifying at any given time. To apply the basic facts about body image, specific patient care problems dealing with alterations in body image will be presented in subsequent chapters.

REFERENCES

BROWN, F. Sexual problems of the adolescent girl, *Pediatric Clinics of North America,* 1972, *19,* 729–764.

ERIKSON, E. *Childhood and society.* New York: W.W. Norton and Co., Inc., 1963.

FAST, J. *The body language of sex, power, and aggression.* New York: M. Evan & Co., Inc., 1977.

FISHER, S. Sex differences in body perception, *Psychological Monographs,* 1964, *78,* 1–22.

FISHER, S. and CLEVELAND, S. *Body image and personality.* New York: Dover, 1968.

HALL, E.T. *The silent language.* Westport: Greenwood Press, 1980.

JAQUES, E. The midlife crisis. In S. Greenspan & G. Pollock (Eds.) *The course of life: psychoanalytic contributions toward understanding personality development* - Vol. III: *adulthood and the aging process.* Washington, D.C.: National Institute of Mental Health, 1980.

JOURARD, S. and LANDSMAN, T. *Healthy personality: an approach from the viewpoint of humanistic psychology.* New York: Macmillan, 1980.

KAPLAN, H. *The new sex therapy: active treatment of sexual dysfunction.* New York: Brunner-Mazel, 1974.

KOLB, L. *Modern clinical psychiatry.* Philadelphia: Saunders, 1982.

MARTEN, L. Self-care nursing model for patients experiencing radical change in body image. *Journal of Obstetrics, Gynecology, and Neonatal Nursing,* 1978, *7,* (6), 9–13.

O'BRIEN, J. Mirror, mirror, why me? *Nursing Mirror,* 1980, *150,* (17), 36–37.

PEPLAU, H. Mid-life crisis, *American Journal of Nursing,* 1975, *75* (10), 1761–1765.

SCHILDER, P. *The image and appearance of the human body.* New York: International Universities Press, Inc., 1958.

SCHONTZ, F. Body image and its disorders, *International Journal of Psychiatry in Medicine,* 1974, *5* (4), 461–471.

WELL, W. and SIEGEL, B. Stereotyped somatotypes, *Psychological Reports,* 1961, *8,* 77–78.

WILLIAMS, P. Children's concepts of illness and internal body parts. *Maternal Child Nursing Journal,* 1979, *8* (2), 115–123.

WOODS, N. *Human sexuality in health and illness.* St. Louis: C.V. Mosby, 1979.

3

||||||||||||||||||||||||||||||||||||||||||||||||||||||

LOSS

INTRODUCTION

Loss is a fundamental human experience that spans the entire life continuum. No one can escape the experience of loss since it is ever present and ever occurring. An individual first encounters loss when he or she is expelled from the comforts of the mother's womb and continues to experience loss in many other forms throughout the life cycle. Loss of hearing, loss of mobility, loss of life-long friends and associates, and even loss of wellness are but a few examples of the losses experienced.

Members of the health care team face loss daily and must continually deal with the diverse reactions experienced by individuals to the various forms of loss. Nurses are confronted with the responsibility of contending with the loss itself, supporting the patient and the family's reaction to the loss, and dealing with the responses to loss expressed by fellow health team members. Although each individual has created his or her own means of coping with loss, the concept of loss has been neglected in many health care curriculums because the major focus of concern deals with preservation and maintenance of life. Since the inability to maintain and preserve life may carry with it the act of personal failure, loss is often ignored.

FORMS OF LOSS

By definition, loss is a condition whereby an individual experiences deprivation of, or complete lack of, something that was previously present. Loss may be sudden or gradual, predictable or unexpected, traumatic or temperate. However, the manner in which each individual views the loss depends upon past experiences with loss, the value placed upon the lost object, and the cultural, psychosocial, economic, and family supports available for dealing with the loss. To adequately understand an individual's response to the loss process, the nurse first must be cognizant of what situations or conditions constitute loss. Loss of a significant other, loss of some part of one's physio-psychosocial well-being, and loss of one's personal possessions are the three major forms of loss which will be presented.

Loss of a Significant Other

The most intense loss is the loss of a significant other (Kalish, 1981). Such a loss may occur by way of separation, divorce, or death. The loss may be permanent or temporary, complete or partial in character.

Loss created by separation is temporary and either complete or partial in character. It is temporary in that an individual has parted or withdrawn from another's company or presence for the time being; however, the possibility and potentiality for seeing or being with the other person does exist. Complete separation can occur in the case of war, imprisonment, or estrangement when no form of personal contact is made by means of letter, telephone calls, or any other forms of communication. Loss by separation becomes partial when personal contact can be made by some form of communication, such as letters to loved ones during vacations or visits and telephone calls made to the hospitalized patient. War, imprisonment, or estrangement also may create partial separations once personal contact is made with the individual(s) involved.

Divorce implies a permanent loss, but it may be complete or partial in character. It is permanent in that both parties are no longer legally or emotionally committed to each other. Complete loss in divorce occurs when the husband and wife go their separate ways without ever seeing or requiring monetary or legal contact with each other. Partial loss occurs when the individuals are required to meet and/or either monetarily or legally contact each other because of visitation rights of children, alimony, child support payments, or property settlements and agreements.

Loss by death is a permanent and complete loss that one experiences as the finale of the life of friends, associates, and loved ones. Never again can one make personal contact with the deceased. Whether death be sudden, as with some myocardial infarctions, or gradual, as with various forms of cancer, the impact is traumatic to the individual who is experiencing the loss.

Loss of a significant other may be the initial crisis that brings the patient to the health care setting, as in the case of a situational adjustment reaction, or may be the precipitating factor that leads to a physiological change, such as ulcer formation. Regardless of its relationship to existing health care problems, the psychodynamics involved must be taken into account when caring for an individual experiencing such a loss (Lambert and Lambert, 1977).

Loss of Physio-Psychosocial Well-Being

The second form of loss is loss of one's physio-psychosocial well-being. As the term implies, this form of loss includes three components: the individual's state of physiological function; the individual's ideas and feelings about himself or herself; and the individual's social roles. Alterations in any one of these three components of the individual's physio-phychosocial well-being do not occur independently. Alterations in any one of the components invariably affect the other two components. For example, if an individual encounters an alteration in physiological function, changes in psychological well-being subsequently may occur (Lambert, 1981). As a result of the physiological alteration, the individual also may be forced to change or alter his or her role(s) in society.

The components of one's physio-phychosocial well-being are intricate and intermeshed. The nurse's assessment of each individual constituent is necessary prior to determining the magnitude of loss. Loss of physiological functions may occur during partial or complete failure of body function and it may be permanent or temporary. Changes in vision and hearing that occur throughout the life cycle may be examples of partial failure of body function. The alteration is not complete because vision and hearing are not entirely lost, but the individual involved is unable to see and hear as well as when he or she was younger. The complete failure of a body function occurs in such instances as total renal failure, cardiac arrest, and paralytic ileus. If these conditions are not rectified, they could terminate in death.

The removal of a body part, such as a limb amputation, or the presence of a chronic illness, such as diabetes mellitus, may demonstrate a permanent loss of physiological function. It must be realized, however, that each individual's experience with a form of permanent loss of physiological function varies. Many individuals who have a permanent form of physiological dysfunction are capable of operating at an optimal level of wellness with the assistance of appropriate health care. By comparison, an alteration in breathing may be a temporary form of loss of physiological function, as in the case of an individual who has an obstructed airway. Once the obstruction is removed, the patient most likely will be able to breathe in his usual manner. Regardless of whether the loss of physiological function is partial or complete, permanent or temporary, it demonstrates a loss that is real to the individual involved.

The second component of one's physio-psychosocial well-being is the loss of some part of one's psychological well-being. In other words, it is an alteration in the individual's concept of his or her ideas and feelings about his or her worth, attractability, and desirability. Such a loss may be permanent or temporary.

A state of permanent loss may be seen in the individual who becomes unable to reestablish feelings of self-worth after removal of a body part. Such an individual may feel incomplete and, therefore, of little or no value to anyone. Subsequent acute and/or chronic emotional upheaval may ensue and intense psychiatric care may be required. On the other hand, a temporary state of loss of self-worth may occur, as in the case of a patient requiring hospitalization for minor surgery. Difficulties in accepting the changes that have occurred in body function or appearance may be experienced and the individual may view himself or herself as inadequate and undesirable. Once an individual who has a disability begins receiving rehabilitation, or a patient is discharged from the hospital after a successful surgery, the feelings of worthlessness and undesirability may suddenly or gradually dissipate. However, the individual who has a permanent disability may fluctuate between feelings of worthlessness and feelings of worth depending upon the present-day situation.

Loss of one's occupation or profession, status in the family setting, position in the community, and even one's sexuality comprise the third and final component of the loss of part of one's physio-psychosocial well-being. Each of these roles is temporary and either partial or complete in character.

Occupational or professional roles are temporary since an individual from the time of his or her first employment to last working days assumes a variety of positions within the chosen occupation or profession. For example, a college president may have begun as a college instructor and through time worked his or her way up the professional structural hierarchy to an administrative position. Similarly, a gas station attendant may have started out pumping gas, but eventually was required to assume the additional responsibilities of changing tires and doing mechanical work on cars. The positions and responsibilities maintained by both the college president and the gas station attendant may suffer partial or complete loss at any given time. To illustrate, if a stressor, such as illness, befalls either individual, his or her job responsibilities may require a partial or possibly a complete removal of accountability. Partial or complete loss of the social role may result. Once the stressor, illness, is removed, total job responsibilities again may be resumed and the state of partial or complete loss of the social role is rectified.

One's position in a family structure is temporary in character since each individual assumes a variety of family roles throughout his or her lifetime. An individual can progress from child to adult head-of-the-house, to parent, and on to grandparent. On the other hand, an individual may progress from child to adult and continue to live with his or her parents as their child. Once the parents become elderly, the child may be required to assume the responsibility for their care and become the adult head-of-the-house.

Family roles also may oscillate between being complete or partial in character. A man in the household, for example, may be the source of total family income. If illness or a work slowdown occurs, other family members may have to assume additional responsibility for the family income. The man may demonstrate a partial social loss if his role as breadwinner is assumed in part by others. If the illness becomes acute and requires lengthy hospitalization and treatment or if the man is laid off from his job, complete loss of the family role of breadwinner may ensue because the man is no longer capable of maintaining total gainful employment.

Community roles, the third part of one's social role, are in a state of constant flux for each individual. They are by character temporary and either partial or complete. An individual can assume any number of roles at any given time during his or her life. One can be the member of a church, the mayor of a town, and the participant in a voluntary fire department. Any one of these roles may last for a considerable length of time, but each role is subject to change and cancellation; consequently, these roles are temporary in character.

If a stressor such as illness or sudden additional family responsibilities occurs, the individual may be required to relinquish some components of his or her community role. Thus, partial loss develops. In the case of incompetent performance or total inability to carry out responsibilities as the result of lack of wellness, an individual may be totally removed from the role with the end result being a complete loss of the community role.

Loss of one's sexuality is the final part of one's physio-psychosocial well-being. Sexual roles have undergone great change during the past two decades. The realization of the importance of human sexuality has become of great concern to society and especially to the health care team. Sexuality consists of four major components and is temporary and either partial or complete in character. These four components are: (1) the presence of maleness or femaleness; (2) the existing feelings the individual holds concerning his or her sexual well-being; (3) the effects that maleness or femaleness has upon his or her daily living; and (4) the presence of reproductivity or nonreproductivity.

The presence of maleness or femaleness is the identification of one's biological sex by oneself and by others. In rare instances, individuals at birth may not be identified as one sex or the other because of genetic malfunctioning. In such cases, further medical studies and examinations may be required before the infant's sex is publicly determined (Money, 1980). In other instances, individuals have decided to change their sex by surgical intervention. Such cases demonstrate that one's biological sex is temporary in form; however, most individuals elect to maintain their "birthed" sex throughout their lifetime.

An individual's feelings about his or her sexual well-being play an important part in the acceptance of sexuality. Is the individual pleased about being a male or a female? Are sexual dysfunctions present? Does the individual have a satisfying sex life? Is the individual involved in sex therapy? These are a few of the questions posed to determine one's feelings about his or her own human sexual response pattern (Kaplan, 1974). It is difficult for an individual to experience complete and satisfying sexuality if personal feelings about it are degrading. For example, if a stressor such as surgery occurs, the patient's sexual well-being may be threatened. Should surgery involve the individual's sex organs or structures close to the sex organs, the feelings of threat may be intensified. Such surgical interventions may include a vasectomy, a hysterectomy, an inguinal hernia repair, or a transurethral resection. Unless the feelings of threat toward sexual well-being are alleviated, the individual will continue to demonstrate a partial loss of sexuality.

Maleness or femaleness plays an important part in one's pattern of daily living and it affects the individual at home, at work, and in the social setting. Although sexual stereotypes are changing, one's biological sex continues to have an effect on the family, work, and social roles that are played. For example, since males have been considered physiologically stronger, it has not been unusual for them to be responsible for lifting heavy objects and maintaining equipment in both the home and work environment. Throughout history the presence of maleness in social settings has granted the individual the privilege to be assertive and directive. By comparison, the female has been deemed the "passive one" and has been responsible for raising children, maintaining the household, and relying upon the male for her social identity. These practices currently are undergoing change and the usage of one's biological sex in the home, at work, and in the social setting are less significant. However, it is still common for a partial loss of sexuality to occur when an individual enters a situation (be it at home, at work, or in the social setting) where members of the opposite sex predominate. For example, career aspirations of a male in home economics often are hindered due to his sexuality. Similarly, the female construction worker frequently is ostracized by her male co-workers. Even the female politician may confront uncooperative behavior from male counterparts based upon sexuality.

Presence of reproductivity and nonreproductivity is the fourth and final component of one's sexuality. Today a number of heterosexual couples are selecting not to reproduce (Woods, 1979). However, the ability to procreate remains a very important issue for most heterosexual couples. Procreation also is an issue with some homosexual couples. Although homosexual couples themselves are physiologically incompatible for reproduction, some lesbian couples have resorted to artifical insemination as an alternative for developing a family. Should either a heterosexual couple or a homosexual couple desire children and be unable to do so, a partial loss of sexuality will be present.

Since selected patterns of sexual activity vary among individuals, as can be seen in the presence of singleness, marriage, extramarital affairs, homosexual and heterosexual relationships, and self-sexual stimulation, what the individual finds sexually satisfying is the important factor. If, however, the individual's sexual experiences fail to provide sexual satisfaction or off-spring, when desired, then a partial loss of sexuality occurs. The complete loss of sexuality cannot develop unless all four components of the individual's sexual well-being are unmet. The chances of this happening are rare although the individual, at any time, may be unable to fulfill three of the components of his or her sexuality: satisfactory feelings toward sexual well-being; positive affects of biological sex upon daily living; and the presence or lack of reproductivity, depending upon desire. However, the presence of maleness or femaleness, the fourth component of sexuality, is ever present; consequently, one aspect of sexuality continually exists and complete loss of sexuality is not established.

Loss of Personal Possessions

The third and final form of loss during adult life is the loss of one's personal possessions. This form of loss may be permanent or temporary and it may be either partial or complete in character.

Personal possessions consist of such items as money, clothing, jewelry, habitation, and country. These possessions often represent an extension of one's being and loss of such items may demonstrate a true personal threat to the individual involved (Sloboda, 1977). Think of how you would feel if someone took or if you misplaced an item that you personally cherish.

Personal possessions may be lost in a variety of ways: robbery, misplacement, destruction, repossession, removal, or expulsion. Permanent loss occurs when the individual's possession is totally unretrievable. Such may be the case in destruction and expulsion. Never again will the individual be able to lay claim to the personal possession. A common example of permanent loss seen in the health care setting is when a member of the health team breaks a patient's dentures, eye glasses, or writing pen, or puts the patient's rosary beads in the dirty-linen chute with the bed sheets.

Loss of a personal possession becomes temporary if at some point the item is retrieved. Temporary loss of a personal possession may be in the form of robbery, misplacement, repossession, or removal. Temporary loss frequently occurs during hospitalization. One of the most ritualistic procedures carried out by nursing personnel that demonstrates temporary loss is removal of the patient's clothing, money, and medications at the time of admission and returning them upon discharge.

Partial loss of a personal possession occurs when some component or part of the possession is lost, such as when an individual misplaces one piece in a set of jewelry or is asked to relinquish all medications except nitroglycerine at the time of hospital admission. Complete loss of one's possessions occurs when the entire item is lost, as in the case of expulsion from one's home or country.

Loss of one's personal possessions is undoubtedly the most frequent form of loss during adult life. Regardless of its frequency, one continues to view this form of loss as a threat both personally and monetarily.

SUMMARY OF FORMS OF LOSS

An individual's adult life is confronted with three forms of loss: loss of a significant other, loss of physio-phychosocial well-being, and loss of personal possessions. These losses vary in their ability to be permanent or temporary and complete or partial. During his or her lifetime an individual may be forced to deal with any number of losses. The manner in which the loss is viewed affects the individual's ability to cope with its presence and its recurrence.

REACTIONS TO LOSS

Regardless of what form of loss an individual encounters, be it death, separation, loss of a body part, or loss of home, a person responds to loss with a sequential set of behaviors. The speed with which he or she progresses through these reactions, the length of time spent dealing with each phase, and the intensity of each response to the loss depends upon many factors. These factors may include the value of the lost object, the rapidity of the occurrence of the loss, experience with similar losses, individual coping abilities, and cultural support systems (Lambert, 1982). The following discussion will consider the three reactional phases—repudiation, recognition, and reconciliation—experienced by an individual attempting to deal with loss. Related nursing interventions will be presented at the end of each reactional phase presentation to avoid repetition in Part II of the text.

Repudiation

An individual's initial reaction to loss is one of shock and disbelief (Engel, 1964). Comprehension and acknowledgment that the loss has occurred are repudiated. The individual refuses to recognize or accept that the loss has occurred. Common statements made by the individual experiencing the loss include: "No, it can't be true." "It's not possible." "I don't believe it."

In an attempt to protect themselves from the stress of the loss, some individuals may intellectualize the loss and proceed to carry out ordinary activities as though nothing had happened; others sit motionless in a dazed state (Engel, 1964). Either reaction prevents conscious access to the complete emotional impact of the loss. When the loss involves the diagnosis of a chronic illness, the individual may respond by refusing to believe the diagnosis and proceed to search for additional medical opinions (Kubler-Ross, 1969). Thus, the individual attempts to protect himself or herself from having to face the overwhelming stress of the loss.

The act of repudiation may last a few minutes, several hours, days, or in some instances even months. However, the use of repudiation for extended periods, such as months, is an exception. Refusal to acknowledge the existence of loss is a temporary defense and eventually is replaced by, at least, partial acceptance of the loss (Kubler-Ross, 1969). Although repudiation is the initial reaction to loss, it must be recognized that the individual also may require its use in later phases of reaction to loss. The act of repudiation simply provides a buffer and allows an individual time to collect his or her thoughts and to mobilize other less radical reactions to stress-producing circumstances.

Various physiological and emotional reactions accompany repudiation. These reactions may include fainting, pallor, excessive perspiration, increased heart rate, nausea, diarrhea, crying, confusion, and restlessness (Gray, 1974). However, the prevalence and intensity of these reactions will vary greatly among individuals experiencing loss. Some individuals may exhibit many of these reactions while others may exhibit few.

In summary, the major function of this initial reaction to loss, repudiation, is to protect oneself against the effects of overpowering stress created by the acknowledgment of the loss. Repudiation allows one time to collect oneself before attempting to face the loss and work toward accepting it.

Nursing intervention during repudiation.   Before initiating nursing intervention when dealing with an individual and his or her family experiencing loss, the nurse must be cognizant of what phase of loss is being demonstrated. This information must then be disseminated among all of the health team members dealing with the individual and with the individual's family in order to avoid conflicts in approach and to facilitate continuity of care.

The nurse's primary role during repudiation is to allow the individual the right to deny (Carlson, 1978) and to facilitate the individual's movement from the stage of repudiation into the stage of recognition. During the individual's movement through this reactional phase the nurse needs to provide a conducive environment for the expression of feelings, to be an active, nonjudgmental listener, and to be a supportive facilitator for the provision of the individual's activities of daily living.

Provision of a private environment conducive to the expression of feelings is imperative. In a private setting the individual is more likely to openly express his or her true feelings. A private environment may be created by the provision of a private room, the usage of a conference room for discussions, or the partitioning off of the individual by way of bedside curtains.

Being an active, nonjudgmental listener is essential to assure the individual that his or her expressed feelings are being accepted and that no value judgments are being made. Agreeing or arguing with the individual about the denial should be avoided, for denial is the only means of coping with the loss at the time. If a patient were to say, "I don't need those medications!", the nurse must avoid responses such as, "I suppose you really don't!" or "You certainly do!" The first response supports denial and the second response is argumentative. Nothing is accomplished by such comments other than increasing the patient's already high anxiety level. It would be more advisable to respond in such a reflective manner as, "You don't believe that you need the medication?" or "You feel this medication will not be useful?" By responding in this manner the nurse requests additional information about the denial of loss and, subsequently, obtains data for deciphering the patient's specific concerns.

In addition to encouraging the individual to express feelings about the loss, the nurse may have to manipulate the environment in order to assist the individual in maintaining the usual activities of daily living. Providing a patient with the opportunity to carry out personal hygiene or prescribed medical therapies and making sure that scheduled clinic appointments are kept are some possibilities. On occasion the individual may be unable to carry out his or her activities of daily living because of the energy expended in denying. In such a case the nurse assumes the responsibility for the individual's care so that the individual is free to continue denial of the loss. Whether the nurse provides the individual with the opportunity for active involvement in activities of daily living or assumes the responsibility for the individual's care, continuity of care and prevention of possible additional losses are assured.

While working with an individual experiencing loss, the nurse must recognize that the individual's family members also require support as they work through their feelings of shock and disbelief. The therapeutic approaches utilized for dealing with an individual in the stage of repudiation also apply to members of the individual's family. Each family member may require separate intervention on the part of the nurse because all family members may not progress through the reactional phases of loss at the same pace. Some family members may repudiate the loss momentarily while others may carry on disbelief about the loss for extended periods of time. The expression of feelings by each family member should be encouraged since it is, as with the individual experiencing the loss, the one means of coping with loss at the time.

In addition, the nurse must determine which family member the remaining members rely upon for emotional support and guidance. Such determination may be made by observing family interactions and subsequently noting who is the family spokesperson and decisionmaker. This individual may require additional support from members of the health care team due to his or her responsibilities within the family structure. Through increased support this family member becomes more capable of facilitating other family members' movement through the reactional phase of repudiation.

Recognition

The second phase in the individual's reaction to loss involves recognition. Generally, within minutes or hours (possibly days or months for some individuals) recognition of the reality of the loss begins. The conscious has been penetrated and the increased awareness of the anguish of loss evolves. Anger is likely to be elicited and projected upon other individuals or circumstances in the environment or directed toward oneself in the form of depression (Engel, 1964). Verbal attack, and aggressive or destructive acts, such as hitting an inanimate object, are various demonstrations of the acting out of anger. In the hospital setting the patient may express anger by refusing medication or treatment. It is not uncommon to hear such verbal accusations as: ''It is your fault that this medicine tastes so bitter." "I'm not going to physical therapy today. They don't know what they are doing. All they do is hurt me!" Regardless of what others do, individuals expressing anger due to loss may continually find fault.

Family and health team members often find it difficult to cope with the verbally abusive, angry individual experiencing loss, since they find it difficult not to take the expressed anger personally. Actually, the outwardly angry individual is not angry at them but at attributes which they represent, for example, wellness, purpose, freedom, vitality, cheerfulness, mobility, and the ability to control their own lives (Gray, 1974).

The individual who expresses anger about his or her loss in the form of depression also may be difficult for family and health team members to deal with. He or she expresses anger by being the "good patient" or by withdrawing into a room and being uncommunicative. Loss of appetite, sleep disturbances, decreased libido, and fatigability are additional manifestations of incipient depression arising due to loss (Schatzberg, 1978). The following statements are often heard: "Don't waste your time nurse. The treatment won't help anyway." "Don't tell my family how I feel. They don't care about me either." The depressed patient may assume a bleak and fatalistic view about the loss and these feelings of helplessness and hopelessness only add to increasing biological vulnerability (Parkes & Brown, 1972; Maddison and Viola, 1968).

After the individual has expressed anger, he or she may make attempts to postpone the loss by negotiating and entering into the *IF* stage. The negotiation may be with a supreme being (Kubler-Ross, 1969), another individual, or with oneself. Common propitiatory attempts involving loss due to chronic illness or impending death may include such statements as: "*If* I can just go to my son's bar mitzvah," or "*If* I could only see the seashore one more time." Negotiations involving loss of a personal possession may be made with oneself and include such statements as: "*If* only I had sent my wallet home with my family, the hospital staff couldn't have lost it," or "*If* I only had put new locks on my doors, they never would have robbed me." It should be noted that negotiating statements inherently include or imply the word *if*. If the negotiation is fulfilled, the individual will most likely make another attempt to negotiate in order to extend further the trauma of dealing with the loss, since the act of negotiating is an attempt to deal with feelings of guilt. The individual may believe that his or her thoughts or actions had something to do with bringing about the loss (Marks, 1976). Not until the individual is ready to face the loss directly will the individual be ready to relinquish the need to negotiate.

Once the individual has dealt with the *IF* stage of recognition, he or she then spends a period of time being preoccupied with the loss object, be it another person, a body part, or an inanimate item. This preoccupation is demonstrated by repetitive verbalization about the object (Engel, 1964). Idealization and any negative aspects about the loss object are repressed (Carlson, 1978) because the individual finds a need to identify with the positive qualities of the loss object. At this point the individual remains unable to replace the loss with a new item or relationship and may establish passive, dependent relationships with old well-established objects (Carlson, 1978). Given ample time and proper assistance, the individual can successfully work through the phase of recognition and be prepared to enter into the final reaction to loss, reconciliation.

Nursing intervention during recognition. In dealing with the stage of recognition, the nurse's primary role is one of assisting the individual in coping with the loss, in maintaining behavioral stability, and in moving from the stage of recognition into the stage of reconciliation. Most likely, anger will be the first behavioral response expressed during this reactional phase. Such anger may be diffuse and the individual will blame anyone or anything for his or her loss. By comparison, the anger may be specific and the person will focus his or her reaction on an identifiable person, place, or thing. In dealing with the individual's expressed anger, the nurse must not join the individual in anger or retaliate against the individual's anger in an attempt to protect one's own ego. For example, the patient says, "Do you have to be so cheerful all the time? Your sweetness makes me sick," and the nurse responds, "Well, excuse me for living!" The nurse's response in this interaction would be considered retaliative and indicative of a personal threat. The nurse would be more appropriate in responding with a reflective statement suggesting that the individual's verbalization indicates angry feelings. Such a reflective statement might be, "My cheerfulness seems to bother you. Let us discuss what is happening with you today." Remember, the individual experiencing loss becomes angry at others' attributes, such as cheerfulness, and not necessarily at other individuals themselves.

An individual may have justifiable reason for anger and must not be reprimanded for expressing it. Instead, the individual should be encouraged to vent verbally his or her feelings. By "talking out" the angry feelings about the loss, the individual is less likely to express anger in a socially unacceptable manner, such as throwing things or striking others. Take the case of the individual whose clothes have been lost by health care personnel during the hospital admission procedure. Does the individual not have justifiable reason for anger? By verbally attacking the individual or by making excuses for the loss, reinforcement of the individual's anger is intensified. A more therapeutic approach would be to say, "Your anger is certainly understandable. We will take appropriate steps in an attempt to retrieve your clothing. I will inform you step.by step of the progress that we are making." Such a response by the nurse acknowledges the existence of the individual's anger, provides the individual concrete information on what attempts are going to be made to alleviate the anger, and provides follow up on health care actions. The nurse then *must* follow through and relay the actions to the individual; otherwise, mistrust may develop and further anger may be incited.

Anger about a loss may be directed toward oneself and be expressed in the form of depression. In the American culture, depression tends to be the most common reaction to loss (Carter, 1976) and often is exhibited by withdrawal, isolation, and feelings of decreased self-worth. When dealing with depression, nurses must be aware that members of the health care team often unconsciously avoid individuals exemplifying this behavior. An atmosphere of personal isolation is created which may be interpreted by the depressed individual as rejection. Angry individuals demonstrating depression should not be avoided, for avoidance may intensify their depression. Instead, they need frequent personal contact and encouragement to express their feelings outwardly rather than expressing anger through internalization. Crying may be a means of such expression and value judgments regarding its use should not be made by the nurse. Privacy for the expression of such emotions should be made available for the individual's use. Removing the individual from the chaos of the environmental surroundings and placing the individual in a quiet, private setting allows the expression of feelings with no reservation or embarrassment. When a private environment is provided for the expression of feelings, the nurse should avoid withdrawing from the situation. Withdrawing from the uncomfortable circumstance may be an easy way out for the nurse, but it is not necessarily a therapeutic maneuver for the individual's benefit. Sitting quietly with the individual as he or she begins to express anger, either in the form of verbal abuse or depression, demonstrates the nurse's acceptance of the individual and helps alleviate the individual's feeling of isolation and rejection. As the individual begins to verbalize feelings of depression about the loss, the nurse should provide appropriate feedback. The nurse can point out to the individual that it is obvious that he or she is depressed, but through time and with assistance the depression will subside. Asking the individual if he or she has ever been depressed and, if so, what actions he or she has taken to deal with the depression may provide avenues for a therapeutic intervention. Identifying what action the health care team can provide in assisting the individual to cope with the loss is another tangible way of dealing with the individual's depression. For example, necessary readjustments in job responsibilities because of an amputation may be disturbing the individual; hence, anger in the form of depression may ensue. With the assistance of social service and occupational therapy, alternatives in dealing with changes in work responsibilities may be developed and, in turn, the need for anger, in the form of depression, may be decreased. Regardless of what means are used in dealing with the individual's depression, it is important for the nurse to point out present positive attributes instead of feeding into the individual's negative feelings. Positive feedback may include making note of the individual's ability to walk farther today than yesterday or commenting on how much the individual's facial color has improved.

When dealing with negotiation, another behavior manifested during the stage of recognition, the nurse's primary responsibility is to guide the individual in looking at the reasons for using such a maneuver. The individual sometimes assumes that he or she must have done something wrong; therefore, the individual may think that he or she is guilty of some grievous act. It is necessary to assist the individual in identifying those acts and thoughts for which the individual believes he or she is guilty. Verbalization is one method that can be used to help the individual identify guilt feelings. The nurse may want to initiate a discussion with the individual by commenting, "You keep saying *if* I only had done thus and such. Do you feel responsible for the loss?" Such a comment may guide the individual's thoughts and verbalizations toward expressing repressed guilt. Once the individual has identified the presence of his or her guilt feelings, the nurse needs to assist the individual in realistically exploring the *reasons* for these feelings. Is the person feeling guilty because he or she believes that society expects it? Is the individual expressing guilt for the purpose of obtaining secondary gains? Did the individual actually do something to warrant his or her feelings of guilt? If the answer to any one of these questions is "yes," the individual may need assistance in working through his or her guilt feelings. In some instances psychiatric therapy may be required to assist with guilt resolution. Above all, the nurse must avoid giving the individual "pat" answers, such as, "Oh, I'm sure everything will work out. It is not your fault!" This response is an abortive attempt to pacify the individual and direct the conversation away from a topic which, no doubt, is making the nurse uncomfortable.

As the individual passes the negotiation phase of recognition and begins to face the loss, intense preoccupation with the positive aspect of the loss object evolves. During this phase of recognition the nurse must allow the individual to vent his or her feelings about all of the positive qualities of the loss object and not expect the individual to establish relationships with new objects at this time. Not until the individual experiencing loss is allowed to be purged of the idealized beliefs about the loss object will the individual be capable of viewing the aspects of the loss more objectively. Only then can the individual begin to relinquish dependent relationships with old well-established objects and begin to organize new relationships with other objects.

The nurse not only must be available to assist the individual, but also must be accessible to the family members as they work through the phase of recognition. As with the stage of repudiation, each member of the family may be at a different level in the phase of recognition. The therapeutic approaches utilized for dealing with an individual in the stage of recognition also are applicable to the individual's family members; however, a few additional considerations must be addressed. The family may require frequent information about their loved one's reaction to loss. Such a maneuver provides the family with the feeling of some control over the situation and, in turn, facilitates in decreasing their anxiety levels about the loss. The family's anxiety level has a grave impact on the individual experiencing loss since family members frequently are the primary support system upon which the individual relies. If the family's anxiety is maintained at an appropriate level, so might the individual's. Second, the family members may provide valuable information and suggestions on how to assist their loved one in dealing with loss; therefore, the family also must be consulted during the planning of nursing care. The nurse should remember that family members usually are most knowledgeable about how their loved one deals with life's stresses and can provide valuable insights into effecting coping strategies. Once the individual and/or the individual's family members have dealt with the shock and disbelief of the loss object and have recognized the realities of the loss experience, they stand ready to begin to deal with the final stage of loss, reconciliation.

Reconciliation

Reconciliation involves reorganization of one's feelings about the loss. Preoccupation with the loss object becomes less and the individual begins to develop a more factual memory of the loss experience. The need for anger and depression no longer exists and idealization of the loss object progresses to a detachment of the object from the self. A gradual interest in new objects evolves and an active participation occurs in developing and fostering new attachments.

When the reconciled loss has involved a significant other, new personal relationships are explored and new interests in others are developed. This activity may be exemplified by the individual's participation in new social or religious organization, increased involvement in family get-togethers, and the development of new one-to-one interactions. Verbalization indicating reconciliation with loss of a significant other may include: "At times I'm sure I will miss my husband now that he is gone, but I'm so relieved that he isn't suffering anymore." or "My baby is going to be in the hospital a long time, but the rest of my family needs me too; therefore, I'm going to spend more time at home. I'm confident that my baby is receiving good care while I'm gone."

When the reconciled loss involves a body part, as in the case of a colectomy or a limb amputation, interest often is directed toward the newly needed appliance or prosthetic device. It is not uncommon for an individual to give a "pet name" to an appliance or device and make statements about it in an attempt to indicate that it is an extension of oneself. Such statements may include, "I have been so concerned about my appearance since my surgery. However with "Charlie" (new prosthetic device) no one can tell that I've had my leg removed." Incorporation of the newly acquired appliance or prosthetic device as part of the self allows the individual freedom to resume personal interactions with limited concerns about how others will view him or her.

Reconciliation of the loss of a personal possession is likely to be demonstrated by the purchase of a replacement and the establishment of an attachment to the newly acquired object. A reconciliatory statement involving such a loss may be, "I really liked the coat I lost, but my new one is just as nice." Final reconciliation involving any loss object is accomplished when the individual accepts the loss and, with no hesitation, is capable of openly ventilating and dealing with all feelings regarding the loss experience.

Nursing intervention during reconciliation. Even when the individual reaches the final phase of loss, reconciliation, the nurse's role is not finished, for during this phase the individual requires encouragement in expressing views about himself or herself and assistance in making plans for the future. The role of the nurse revolves around urging the individual to express his or her personal feelings now that the loss has been resolved. In what way does the individual see himself or herself now that he or she has experienced loss? How has the loss been incorporated into his or her body image? In what way has the individual assimilated the role of his or her present state of illness?

It is during this phase of loss that family members may require additional information about the individual's actions in order to prepare them for complete reintegration of the individual into the family settings. Family members also may need the opportunity to vent their personal feelings about the individual's present reaction to the loss. Not all family members are in the same phase of loss reaction and, therefore may experience difficulty in understanding how the individual has come to accept the loss. The individual's reconciliation with loss does not inherently imply reconciliation by family members. Family members may require guidance in planning how they will interact with the individual in regard to the loss experience. This guidance should include the identification and discussion of potential difficulties that may arise due to family members' differences in loss resolution so that unnecessary conflicts can be prevented.

During the phase of reconciliation the nurse also may be required to assist the individual experiencing loss to plan and institute actions for his or her future. An individual experiencing loss of a significant other may express desire for companionship. The nurse may suggest various places, organizations, or ways of meeting new people. If the loss is caused by illness, the individual may require guidance in planning alternate ways of incorporating therapies into his or her busy work schedule. An individual experiencing loss of a personal possession may request nothing more than guidance in how to obtain a replacement for the loss object. Regardless of the kind of loss each individual experiences, his or her needs for future planning vary and these examples are but a few ways in which the nurse can intervene.

SUMMARY OF REACTIONS TO LOSS

An individual encountering loss progresses through three reactional phases—repudiation, recognition, and reconciliation—when dealing with a loss experience. All three phases must be worked through before the individual can be acknowledged as having successfully dealt with the loss experience. The nurse must be aware that an individual experiencing loss may undergo the entire process of loss each time a new loss is encountered. Therefore he or she needs to successfully deal with each loss as it occurs since prior losses and how they have been resolved will influence an individual's ability to cope with the present loss (Kubler-Ross, 1969). The nurse plays a vital role in assisting the individual and his or her family as they each work through each reactional phase of the loss experience. The interventions the nurse uses should facilitate progressive movement from repudiation through reconciliation and should relate to the reactional phase being experienced.

REFERENCES

CARLSON, C. Grief. In C. Carlson and B. Blackwell (Eds.). *Behavioral concepts and nursing interventions*. Philadelphia: Lippincott, 1978.

CARTER, F.M. *Psychosocial nursing: Theory and practice in hospital and community mental health*. New York: Macmillan, 1976.

ENGEL, G. Grief and grieving. *American Journal of Nursing,* 1964, *64* (9), 93–98.

GRAY, R. Grief, *Nursing '74,* 1974, *4* (1), 25–27.

KALISH, R. *Death, grief, and caring relationships*. Monterey, Calif.: Brooks/Cole, 1981.

KAPLAN, H. *The new sex therapy: Treatment of sexual dysfunction*. New York: Brunner /Mazel, 1974.

KUBLER-ROSS, E. *On death and dying*. New York: Macmillan, 1969.

LAMBERT, C. and LAMBERT, V. Divorce: A psychodynamic development involving grief, *Journal of Psychiatric Nursing and Mental Health Services,* 1977, *15* (1), 37–42.

LAMBERT, V. Factors affecting psychological well-being in rheumatoid arthritic women. (Doctoral dissertation, University of California, San Francisco, 1981). *Dissertation Abstracts International,* 1982, *40* (10), 4017B.

MADDISON D., and VIOLA, A. The health of widows in the year following bereavement, *Journal of Psychosomatic Research,* 1968, *12,* 297–306.

MARKS, M.J. The grieving patient and family, *American Journal of Nursing,* 1976, *76* (9), 1488–1491.

MONEY, J. *Love and love sickness: The science of sex, gender differences, and pair-bonding,* Baltimore: The Johns Hopkins University Press, 1980.

PARKES, C.M. & BROWN, R. Health after bereavement: a controlled study of young Boston widows and widowers. *Psychosomatic Medicine,* 1972, *34,* 449–461.

SCHATZBERG, A. Classification of depressive disorders. In J. Cole, A. Schatzberg, and S. Frazier (Eds.), *Depression: Biology, psychodynamics, and treatment*. New York: Plenum, 1978.

SLOBODA, S. Understanding patient behavior, *Nursing '77,* 1977, *7* (9), 74–77.

WOODS, N. *Human sexuality in health and illness*. St. Louis: C.V. Mosby, 1979.

part II: coping with specific physical illnesses

4

AMPUTATION

INTRODUCTION

Amputation surgery has been in existence since the beginning of mankind. Archeologists have found skeletal remains with amputed bone stumps dating as early as the Neolithic period (Rang and Thompson, 1981). The term amputation is derived from the Latin, *amputatio,* and means "cutting around." Originally the term amputation was used to describe the removal of limbs or portions of limbs by a knife. Now it also is used to describe the removal of such appendages as a breast or testicle.

During the past quarter of a century considerable progress has been made in medicine and surgery related to amputations. With the advent of antibiotics, vascular surgery, and effective control of diabetes mellitus, the necessity for the amputation of limbs and appendages has decreased (Larson and Gould, 1978). Although improvements in medicine and surgery have decreased the number of amputations, adaptation to amputation remains a prevalent health care problem.

CAUSES FOR AMPUTATIONS

There are four major causes for amputations: trauma, disease, tumors, and congenital disorders (Larson and Gould, 1978). In the category of trauma, amputation is required as a result of crushing or of extensive lacerations of the vascular and nervous structures in the extremity, thus rendering the extremity unsurvivable and in need of removal. Trauma generally involves individuals in the age group of twenty years to fifty-five years and is the most common cause for amputation of a lower extremity (Tooms, 1980).

The second cause for amputation, disease, comprises the greatest number of amputations (Kay and Newman, 1975). This category may include such maladies as extensive osteomyelitis, atherosclerosis, and arteriosclerosis, with diabetes mellitus often accompanying the two vascular disease processes. According to Warren (1975), at least three fourths of all amputations are brought about by vascular changes. Since vascular changes are enhanced by the aging process, people in the age category of fifty years and older constitute the largest percentage of individuals undergoing an amputation (Kerstein, Zimmer, Dugdale, and Lerner, 1975), with men experiencing nearly three fourths of all amputations (Tooms, 1980).

Tumors, the third cause for amputation, comprise a small percentage of the total number of amputations. Tumor related amputations are most prevalent in the second decade of life and generally are performed to prevent the spread of the lesion (Fernie, 1981).

The fourth cause of amputation, congenital disorders, also makes up a small percentage of the total number of amputations. Congenital disorders may consist of the absence of or severe malformation of a limb at birth resulting from faulty embryonic development. When a malformed limb does not respond to corrective therapy, its removal may be necessary to improve the function of the child (Gillespie, 1981).

In summary, amputations can occur at any age and involve upper or lower extremities or appendages. The level of amputation may be proximal, distal, or involve total loss of structure. The amputee most frequently seen is a male, fifty years of age or older, stricken with peripheral vascular changes, who has lost a lower extremity. Regardless of whether the amputation is brought about by trauma, disease, tumors, or congenital malformation, the individual is faced with experiencing the illness role, the impact of loss, and an alteration in body image.

IMPACT OF AMPUTATION

Psychological Impact

The psychological impact of amputation on an individual is often underrated by members of the health team. In today's society the individual who is a highly mobile, physically attractive, independent achiever is admired. Communication media reinforce this concept in their advertisements for products that increase one's mobility, enhance one's beauty, and develop one's capabilities. For these reasons, the loss of a limb may signify more than just the relinquishing of a body part. Amputation may be viewed as the end of mobility, the loss of the capability for self-achievement, and the destruction of physical attractiveness.

When the individual first encounters the thought of an amputation, the initial reaction, as pointed out in Chapter 1, may include acute fear of impending death followed by a feeling of relief that he or she is alive. Such a reaction tends to be short-lived and occurs most frequently in individuals who have suffered a traumatic amputation, such as military personnel during wartime (Jeglijewski, 1973). However, this does not imply that individuals encountering an amputation brought on by disease, tumors, or congenital malformation may not experience the same reaction. The fear of surgical intervention to remove the limb or appendage can carry connotations of possible death for many people.

While the individual is experiencing the immediate fear of death, the individual must be allowed to verbalize these feelings. How does the fear of death affect the individual? What are the individual's uppermost thoughts and concerns? As discussed in Chapter 3, a judgmental approach should be avoided as the individual expresses his or her feelings. Value judgments conveyed by the nurse may hinder the individual's desire for expression. In addition, statements that change the subject should not be used, since the individual has a need to express these frightening thoughts. The use of statements that redirect the topic is often a defensive maneuver on the part of the nurse to avoid an uncomfortable subject, such as death.

The individual's first reaction to the thought of an amputation may well be one of repudiation. However, with individuals encountering acute fear of impending death, repudiation may constitute the second emotional reaction to amputation. Repudiation is demonstrated by not believing that the limb or appendage will actually be removed and/or maintaining a state of disbelief even after the amputation has occurred. This happens despite the immediate intellectual observation that the body part is gone. The amputee may demonstrate repudiation in such forms as refusing to look at the stump or attempting to ambulate without appropriate aids in the case of a lower limb amputation. Repudiation, like the acute fear of impending death, is generally short-lived. Some individuals, however, may use it for extended periods of time and require long term psychiatric intervention to achieve resolution.

As delineated in Chapter 3, family members also may experience repudiation. Their disbelief may be manifested in such ways as refusing to sign a consent form for the amputation (as in the case of the parents of a child who has a malformed, untreatable extremity) or simply refusing to touch the loved one's stump. As the amputee must be assisted during the act of repudiation, so must the family members since their feelings may well affect the amputee's ability to deal with the loss.

The nurse must keep in mind that the act of repudiation is one way the individual and the family can cope with the experience of amputation at this point in their lives. Therefore, both the individual and the family must be allowed to express their denial of the loss. The nurse, however, must not join in the expression of this denial. For example, if the individual is experiencing peripheral vascular disease and requires an amputation because gangrene has set in, yet refuses the surgical removal of the limb because he or she feels that with time circulation will improve, the nurse must avoid supporting this decision. The individual requires assistance in exploring why he or she believes that circulation will improve and also what consequences may occur if the limb is not removed. By directing the individual's attention to the reality of the situation, but still allowing the expression of denial, the nurse is more likely to help the patient in making the best decision for his or her particular situation.

The stage of recognition, as discussed in Chapter 3, is the second reactional stage that the amputee enters. It is during this stage that anger, negotiation, and depression are demonstrated as the patient attempts to cope with the amputation. The amputee's anger may be directed toward those in the environment, including the health team and family members. Statements demonstrating anger may include: "You don't know what it is like to have a leg missing, so don't tell me I'll walk again." "You never wrap my ace bandage right. Don't you know anything?" The necessity for projecting blame elsewhere may exist regardless of what others do. It is the one way the amputee attempts to cope with the loss. When the individual begins to express anger, he or she should be encouraged to do so without retaliative measures from others. The nurse must remember that the amputee sees others as mobile, self-sufficient, and physically attractive individuals. Questioning whether he or she has these attributes is not uncommon in the amputee. The expression of anger usually is directed toward these attributes held by others and not necessarily at others personally.

A growing awareness that the amputation has occurred will often elicit feelings of guilt. The amputee may feel that he or she contributed to the need for the amputation or that he or she did something for which the amputation is a punishment. The belief that an act of his or hers could have changed the situation may arouse acts of negotiation in an attempt to deal with these feelings of guilt. For example, the negotiating amputee might say: "If only I had not been driving in rainy weather, I wouldn't have had the accident and ended up like this (pointing to the stump)." "If I promise to move around in bed more, will you stop making me try to walk?"

To deal with the individual's guilt feelings it is necessary to engage in frank discussion before the amputation about the pathological processes that necessitate the amputation and the expected course of progression postoperatively. This discussion is the responsibility of *all* members of the health team, with particular emphasis on the physician and the nurse. During the discussion about the disease process the individual needs reassurance that the condition is something over which the individual has had no control. The individual should be informed that there is no reason to feel guilty about not coming for medical assistance sooner or for not carrying out measures that could have avoided the need for the amputation. In other words, the individual's guilt should be dealt with *before* the amputation instead of weeks later so that the overall rehabilitative process will not be delayed.

It is imperative that family members be included, as much as possible, in all explanations. Fear of the unknown is diminished by providing the individual and the family with information about the condition necessitating the amputation and about the expected course of progress during the postoperative period. Being aware of what their loved one faces provides family members with important data. It also provides the family with a better understanding of their loved one's personal needs while they are providing moral support. Subsequently the intensity of the individual's and family's depression about the loss of the limb may be held to a minimum.

Depression, generally a short-lived reaction, follows anger and guilt. Nurses may unintentionally inhibit the amputee's expression of anger and guilt and instead encourage the patient to be submissive and cooperative to the point of dependence. The individual who is basically a dependent person may relish the idea of having someone else care for his or her needs, since this relieves the individual of the responsibility. Extreme mood swings tend to be the exception rather than the rule and most emotionally well-balanced individuals will not experience severe degrees of depression. Nonetheless, some individuals may experience great difficulty in coping with the amputation and demonstrate deep-seated depression requiring intense psychiatric therapy.

As the amputee enters the stage of reconciliation, he or she begins to view the prosthetic device, if the amputee has one, more as a part of his or her body image than as an extemporaneous piece of equipment. The amputee assumes greater responsibility and pride in caring for both the stump and the prosthetic device. No longer does the amputee shy away from social interaction and work responsibilities. The amputee who has reconciled the loss of a limb or appendage is now capable of resuming a life-style close to that which he or she had before the amputation. The amputee's life-style will never be exactly the same, but the reconciled amputee adapts to these necessary alterations and functions at his or her optimal level.

A general guide for the nurse to use in attempting to determine whether the individual is beginning to work toward the resolution of the amputation is to note his or her attempts to move about and to resume social interaction and work responsibilities. The nurse's primary responsibility to the amputee in the stage of reconciliation is one of supporting the individual's achievements and expressing positive feedback on the individual's accomplishments (Walters, 1981). The amputee also needs to verbalize his or her feelings now that he or she has learned to function with the loss. Only when the amputee can comfortably talk about the loss and view postamputation accomplishments and failures in a realistic manner will he or she achieve reconciliation.

Somatic Impact

After an amputation most individuals experience the phenomenon of the phantom limb. The amputee describes the phantom limb phenomenon as a sensation of the lost limb's continuing presence. Although the extremity is perceived as being whole, the amputee is most aware of the distal portions of the phantom limb, the toes and fingers. This is because fingers and toes have more nerves and cortical representation than any other body part (Williams and Warwick, 1980). The phantom phenomenon usually is experienced immediately after surgery and may persist from six months to twenty years after the amputation (Frazier and Kolb, 1970). Since an individual has built up over the years a detailed mental picture of each body part, just as he or she has built up mental pictures of his or her surroundings, it is not amazing to find that image persisting even though the body has undergone drastic change (Parkes, 1976).

As can be expected, phantom phenomenon is not present in the individual who has a congenitally absent limb or in early childhood amputation, since, as discussed in Chapter 2, the body image is minimally developed before the age of six years. Adults experiencing anesthesia to the limb for extended periods before the amputation do not encounter the phantom phenomenon (Frazier and Kolb, 1970). This can be attributed to the fact that the individual has had time to reestablish a body image void of the limb prior to its amputation.

The amputee may actually experience pain in the phantom limb. The pain can vary in severity from a mild, tingling sensation to a cramplike or burning pain. According to the research conducted by Sherman and associates (1984), approximately 80 percent of all amputees experience significant amounts of phantom pain.

The nurse, in caring for the amputee, must not confuse phantom limb pain with stump pain. Stump pain does not occur immediately after surgery. It takes time to develop, occurs at the site of the surgical intervention, and can be brought on by touching the stump (Riding, 1976). Phantom limb pain, however, can be experienced at any time in the zone of the former limb.

Phantom pain is believed to be elicited by pain referred from somewhere else in the body such as the low back or the stump (Sherman and Tippens, 1982). Although many methods of treatment for phantom pain have been attempted, none has been universally successful (Larson and Gould, 1978; Sherman, Sherman, and Gall, 1980). Some methods have included nerve blocks, reamputation, biofeedback training, and hypnosis. Successful treatment of phantom pain depends upon the ability of the nurse and other health care providers to identify the source of pain referral and to deal with it appropriately.

The likely existence of phantom limb phenomenon and phantom pain after amputation should be explained to the individual and the family *before* the surgical intervention. The sensations should be described to the individual and the family because they must be made aware that these sensations are normal (Parkes, 1975). Failure to carry out appropriate counseling on phantom phenomenon and phantom pain may lead to an anxiety-ridden amputee who feels that he or she has "gone off the deep end." The amputee may not wish to describe these phantom sensations due to believing that others may perceive him or her to be emotionally disturbed. Hence, preoperative explanation of the phantom phenomenon is imperative.

In addition to the phantom phenomenon and phantom pain, one's altered body structure constitutes part of the somatic impact of amputation. The trauma of amputation greatly changes the body image and no longer are the body boundaries the same. The amputee now is forced to reassess body boundaries. The kind of impact amputation imposes upon one's body image is greatly affected by the stage of development that one is experiencing at the time of the loss of limb or appendage. For example, as discussed in Chapter 2, the young adult (eighteen years to forty-five years of age) is in the stage of intimacy versus isolation (Erikson, 1963). It is at this point in life that the individual is ready to merge his or her identity with others and to identify the body as a major factor in relating to others. The young amputee who has accepted the alteration in body structure brought about by the removal of a limb or appendage is capable of merging his or her identity with others and developing a sense of intimacy. However, the young adult experiencing the loss of a limb or appendage may view his or her physical body as less than acceptable since Western society places a great deal of emphasis upon physical attractiveness (Woods, 1979). If the individual thinks that he or she is less than adequate because of his or her physical appearance, the individual may fail to establish a state of intimacy with others and may retreat into isolation.

As presented in Chapter 2, the male is a low-barrier individual and defines his role in terms of achievement based upon body function (Fisher, 1964). Thus, he may view his amputation as an assault that hinders his performance and ability to achieve. The female, on the other hand, is a high-barrier individual and identifies her role more specifically with her body and its functions (Fisher, 1964). Consequently, a female amputee may view her loss as an assault that affects her ability to carry out her "feminine role." Regardless of whether the amputee is male or female, the maximum regular contour consistent with the body wall has been reached as a young adult (Fisher and Cleveland, 1968).

The impact of an amputation is somewhat different in adulthood (forty-five years to sixty-five years of age). During this developmental stage the individual directs energy toward establishing and guiding future generations with the hope of improving society (Erikson, 1963). The presence of an amputation is likely to alter this goal and instead of being generative, the adult may enter a state of stagnation. Fear of old age often becomes uppermost in one's mind. The amputation may be viewed as an additional or unwanted bodily change related to old age. By comparison the adult amputee who has incorporated the loss of limb into his or her body image is capable of establishing and guiding future generations.

The amputee in the final stage of life, maturity (sixty-five years of age and over), views the presence of loss differently. Since frequent thoughts of death occur during this stage, the existence of an amputation may be seen as the prelude to the termination of life. Hence, the mature adult may enter a stage of despair (Erikson, 1963) with a feeling of having little to offer others. As with the young adult and the adult, the mature adult who has successfully incorporated the alteration in body structure into his or her body image is capable of deriving satisfaction from life's experiences and accomplishments, and accepting the triumphs and disappointments of the past.

The nurse's role in dealing with altered body image revolves around assisting both the amputee and his or her family in accepting the amputee's new image. In this regard, six points of health care are important. First, the amputee and his or her family need reassurance that one can lead a functional and productive life regardless of the presence of a prosthetic device. Second, if possible, the amputee and the family should be introduced to another amputee of similar age, kind of amputation, and medical condition who has accomplished a readjustment in body image. This can be done through involvement in social support groups for the physically handicapped. Such interactions provide the amputee and the family with evidence that the incorporation of loss of limb into the body image is possible. Third, the amputee and the family should be informed that it takes several weeks to become accustomed to the prosthetic device and that initially the device will feel heavy and cumbersome. Provision of such information can facilitate the amputee's adjustment to the prosthesis. Fourth, the amputee and the family should be told that a training period in the use of the prosthesis will be provided in order to prevent inappropriate use of the artificial limb. Fifth, the amputee and the family should be instructed that no cosmetic prosthesis is completely natural in appearance. Realistic expectations related to cosmetic appearance of a prosthetic device can facilitate successful incorporation of the device into the body image. Sixth, the lower limb amputee and his or her family should be told that a change in gait is to be expected. Understanding that one's pre- and postamputation gait will not be identical can prevent frustration and subsequently facilitate mastery in the use of the prosthetic device.

Nursing's focus in facilitating the readjustment of the amputee's body image is honesty, good preoperative teaching, reinforcement of teaching in the postoperative period, incorporating the family into the entire rehabilitative process, and listening to what the amputee has to say. Only then can the amputee come to accept satisfactorily a change in body structure.

Sexual Impact

The way an individual perceives the body may influence his or her sexual self-concept and sexual behavior (Woods, 1979). The amputee who feels unattractive or unlovable may feel inadequate in a sexual relationship. As pointed out by Parkes (1976), limbs often are viewed as a component of sexual attractiveness and sexual self-image. Therefore, the female lower limb amputee may consider herself as less attractive to males who are sexually aroused by women's legs. By comparison, the male amputee may equate the loss of a limb or appendage with castration and subsequently believe his manhood has been threatened (Cummings, 1975).

The amputee may "act out" sexually in an attempt to test personal sexual image, to gain control of a situation that fosters dependence, and/or to attract attention from those in the environment. The wearing of revealing garments and the use of seductive statements are two possible manifestations suggesting the female amputee's attempt to test her sexual image. In an attempt to maintain masculinity, the male amputee may "act out" with such aggressive behavior as ramming doors with his wheelchair or balancing precariously on its rear wheels (Compton, 1973). Other means used to uphold an image of virility and "manliness" may be the displaying of pinup pictures, carrying out seductive, flirtatious acts toward female nurses, or outright exhibitionism.

Often the nurse's immediate reaction toward acts with sexual overtones is to retreat and avoid. In dealing with sexual acting out from either a male or female amputee, the nurse must set firm limits, neither going along with the flirtatious acts nor rejecting them. For example, the nurse could say, "I would rather you not touch me. It makes me uncomfortable. However, I will still come and talk to you whenever you desire." This helps set limits, but it does not express rejection. In addition to setting limits, the nurse should assist the amputee in exploring such behavior and encouraging verbal expression of feelings. The nurse may respond, "Your sexually aggressive behavior is not appropriate. I'd much rather talk to you about how you're feeling right now. It must be frustrating to be in the hospital not knowing how people will respond to you sexually." Such phrases aid in guiding the amputee's actions into words, showing empathy and understanding, demonstrating acceptance, and facilitating overall communication while providing guidelines for what is and is not acceptable behavior.

In addition to having a threatened sexual image, physical problems of carrying out the sex act may occur. The mechanics of positioning during sex play and intercourse most likely will need to be altered. For the lower limb amputee, it generally is desirable for the nonamputee to assume the superior position. An upper extremity amputee, when using sidelying positions, will find that keeping the unaffected arm free is most conducive to carrying out the sex act (Cummings, 1975). Regardless of the level or location of the amputation, the amputee and sex partner will need to experiment with various positions and techniques to find those which are mutually satisfying for their particular sexual relationship.

Another physical problem that tends to be encountered is an increase in phantom pain after orgasm in the male amputee and during orgasm in the female amputee (Riding, 1976). Unless the amputee is made aware of this phenomenon, guilt feelings are likely to be aroused, since the amputee may believe that engaging in sex is "bad." In addition, the amputee's sexual enjoyment may be diminished. Unless both the amputee and sex partner are aware of the occurrence of phantom pain during sex, additional strains will be placed upon their sexual relationship.

The nurse, however, must be aware that the amputee's sexual dysfunction may not be directly related to the amputation. Alterations in sexual function may have been present before the amputation or may be related to various disease entities, such as neurological conditions or endocrine disorders (Siemens and Brendzel, 1982). If the nurse detects, in the amputee or the sex partner, expressions of dismay about any aspect of their sexual activity (i.e., required position changes or decreased libido), referral for sex therapy is in order.

Occupational Impact

One's identity with an occupation is important since it provides the sense of doing or of having accomplished something constructive and worthwhile. This is demonstrated by the frequency with which one is asked, "What do you do for a living?" Now that the amputee has suffered the loss of a limb or appendage, he or she may ask "What has become of me? What am I going to do now?"

Depending upon the individual's prior occupation, either minor or major work adjustments may be necessary. A minor adjustment could include placing left-handed banisters along the staircases at work for the individual who has a right arm amputation. A major occupational adjustment might include completely changing jobs. If, for example, the individual's job requires the use of two functional hands, an upper extremity amputee will need occupational training for a new job. Having to change jobs can prove stressful to the amputee. Therefore, the nurse's role at this time will be one of listening and providing guidance and support to the amputee as he or she expresses fear about changing or modifying occupational endeavors. The discussion should be directed toward identifying the positive attributes of the amputee and praising all accomplishments he or she has made.

One of the most important factors affecting an individual's ability to cope well with life as an amputee is the capacity to work (Parkes, 1975). As discussed in Chapter 3, the role of breadwinner is an important component of one's physio-psychosocial well-being. Due to the loss of a limb, the family breadwinner is likely to view his or her role as endangered and, in turn, may imagine that family affections are diminishing. The amputee's belief that family affections are waning may be incited by the fact that family members are being required to assume some of the responsibilities of breadwinner while the amputee is readjusting to a new occupational role. The amputee perceives a loss in status in the family structure due to the additional responsibilities he or she has placed on family members. In addition, the amputee might fear that a lowered standard of living will occur because he or she may not be able to cope with the alteration in work status. The loss of limb may be perceived as the end of occupational pursuits and the beginning of premature, sedentary retirement.

Providing support and acceptance as the amputee attempts to reconquer simple physical tasks is a major role for family members. Since family members are the ones most directly affected (aside from the amputee) by the occupational readjustments, provisions should be made for them to verbalize their feelings about the impact of the amputation on occupational changes and to examine financial alternatives. In some situations family members and the amputee may need to be directed to appropriate sources (i.e., social workers) for financial counseling. As with the amputee, the family members should be encouraged to focus on the positive accomplishments made by the amputee during his or her rehabilitative program. Frequent expressions of encouragement, stating that the amputee is a worthwhile and contributing member to the family, are necessary. The amputee's readjustment to a different occupation is not always rapid or easy, and patience on the part of the family and health care team is imperative.

Social Impact

What one is to oneself and to others constitutes one's social identity. In other words, the inward assurance of expected recognition from oneself and from individuals of personal importance, such as family, friends, and associates, makes up one's identity in society.

When the new amputee leaves the protective environment of the hospital and enters the world again, he or she must reestablish his or her social identity. This identity must incorporate the changed physical appearance as well as the required adaptations to daily living.

To deal with the altered physical appearance, the amputee must be made aware that some individuals in society may stare, make comments about the missing limb, or ask numerous questions about the amputation. Amputees have commented that one of their most difficult social encounters is when an innocent child says, "Mommy, look, why does that man have only one leg?" The amputee must realize that some individuals are not probing to be personal but that they are actually uncomfortable and unable to handle the presence of an amputee. Their own anxiety and insecurity are demonstrated by their probing. It is vital to encourage the amputee before and after reentering society to discuss how he or she may feel about such a situation and how he or she may handle the incident. Engaging amputees in sharing their individual social experiences and how they dealt with them often proves helpful. Society's reactions are reality and the amputee needs assistance in facing and dealing with these realities.

To deal with effective incorporation of required adaptations to daily living, the amputee needs assistance and guidance in feeling competent with use of supportive aids such as handrails, special driving devices, and the prosthetic device (if one is prescribed). The amputee who feels competent and comfortable in utilizing equipment or devices that enhance independence is more likely to seek out and engage in social interactions.

In addition to the competent use of aids and devices which enhance independence, the amputee needs to be directed toward a *role* of self-sufficiency since reentering society demands a certain degree of independence. Carrying out one's personal hygiene and transfer techniques are but two examples manifesting a role of self-sufficiency. As the lower limb amputee learns to ambulate with a prosthesis, the family, the nurse, and other members of the health team must avoid overprotection. If the patient falls while attempting ambulation, the nurse should ask if he or she needs assistance instead of running immediately to help. Immediate assistance in such an incident is not only degrading, but it fosters dependence on the part of the amputee.

The amputee needs reassurance that many preamputation activities can be reestablished. Amputees have engaged in such sports as scuba diving, snow skiing, sky diving, and horseback riding. The amputee's personal drive to succeed and the family's support and understanding are vital in his or her reestablishment of preamputation activities.

If there were family problems before the amputation, the loss of a limb may be the final crisis that disrupts the family structure. In this case, psychiatric therapy may be needed for the amputee and the family since disruption of family structure may be interpreted by the amputee as further rejection. When the amputee feels rejection, he or she encounters difficulty in reestablishing a strong social identity.

Each amputee redevelops his or her social identity at a different pace. However, preparing the amputee for situations that might be encountered, allowing the amputee to verbalize feelings about how others react to him or her, fostering independence, and providing encouragement for all forms of progress can facilitate the reestablishment of a social identity.

SUMMARY

Amputation surgery is brought about by four major causes: trauma; disease; tumors; and congenital disorders. Nearly three fourths of all amputations are brought about by peripheral vascular changes, thus making disease the most frequent cause of amputation. The greatest percentage of amputees are males fifty years old and older.

Amputation imposes a great impact upon both the individual involved and his or her family. The impact of amputation affects the amputee's psychological well-being, somatic identity, sexuality, occupational identity, and social role. The amputee experiences loss, body image alteration, potential threats to sexuality, possible job alterations, and social reacceptance. Therefore, the psychosocial impact of amputation should never by underrated by members of the health care team. The major role of the health care team is to prepare the individual and the family for alterations in daily living which are likely to occur and to assist them in dealing with each of these changes.

Patient Situation   Mr. A. K., a fifty-five-year-old truck driver, has been a diabetic for the past thirty years. Because of chronic vascular changes that have accompanied his diabetes, a right lower limb amputation has been performed. Mr. A. K. is married and the father of two children. His elder child, a daughter, is married and his younger child, a son, is a sophomore in a local city college. Mr. A. K. is two days postamputation and demonstrates problems affecting his psychological well-being, somatic identity, sexuality, occupational identity, and social role.

Following are Mr. A. K.'s nursing care plan and patient care cardex dealing with the above mentioned areas of concern.

NURSING CARE PLAN

Nursing Diagnoses	Objectives	Nursing Interventions	Principles/Rationale	Evaluations
Psychological Impact Unreconciled loss manifested by anger directed at health care team and family members.	To decrease Mr. A. K.'s anger.	Encourage the expression of feelings by using open-ended statements such as, "You seem upset today."	Expressing feelings may assist the amputee in identifying what is causing the anger.	The nurse would observe for: Changes in Mr. A. K.'s expressions of anger.
	To demonstrate acceptance of Mr. A. K.	Avoid retaliative acts and statements when Mr. A. K. expresses his anger.	Retaliative acts and statements may further upset and anger the amputee. Retaliative acts may be interpreted by the amputee as rejection by health team members and family members. Retaliative acts may be the family and health team members' projection of their own anger.	Mr. A. K.'s ability to express himself freely without fear of retaliation from others.
	To support Mr. A. K.'s family during his expressions of anger.	Act as a sounding board for family members so that they might express their feelings of frustration when Mr. A. K. "strikes out" at them in anger.	A family frustrated by acts of anger directed at them by a loved one may be unable to provide necessary support to the loved one.	The family's ability to cope with Mr. A. K.'s anger.
		Provide explanations to Mr. A. K.'s family about reasons for his anger.	Expressions of anger are often directed at attributes, such as mobility, which others represent and not necessarily at others personally. Anger expressed in the form of blaming others is one way the amputee attempts to cope with his loss.	

Somatic Impact				The nurse would observe for:
Body image alteration manifested by presence of phantom limb phenomenon and phantom pain.	To enhance Mr. A. K.'s and his family's understanding of phantom limb phenomenon.	Describe phantom limb phenomenon to Mr. A. K. and his family as the sensation at the amputated site that the limb is still present. Mention that the sensation is present in the majority of amputees and lasts anywhere from six months to twenty years.	Realizing that such a phenomenon exists and is experienced by the majority of amputees decreases the anxiety of both the amputee and his family.	Anxiety and fear expressed by Mr. A. K. and his family related to the presence of phantom phenomenon and phantom pain.
	To enhance Mr. A. K.'s and his family's understanding of the difference between phantom limb and stump pain.	Describe the difference between phantom limb pain and stump pain to Mr. A. K. and his family. Describe stump pain as: 1. pain that does not occur immediately after surgery. 2. pain brought on by touching the stump. 3. pain that occurs at the site of surgical intervention. Describe phantom limb pain as: 1. pain in the phantom limb that often is elicited by an emotionally charged situation such as anger or talking about the amputation.	By knowing the difference between phantom limb pain and stump pain, the amputee is better prepared to determine when pain medication is necessary for his stump pain.	Inappropriate use of pain medication (use of pain medication for phantom limb pain rather than stump pain).
			By realizing that phantom limb pain can be brought on by emotionally charged situations, the amputee and his family are better able to recognize and avoid such situations.	Identification and avoidance of situations by Mr. A. K. and his family which elicit phantom limb pain.

(cont.)

NURSING CARE PLAN (cont.)

Nursing Diagnoses	Objectives	Nursing Interventions	Principles/Rationale	Evaluations
Body image alteration manifested by fear that body structure change is related to aging.	To assist Mr. A. K. in dealing with his fears of body change.	Encourage Mr. A. K. to verbalize his fears about how he views the amputation as an unwanted body change related to aging. The use of open-ended statements such as, "It must be frightening to lose a limb and not know what the future holds for you" may be helpful.	Verbalization about a fear tends to decrease the fear. Verbalization about a fear often assists the individual in identifying ways of dealing with the fear.	The nurse would observe for: Verbalization alluding to how Mr. A. K. views his body change.
		Provide privacy during Mr. A. K.'s discussions about his fears of body change related to aging.	Privacy enhances the likelihood that the amputee will express feelings freely.	Mr. A. K.'s uninhibited verbalization of fears.
	To assist Mr. A. K. in analyzing the positive aspects of his life.	Assist Mr. A. K. in identifying and discussing those aspects of his life that he finds positive and supportive.	Recognizing the positive and supportive aspects of the amputee's life may provide a reason to be generative. Identifying and discussing positive aspects of life prevents a state of stagnation by the amputee.	Mr. A. K.'s verbalization of hopeful feelings and plans for the future.
Sexual Impact Unreconciled sexual identity manifested by inappropriate sexual statements and behavior toward female staff.	To alter Mr. A. K.'s inappropriate behavior.	Provide Mr. A. K. with limits for his behavior while never going along with nor rejecting his inappropriate behavior (i.e., inform him that you find his behavior unpleasant, but reassure him that you accept *him.*)	Providing a sexually aggressive individual with well-defined limits for inappropriate behavior, yet expressing acceptance of the patient as a person, aids in decreasing inappropriate sexual behavior.	The nurse would observe for: A decrease in Mr. A. K.'s inappropriate sexual statements and behavior.

Occupational Impact Unreconciled financial concerns manifested by expressed concern about an alteration in the family standard of living.	To enhance Mr. A. K.'s feelings of self-worth.	Encourage Mr. A. K. to examine his behavior.	Looking at one's own behavior aids in identifying ways of dealing with the behavior.	Mr. A. K.'s positive expression about his self-worth.
		Encourage Mr. A. K. to express his feelings.	Verbalization aids in decreasing anxiety and helps in identifying ways of dealing with feelings.	The nurse would observe for: Expressed satisfaction by Mr. A. K. of possible solutions of his financial concerns. Increased communication between Mr. A. K. and his family concerning their financial situation.
	To assist Mr. A. K. in examining his concerns about the family's financial status.	Encourage Mr. A. K. to discuss his concerns about his family's financial security with his wife and children. Notify social service about Mr. A. K.'s expressed concern.	Financial concerns affect the entire family; therefore their knowledge and input in developing a solution is imperative. Social service is a component of the health team prepared to assist the amputee and the family with financial concerns.	
Social Impact Potential social isolation manifested by expressed concern about how society will accept his altered physical structure.	To assist Mr. A. K. in dealing with his concern about society's acceptance of his altered physical structure.	Encourage Mr. A. K. to continue to verbalize his concern about his family's financial status.	Internalizing a concern can lead to undue anxiety.	Decreased anxiety in Mr. A. K. about family financial concerns.
		Encourage Mr. A. K. to verbalize how he may react and deal with people staring at him, commenting about his lost limb, or asking probing questions about the amputation.	Verbalizing feelings about social acceptance and possible ways of dealing with these feelings assists the amputee in preparing for a potentially traumatic social reality.	The nurse would observe for: Open expression by Mr. A. K. about his feelings and his possible reactions to society's response to his altered physical structure.
		Encourage Mr. A. K. to express his concerns about society's acceptance of him with his family.	Family members who are cognizant of a loved one's concerns are better prepared to provide support during a traumatic situation.	Supportive statements from the family related to society's acceptance of Mr. A. K.'s altered physical structure.

PATIENT CARE CARDEX

PATIENT'S NAME: _____Mr. A. K._____

AGE: _____55 years_____

MARITAL STATUS: _____Married_____

SIGNIFICANT OTHERS: Wife and two children (one married and one

attending local college)

MEDICAL DIAGNOSIS: _____Right lower limb amputation_____

SEX: _____Male_____

OCCUPATION: _____Truck driver_____

Nursing Diagnoses

Psychological: Unreconciled loss manifested by anger directed at health care team and family members

Somatic: Body image alteration manifested by presence of phantom limb phenomenon and phantom pain. Body image alteration manifested by fear that body structure change is related to aging.

Nursing Approaches

1. Encourage the expression of feelings by use of open-ended statements (i.e., "You seem upset today").
2. Avoid use of retaliative acts and statements when patient expresses anger.
3. Act as sounding board for family so that they might express their feelings of frustration when patient "strikes out" at them in anger.
4. Provide explanations to family about reasons for patient's anger.

1. Describe phantom limb phenomenon to patient and family.
2. Mention that phantom limb phenomenon is present in the majority of amputees and lasts anywhere from 6 months to 20 years.
3. Describe difference between phantom limb pain and stump pain to patient and family.

Describe stump pain as:

(a) pain that does not occur immediately after surgery.

(b) pain brought on by touching the stump.

(c) pain that occurs at the site of surgical intervention.

Describe phantom limb pain as:

(a) pain in the phantom limb which often is elicited by an emotionally charged situation such as anger or talking about the amputation.

4. Encourage to verbalize fears about how he views the amputation as an unwanted body change related to aging.

5. Provide privacy during discussions about fears of body change related to aging.

6. Assist in identifying and discussing those aspects of life which are positive and supportive.

Sexual: Unreconciled sexual identity manifested by inappropriate sexual statements and behavior toward female staff.

1. Provide with limits for behavior while never going along with nor rejecting inappropriate behavior (i.e., inform that you find behavior unpleasant, but reassure that you accept *him*).

2. Encourage to examine behavior.

3. Encourage to express feelings.

Occupational: Unreconciled financial concerns manifested by expressed concern about alteration in the family's standard of living.

1. Encourage to discuss concerns about family's financial security with family.

2. Notify social service about expressed concern.

3. Encourage to continue to verbalize concern about family's financial situation.

Social: Potential social isolation manifested by expressed concern about how society will accept his altered physical structure.

1. Encourage to verbalize how he may react and deal with people staring at him, commenting about lost limb, or asking probing questions about the amputation.

2. Encourage to express with family concerns about society's acceptance of him.

REFERENCES

COMPTON, C. War injury: identity crisis for young men, *Nursing Clinics of America,* 1973, *8,* (1), 52–66.

CUMMINGS, V. Amputees and sexual dysfunction, *Archives of Physical Medicine and Rehabilitation,* 1975, *56* (1), 53–66.

ERIKSON, E. *Childhood and society.* New York: W.W. Norton and Co., Inc., 1963.

FERNIE, G. The epidemiology of amputation. In J. Kostrik (Ed.), *Amputation surgery and rehabilitation: The Toronto experience.* New York: Churchill Livingstone, 1981.

FISHER, S. Sex differences in body perception, *Psychological Monographs,* 1964, *78,* 1–22.

FISHER, S., and CLEVELAND, S. *Body image and personality.* New York: Dover, 1968.

FRAZIER, S., and KOLB, L. Psychiatric aspects of pain and the phantom limb, *Orthopedic Clinics of North America,* 1970, *1* (2), 481–490.

GILLESPIE, R. Congenital limb deformities and amputation surgery in children. In J. Kostrik (Ed.), *Amputation surgery and rehabilitation: The Toronto experience.* New York: Churchill Livingstone, 1981.

JEGLIJEWSKI, J. Target: outside world, *American Journal of Nursing,* 1973, *73* (6), 1024–1027.

KAY, H., and NEWMAN, J. Relative incidence of new amputations, *Orthotics & Prosthetics,* 1975, *29,* 3–16.

KERSTEIN, M., ZIMMER, H., DUGDALE, F., and LERNER, E. What influence does age have on rehabilitation of amputees? *Geriatrics,* 1975, *30* (12), 67–71.

LARSON, C., and GOULD, M. *Orthopedic nursing.* St. Louis: C.V. Mosby, 1978.

PARKES, C.M. The psychological reaction to loss of a limb: the first year after amputation. In J.G. Howells (Ed.), *Modern perspectives in the psychiatric aspects of surgery.* New York: Brunner/Mazel, 1976.

PARKES, C. Reaction to loss of limb, *Nursing Mirror,* 1975, *140* (1), 36–40.

RANG, M., and THOMPSON, G. History of amputations and prostheses. In J. Kostrik (Ed.), *Amputation surgery and rehabilitation: The Toronto experience.* New York: Churchill Livingstone, 1981.

RIDING, J. Phantom limb: some theories, *Anaesthesia,* 1976, *31,* 102–106.

SHERMAN, R., SHERMAN, C., and GALL, N. A survey of current phantom limb pain treatment in the United States, *Pain,* 1980, *81,* 85–99.

SHERMAN, R., SHERMAN, C., and PARKER, L. Chronic phantom and stump pain among American veterans: results of a survey, *Pain,* 1984, *18,* 83–95.

SHERMAN, R., and TIPPENS, J. Suggested guidelines for treatment of phantom limb pain, *Orthopedics,* 1982, *5* (12), 1596–1600.

SIEMENS, S., and BRENDZEL, R. *Sexuality: nursing assessment and intervention.* Philadelphia: Lippincott, 1982.

TOOMS, R. Amputation. In A. Edmonsen and A. Crenshaw (Eds.), *Campbell's operative orthopedics.* St. Louis: C.V. Mosby, 1980.

WALTERS, J. Coping with a leg amputation, *American Journal of Nursing,* 1981, *81* (7), 1349–1352.

WARREN, R. Amputation in the lower limb, *Surgery Annual,* 1975, *7,* 331–346.

WILLIAMS, P., and WARWICK, R. (Eds.), *Gray's anatomy.* Philadelphia: Saunders, 1980.

WOODS, N.F. *Human sexuality in health and illness.* St. Louis: C.V. Mosby, 1979.

5

MASTECTOMY

INTRODUCTION

Approximately 115,000 women are diagnosed each year as having cancer of the breast (Silverberg, 1983). In other words, one out of every thirteen women in the United States will be affected by breast cancer at some time during her life. The majority of cases of breast cancer have been found in women over the age of forty-five years, with the incidence increasing with age. Studies reveal that cancer occurs most frequently in the outer quadrant of the left breast in women who have not borne or breast-fed infants (Savlov, 1978). However, cancer of the breast diagnosed in a localized stage has been treated successfully with five-year survival rates for white females (88 percent) and black females (79 percent) (Silverberg, 1983).

Although cancer of the breast remains the leading cause of cancer deaths in women, it must not be forgotten that males also are susceptible to tumors of the breast. Tumors of the male breast, however, are not as common as those that occur in the female organ. In addition, males affected by tumors of the breast tend to be slightly older than females so affected (Silverberg, 1983).

When an individual first detects the presence of a lump in the breast, nursing intervention is required. The nurse's role involves assisting the individual in: obtaining appropriate medical evaluation; dealing with the impact that the detection of a lump has upon one's life; being cognizant of the possible ramifications of a mastectomy, and utilizing appropriate support systems. This chapter will deal with the impact of mastectomy on both the female's and male's psychological well-being, somatic identity, sexuality, occupational identity, and social role.

SIGNIFICANCE OF DISCOVERY AND DIAGNOSIS

The female breast is a symbol of motherhood both from a nutritious and nurtural point of view. The infant can be fed by the female breast or the child can be cuddled close to the breast in a protective manner. The importance of the breast to the female becomes apparent during adolescence when the young girl focuses a great deal of attention on the development of her bustline and goes to great effort to draw attention to her new identifiable mark of femininity. The attention may be brought about by the clothing she wears or by the posture she maintains. The breast also plays a role in sexual stimulation and it may assume an important role in sex play for both sexes.

The presence of a lump in the breast, in the majority of cases, is found during bathing, dressing, examination by the individual, or during manipulation of the breast by the sex partner. Discovery of a lump in the breast often elicits an immediate reaction of concern for life (Katz, Weiner, Gallagher, and Hallman, 1976). A palpable lump denotes the possible presence of cancer with the fear of impending death being uppermost in the individual's mind, since many individuals equate the word cancer with death. The individual's response may be one of repudiation, as presented in Chapter 3, and may be demonstrated by such a statement as, "No, this can't be happening to me." Repudiating the existence of the lump or the fear of a possible mastectomy is likely to lead to the individual's delay in seeking medical treatment.

Once the presence of the lump has been noted, the individual questions how others will respond to the presence of the lump and is concerned about the possibility of a mastectomy. A mother may be concerned about the welfare of her children should she require a mastectomy as a result of the breast lump. The model will fear the effects that a mastectomy may have upon his or her career since clothing, such as a low-cut evening dress or a tight-fitting T-shirt, often accentuates the chest area.

The mastectomy candidate may wonder how his or her sex partner will respond to the results of the surgery. In today's society the impact of mastectomy on the sex partner frequently is overlooked. Generally, he or she is the first person called upon to provide psychological support to the mastectomee, yet little support and understanding are provided by the health care team to the sex partner. The sex partner has need for support and understanding. The fear of whether the loss of a partner will occur, what needs the mastectomee may have which require assistance, and how the partner will react to the surgical experience are but a few of the concerns expressed by the mastectomee's sex partner. A sex partner who is uncertain and full of conflicting emotions may project an attitude of rejection, the very attitude most feared by the mastectomee. The health care team must provide the sex partner with information regarding the surgical procedure, an opportunity to ventilate feelings, and guidance concerning his or her possible reactions to the outcomes of the mastectomy.

Information about the surgical procedure can be dealt with by explaining to the sex partner what pre- and postoperative experiences the mastectomee will experience as well as what portions of the breast and surrounding structures will be removed. Guidance concerning the sex partner's reaction to the outcome of the mastectomy will need to focus on the fact that the sex partner may find the surgical scar distasteful but that this reaction is a normal response to the visible loss of a body part of a loved one. The sex partner's honesty about his or her feelings with self and the mastectomee should be encouraged since dishonest behavior on the part of the sex partner may be perceived as rejection by the mastectomee. Such interventions will facilitate the sex partner's ability to cope with the demands placed upon him or her. If adequate preparation and support are not provided for the sex partner, he or she may be ill-prepared to cope with the demands of the situation.

IMPACT OF MASTECTOMY

Psychological Impact

When the individual first discovers that the breast has been removed, the act of repudiation occurs. Repudiating the loss of the breast generally lasts from a few minutes to several days. In some cases, however, the use of repudiation may extend for months. As with any loss, repudiation is the "buffer" that allows the individual time to activate thoughts and mobilize other means of coping with the loss.

After the stage of repudiation, the mastectomee enters the stage of recognition and it is during this emotional stage that anger, depression, or negotiation may be elicited. The most common emotional reaction of the mastectomee during this stage of loss is depression (Maguire, 1976). Most female mastectomees experience depression within a week or so after the operation. This depression may last as long as several months. The woman feels that her life is ended and that no one understands how she feels. Every time she bathes, undresses, or looks in a mirror, she is faced with the fact that a potentially fatal disease may be present. Some women may demonstrate their depression by insomnia, frequent expressions of hopelessness and despair, inability to concentrate, or failure to carry out necessary household or work responsibilities. They may retreat to bed and assume the illness role as discussed in Chapter 1. These women often view themselves as worthless and noncontributing members of society and may make such statements as: "What good am I to myself and my family now that I'm not a whole person. I can't even carry out my usual duties since I've had surgery."

The male mastectomee also can go through a stage of depression after the loss of a breast. It must not be forgotten that male mastectomees also are reminded that they may have a potentially fatal disease each time they touch or view their chest area.

To deal with the depression expressed by both the male and female mastectomee, the use of group sessions consisting of individuals in similar stages of loss has proven effective (Schmid, Kiss, and Hibert, 1974). Mastectomees, thus, are able to empathize and provide support to one another during this period. Empirical evidence has shown that "support" is of crucial importance when one is faced with a stressful experience (Morris, 1979; Northouse, 1981; Nuckolls, Cassel, and Kaplan, 1972) such as the loss of a breast.

Crying plays an important role for the female mastectomee in dealing with her depression. It serves as an alternate means of expression when verbalization of feelings is difficult. At no time should the individual be reprimanded for crying or should the presence of crying be interpreted as a sign of weakness. Privacy should be provided during crying and the individual should be reassured that there is nothing wrong with expressing one's feelings in the form of tears. Family members, if present during the mastectomee's crying, may feel embarrassed and encourage the woman not to cry. It is the nurse's responsibility to explain: "Crying is one way of relieving pent-up frustrations and your wife/mother needs to cry at this time in order to express her feelings about her mastectomy."

To assist family members with their feelings of discomfort during the mastectomee's crying, the nurse should encourage them to provide support in the form of listening, holding her hand, or simply touching the woman's arm in an expressive, gentle manner. In addition, the nurse may find it helpful to discuss with family members their feelings about crying after the incident is over. Encouraging the family to identify and describe why the mastectomee's crying makes them uncomfortable will assist the family in dealing with their own feelings. Verbalization of this issue allows the family the opportunity to examine the reality of their feelings and to acknowledge the fact that it is alright to have such feelings.

Men are less likely to express their depression in the form of crying because of the societal "taboos" for such behavior in males. The nurse is more likely to observe the male mastectomee retreat into his room, remain uncommunicative, or play the role of the "good patient." It is imperative for the nurse to encourage him to verbalize how he feels about himself. A leading statement such as, "You seem 'low' today," may initiate verbalization and facilitate the expression of suppressed feelings. As the mastectomee expresses his feelings of decreased self-worth, the nurse needs to assist him in identifying his strengths and in investigating with him how he can integrate these strengths into his ability to deal with his specific situation.

Feelings of guilt also may be expressed by the mastectomee during the stage of recognition. Guilt feelings are likely to be incited by misconceptions about cancer. Common misconceptions include the belief that cancer is inherited, contagious, or caused by a blow or injury to the breast. Misconceptions about cancer require clarification and the nurse must take an active role in providing accurate information. Reassurance that the presence of cancer is not punishment for some wrongdoing on the part of the mastectomee should also be provided.

When the mastectomee enters the final stage of loss, reconciliation, he or she is ready to reenter society with a note of confidence. No longer does the mastectomee feel a need for isolation from social interaction or work responsibilities. A feeling of self-worth is reestablished and the need to resume the role of a contributing member of society again becomes apparent. It must not be overlooked, however, that the mastectomee continues to live with the fear of possible metastasis and possible loss of the other breast. Therefore, fluctuations in psychological well-being do occur and the mastectomee may move back and forth between the stages of repudiation, recognition, and reconciliation.

Somatic Impact

The breast is an important part of one's body image. As discussed in Chapter 2, this image is not necessarily an objective or accurate picture of oneself, but rather an accumulation of thoughts that one has about oneself. Loss of any body part, such as a breast, disrupts one's body image and, with it, the sense of naturalness and wholeness. The female mastectomee views her breasts as a symbol of her femininity (Carroll, 1981). Now that a breast is gone, is her femininity gone? This question may be mulled over and over by the female mastectomee. The male mastectomee, by the same token, may equate the removal of a breast with castration since his masculine physique has been altered. He may now view his manly appearance as being inferior.

The somatic impact of a mastectomy is affected by the individual's stage of development at the time of the loss. The majority of female mastectomees are in the stage of adulthood (forty-five to sixty-five years of age) with the major focus of interest being directed toward establishing and guiding future generations (Erikson, 1963). When a woman has lost a breast she may feel that her ability to "mother" and guide future generations is no longer present. Instead of becoming generative, she may withdraw from others, become self-absorbed, and enter a stage of stagnation.

In addition to the task of generativity during the stage of adulthood, the female is concerned about maintaining an attractive physical appearance. She often identifies, in an exaggerated manner, each single physical change related to aging. The loss of a breast may be viewed by the female mastectomee in the stage of adulthood as an additional unwanted bodily change related to the aging process. Consequently, she may feel resigned to old age. Since she feels unattractive physically and incapable of achieving the task of generativity, chronic defeatism and depression may result and the woman isolates herself in self-pity.

Male mastectomees tend to be older than female mastectomees (Silverberg, 1983) and are more likely to be in the stage of maturity (sixty-five years of age and older) when frequent thoughts of death occur (Erickson, 1963). If feelings of despair are present, the occurrence of a mastectomy may add additional despondent thoughts of impending death. In addition, the male mastectomee may be unable to derive satisfaction from his life's experiences and accomplishments, especially if he has not developed a strong sense of self-worth. The presence of the mastectomy may add to his decreased feelings of self-worth. Consequently, he manifests his feelings of despair in expressions of disgust. Regardless of the developmental stage demonstrated by the individual at the time of the mastectomy, body boundaries have been altered and the individual is forced to readjust his personal mental picture of his body structure.

How the mastectomee believes significant others view him or her is of vital importance. The mastectomee is concerned about how the sex partner will react to the missing breast and to the large scar that exists. "Will my sex partner be repulsed by the appearance of my chest wall?" "Will my sex partner replace me with someone else because of the change in my body structure?" To assist the mastectomee in dealing with such feelings it is advisable to have the sex partner take an active part in dressing changes prior to the mastectomee's leaving the hospital (Northouse, 1981). Early visual and tactile involvement by the sex partner can assist in demonstrating to the mastectomee that he or she is still accepted by significant others.

Following a mastectomy, lymphedema of the extremity on the affected side may occur, rendering that extremity larger than the extremity on the nonaffected side (Golemastic, Delikaris, Balarustsos, and Karamonakos, 1975). Hence, special precautions of arm and hand care are necessary. These precautions include such things as wearing rubber gloves when gardening or using harsh detergents, wearing thimbles when sewing, using electric razors when shaving under the arm, and avoiding injections, infusions, and finger pricks in the affected arm. In addition, since the extremity on the affected side may be larger than on the nonaffected side, the individual should be encouraged not to wear constrictive sleeves, restrictive jewelry, or a tight bra strap on that side. The mastectomee may be concerned about how the enlarged arm appears to others and may remark, "This enlarged arm makes me look like a freak." The nurse will want to investigate with the mastectomee alternatives for dealing with the enlarged arm. Alternatives can include assisting the mastectomee with clothing selections which do not accentuate the appearance of one's arm and/or which provide loose fitting, three-quarter length sleeves.

Numbness and tingling along the inner aspect of the arm on the affected side are likely to occur in most patients. The fact that peripheral nerves are cut during the surgery helps explain the occurrence of this sensation. As the peripheral nerves regenerate, sensation gradually resumes. In some instances, mastectomees will have permanent residual loss of sensation in the arm on the affected side. The individual must be advised of these changes before surgery in order to avoid undue anxiety after surgery that something went wrong. With the presence of numbness and tingling the mastectomee must reestablish body boundaries. Not only is a breast missing, but sensation in the arm on the affected side also is altered.

Phantom breast syndrome, often an issue overlooked by nurses, is not uncommon in the mastectomee. Pain is the most common phantom sensation; itching, numbness, nipple contraction, burning, cramp-like feelings, and soreness can also be experienced (Jamison, Wellisch, Katz, and Pasnau, 1979). These phantom sensations may involve the entire breast or be confined to specific regions of the breast. Although phantom breast syndrome may not be so vivid as that felt in limb amputations, nonetheless the sensation that the missing breast still is present does occur in many mastectomees. Phantom breast syndrome, as does phantom limb phenomenon, yields a more vivid phantom in the proximal area of the appendage. Thus, the nipple is the single most common area felt in the phantom breast. Research has shown that phantom breast syndrome tends to be more prevalent in young mastectomees who perceive that they have not received much emotional support from their surgeons and who perceive that most of their emotional difficulties are secondary to the mastectomy (Jamison, Wellisch, Katz, and Pasnau, 1979). The mastectomee must be made aware that phantom breast syndrome can occur after surgery and that its presence is not an unusual phenomenon. If the mastectomee is not forewarned of the possibility of this syndrome, the presence of the phantom sensations may be interpreted as a possible postsurgical complication.

The breast prosthesis plays a major role in the female mastectomee's reestablishment of body image. It is advisable for a lightweight soft prosthesis to be provided soon after the surgical dressings are removed. Although the initial prosthesis is temporary, it helps raise the woman's self-image while she is vulnerable to feelings of depression (Siemens and Branzel, 1982). It is possible to wear a lightweight prosthesis as early as the second or third postoperative day as a result of contemporary suction techniques and lightweight dressings. A permanent prosthesis should not be fitted until the wound has healed completely. Various prostheses are available which vary in cost. They may be silicone-gel, oil-filled, granule-filled, or air-filled (Winkler, 1977). The woman's selection should be based upon cost, comfort, and what she finds most suitable to restore her figure. The sex partner may wish to take an active role in helping in the selection of the prosthesis. Some prosthetic devices assume a very humanlike texture and may be found desirable by the sex partner. If the woman wants information about breast prostheses, the nurse should direct her to surgical appliance firms, women's wear departments, and drugstores. A list of establishments that carry permanent breast prostheses can be obtained through the American Cancer Society.

If surgically feasible, the mastectomee may want to consider breast reconstruction in lieu of a breast prosthesis. With the many advances in techniques of reconstructive mammoplasty in recent years, the mastectomee has the alternative of having a breast reconstructed that has reasonable contour and consistency. The option of having a reconstructive mammoplasty can be discussed preoperatively by the individual and the surgeon. If during the course of the operation the physician finds that it is possible to begin mammary reconstruction, the surgical procedure can become one aspect of the entire surgical maneuver. It must be pointed out, however, that not all mastectomees are good candidates for reconstructive surgery. In addition to physiological considerations required for a reconstructive mammoplasty, such as the likelihood of not developing recurrence or metastatic disease, certain psychosocial considerations must be approached. These considerations include the mastectomee's awareness of: the time that must be invested in repeated hospitalizations; the mental strength required to endure more surgery and associated risks; and the limitations of reconstructive surgery (Long and Molbo, 1983). Breast reconstruction can provide a positive effect upon the mastectomee's reestablishment of body image, since the chest area now has a closer resemblance to its premastectomy state. Research has shown that reconstructive surgery tends to decrease the mastectomized individual's feelings of dependence and mutilation (Goin and Goin, 1981).

When the mastectomee returns for the first postoperative checkup, the individual should be instructed and advised on the technique for breast self-examination. Pictorial pamphlets are helpful and can be obtained from the American Cancer Society. Introducing this procedure may elicit some feelings of anxiety, since it reminds the mastectomee that recurrence of the cancer is possible. The individual should be encouraged to verbalize these feelings since suppression and internalization of such feelings may lead to depression. As the mastectomee verbalizes his or her feelings about breast self-examination, the importance of early detection of any mass must be stressed.

Sexual Impact

A mastectomy is one of the most prevalent sexually threatening experiences. For the mastectomee a normally visible organ has been either partially or totally removed and there remains an altered chest structure. The sexual significance of the breast to the individual plays a major role in the process of adaptation to the loss of a breast. The value assigned to the lost breast by the individual is of personal importance. If the individual is greatly concerned with bodily appearance, the loss of a breast is more threatening to the self-image than the individual who is not so concerned with bodily appearance. A patient of either sex who perceives himself or herself as mutilated because of the mastectomy is likely to feel that he or she is unacceptable both to society and to significant others, especially the sex partner. Many a woman has actually moved out of her bedroom into a guest bedroom in an attempt to prevent her sex partner from viewing her altered body structure.

Females whose breasts were either very large or very small are likely to be especially sensitive about the altered appearance of their breasts. To add to the trauma of the mastectomy, these women can encounter difficulty in obtaining an adequate prosthesis without the assistance of a skilled prosthetist. Very large breasted women may have difficulty in obtaining a prosthesis of adequate weight to resemble the remaining breast. Women with very small breasts often experience problems both in obtaining a prosthesis of representative size and in keeping the prosthesis in place, since it is relatively lightweight.

The presence of the breast plays an important part in sex play in many relationships. If the individual finds breast stimulation both desirable and essential in foreplay, the absence of a breast could affect sexual satisfaction. The presence of the breast also can serve as a source of sexual excitement for the sex partner. Seeing and touching the breast may have provided sexual pleasure for the sex partner. Now that the breast is gone the sex partner may interpret its absence as interference with his or her own sexual satisfaction.

An individual may feel that personal sexual identity is dependent upon the sexual image projected by one's sex partner. Thus, the presence of a mastectomy may be perceived by the individual as a threat to one's personal sexual image. If an individual is revulsed by the appearance of the mastectomy, personal sexual satisfaction may be threatened. Unless the individual is assisted in expressing these feelings, extreme guilt may be aroused as a result of the uncontrollable thoughts. If the individual attempts to hide such feelings, the sexual enthusiasm displayed by the sex partner will probably decrease. This decrease in sexual enthusiasm, in turn, can be interpreted by the mastectomee as rejection. It is advisable that the mastectomee and sex partner share their fears and emotions with each other and avoid the pretense of being unaffected by the operation. The sex partner should make it clear to the mastectomee that any hesitant response does not imply rejection, but rather an expression of empathy. The sex partner must be encouraged to express to the mastectomee that he or she does not desire separate sleeping accommodations. Allowing the mastectomee to retreat to another bedroom is not being helpful and can lead to marital and sexual problems (Maguire, 1975). To aid in the expression of acceptance of the mastectomee by the sex partner, resumption of intercourse as soon as possible is suggested. When intercourse takes place early in the postoperative period, the chances for the development of a sense of impairment and valuelessness by the mastectomee are decreased and may be viewed as proof of continued affection by the sex partner. To facilitate the comfort of the sexual act during the early postoperative period, it is advisable that the sex partner assume a superior or lateral position, with the mastectomee's surgical area free from contact (Witkin, 1978). However, the couple may choose any position as long as it proves comfortable for both individuals.

The issue of whether marital stability will be affected by the loss of a breast is often present in the mind of the mastectomee. A Gallup poll conducted among women indicated that an already happy marriage would not be endangered by a mastectomy, but many of the women felt that a mastectomy would interfere with the establishment of a new sexual relationship (Women's attitudes regarding breast cancer, 1974). As may be expected, couples who have encountered sexual and/or marital discord prior to the mastectomy often continue to experience difficulties. In some instances, the mastectomy may be used as an excuse for avoiding intercourse in sexually unsatisfying or unpleasant relationships. In this case, the surgical intervention is used as a means of avoiding an unpleasant situation, the sexual experience. It is advisable to assess the sexual relationship preoperatively by way of a sex history (Kaplan, 1974). If difficulties are identified, counseling may be needed in an attempt to minimize the strain that will be placed upon the relationship as a result of the mastectomy.

Occupational Impact

The occupational impact that a mastectomy will have upon an individual varies. For some, a mastectomy may end a career. For others, no alterations in occupational pursuits will occur. No doubt, the individual affected the most by the existence of a mastectomy is one who must rely heavily upon natural body appearance for occupational reasons. Models, for example, may encounter changes in work assignments or complete loss of employment should a mastectomy be performed. The appearance of the body in clothing with varying degrees of exposure is an occupational necessity for most models. For example, the female model who frequently wears evening gowns with plunging necklines or wears blouses designed to enhance the "natural" look may find the presence of a mastectomy a hindrance. In such a situation, if possible, the surgeon is encouraged to use a transverse incision because it avoids scars in the neck, shoulder, and apex of the axilla (Burdick, 1975). Not only is the transverse scar more cosmetic, but later breast reconstruction with a Silastic implant is more feasible. With the modern techniques of reconstructive mammoplasty, a number of individuals have been able to resume their modeling careers with minimal difficulty.

Many individuals may be concerned about their ability to resume activities involving the arm on the affected side. The mastectomee should be reassured that motion of the arm on the affected side will be regained with the consistent use of arm exercises that are taught for use in the postoperative period. However, the mastectomee must be instructed not to lift heavy objects, carry heavy packages, or move furniture during a six to eight week period immediately following the surgery. Assistance with these activities is important to prevent trauma and undue stress to the surgical site and to allow the remaining muscle masses an opportunity to strengthen. In addition to routine arm exercises that may be prescribed for the mastectomee, various activities of daily living are beneficial in exercising the arm on the affected side. Making beds, sweeping, shampooing the hair, cleaning windows and mirrors, playing the piano, painting (household and artistic), typing, cutting with scissors, gardening (with gloves), and driving the car are but a few activities that develop strength in the arm on the affected side. These activities also may not seem so monotonous to the individual as routine arm exercises.

The mastectomee must be encouraged by health team members and family members to resume premastectomy activities as soon as possible, whether it be at home or with a career. Resuming activities done prior to the mastectomy or finding new ones not only provides physical benefits but psychological benefits as well.

Social Impact

The influence that the removal of a breast has upon the mastectomee's social interactions must be examined to ensure effective social reintegration. After a mastectomy, social contacts with individuals outside the marital relationship are most vulnerable to decay. The mastectomee may withdraw from others and avoid contact with family members, friends, or acquaintances due to embarrassment or shame. Therefore, firm yet gentle, encouragement to be with others is necessary for reestablishment of social status. If the mastectomee enjoys golf, bowling, swimming, or tennis, he or she should be encouraged to take an active part with family or friends. The mastectomee's initial limitations should be recognized and positive reinforcement for improvements in performance should be extended. Unless family members are prepared preoperatively for the possibility of the mastectomee's withdrawal and avoidance of others, feelings of anger and frustration may result. It is vitally important for family members to realize that the time immediately after the mastectomy is a difficult period of adjustment for both the mastectomee and the family.

A mastectomee who is unattached emotionally to another's affections prior to the surgical procedure may express concern about setting up a new relationship now that a breast has been lost. The fear of possible rejection is a major concern. Discussing this concern with members of the health team and other mastectomees may prove helpful. The mastectomee needs to be encouraged to express how he or she will deal with the situation should it arise. Generally, the mastectomee is advised not to discuss the fact that a breast has been removed until the relationship is comfortable and the mastectomee does not feel threatened about discussing the issue. In addition, the seriousness of the relationship plays a major role in the mastectomee's decision of whether or not the new acquaintance should be told about the missing breast.

Clothing concerns are of vital importance to the mastectomee's social reintegration. With the advent of breast reconstruction, many female mastectomees do not find it necessary to alter their premastectomy clothing. However, should clothing alterations be required due to extensive surgery, it may prove helpful to have a seamstress provide suggestions. Halter neck dresses require minimal adjustments other than building up under both arms to produce a balanced look. Bathing suits can be worn with ease as long as they are built up under the arms. Some designers have created swimwear that is exclusively for the mastectomee. Strapless evening gowns can be converted into halter top gowns or provided with shrug attachments by using contrasting material. Some strapless dresses may not require alterations if they are well boned and have high support under the arms. The female mastectomee will find that most of her clothing can be worn without alterations. Above all, the female mastectomee must be encouraged to stand erect with head and shoulders back since one's personal appearance is enhanced by excellent posture.

The male mastectomee will encounter fewer required alterations in clothing. One of the major clothing concerns expressed by the male mastectomee is appearance in swimwear. Now that a breast has been removed, he may find the appearance of his trunk displeasing for public viewing. In this case, he can be encouraged to wear a tank-top with his swim trunks so that his scar is covered in a fairly unobvious manner.

Without necessary support and understanding with clothing needs, the mastectomee can easily drift into carelessness in personal appearance and into wearing sloppy clothing in an attempt to conceal the missing breast. This only further undermines one's morale and, in turn, prolongs adequate reestablishment of the social role.

SUMMARY

In the United States approximately one out of every thirteen women will be affected by breast cancer at some time during her life. Women most frequently affected are over forty-five years of age and have not borne or breast-fed children. Cancer of the breast remains the leading cause of cancer deaths in women. If diagnosed when in a localized stage, breast cancer is treated with considerable success.

It must not be forgotten that males also are susceptible to breast cancer. Tumors of the male breast are not so common as those occurring in the female breast and the male involved tends to be slightly older than the female affected by cancer of the breast.

The presence of a breast lump is usually found by the individual involved or by the sex partner. At the time of discovery the most frequent thought of the individual involved is the fear of impending death. Many individuals equate the word cancer with death. Repudiation of the existence of the lump and fear of a possible mastectomy are two major reasons for delaying the individual's move to seek medical attention.

The presence of a mastectomy imposes a great impact upon both the individual affected and his or her family. The impact of a mastectomy affects the mastectomee's psychological well-being, somatic identity, sexuality, occupational identity, and social role. The mastectomee is faced with learning the illness role during the initial impact of the mastectomy and goes on to experience loss, body image alterations, and social readjustment. Therefore, the psychosocial impact of a mastectomy must never be underrated by members of the health care team. The major role of the health care team is to prepare the individual and his or her family for alterations in daily living which may occur because of the impact of the mastectomy. The health care team also should assist the individual in dealing with each of these changes.

Patient Situation   Ms. R. M. is a forty-nine-year-old married woman with three children, ages twenty, eighteen, and thirteen. Mr. R. M. is an executive for a large business firm and is required to do a great deal of entertaining. Consequently, Ms. R. M. is kept busy planning social events with her husband. In addition to her social entertaining, she enjoys playing tennis at the country club.

Ms. R. M. detected a lump in her breast one day while bathing. A biopsy determined that the lump was cancerous; subsequently, a mastectomy was performed. During her hospital stay the nursing staff felt that it was advisable for a community health nurse to visit Ms. R. M. after discharge. Ms. R. M. is now three weeks postmastectomy and the community health nurse has identified problems affecting Ms. R. M.'s psychological well-being, somatic identity, sexuality, occupational identity, and social role.

Following are Ms. R. M.'s nursing care plan and patient care cardex dealing with the above mentioned areas of concern.

NURSING CARE PLAN

Nursing Diagnoses	Objectives	Nursing Interventions	Principles/Rationale	Evaluations
Psychological Impact Depression manifested by frequent expressions of hopelessness and despair.	To decrease Ms. R. M.'s depression.	Encourage Ms. R. M. to express her feelings to her husband and children.	Expressing feelings may assist the mastectomee in identifying what is causing the depression.	The nurse would observe for: Ms. R. M.'s increased verbalization about feelings to her husband and children.
	To demonstrate acceptance of Ms. R. M.	Encourage Ms. R. M. to become involved in mastectomee group sessions.	Groups of mastectomees are able to empathize and provide support to one another since they are experiencing or have experienced similar problems.	Ms. R. M.'s involvement in mastectomee groups.
		Encourage Ms. R. M. to become involved in her premastectomy activities.	Becoming involved in premastectomy activities demonstrates to the mastectomee that she is still a contributing member of society.	Ms. R. M.'s involvement and increased enjoyment in premastectomy activities. Ms. R. M.'s ability to express herself without fear of rejection from others.

To assist Ms. R. M.'s family in ways of dealing with her depression.	Encourage Mr. R. M. and the children to take an active part in getting Ms. R. M. involved in her premastectomy activities.	Mastectomees are more likely to become involved in activities when family members are encouraging and supportive.	Active involvement of Ms. R. M.'s family in dealing with her depression.
	Encourage Mr. R. M. and the children to compliment Ms. R. M. on any accomplishments made in her involvement in premastectomy activities.	Positive feedback for accomplishments facilitate feelings of self-worth.	
	Encourage Mr. R. M. and the children not to reprimand her for crying.	Demonstrations of disgust toward a crying mastectomee can be interpreted by the mastectomee as rejection.	
	Explain to Mr. R. M. and the children the need for Ms. R. M. to cry.	Crying is a means of expressing feelings in the open and family members who understand this are more capable of providing necessary emotional support.	
	Encourage Mr. R. M. and the children to sit with Ms. R. M. as she cries and to make body contact by holding her hand or touching her arm.	Body contact and human presence are means of demonstrating acceptance.	

(cont.)

NURSING CARE PLAN (cont.)

Nursing Diagnoses	Objectives	Nursing Interventions	Principles/Rationale	Evaluations
Somatic Impact Fear of body image alteration manifested by expressed concern that bustline will not have a normal appearance.	To decrease Ms. R. M.'s fear about an abnormal appearance of her bustline.	Encourage Mr. R. M. and the children to allow Ms. R. M. to verbalize her concerns about her appearance.	Verbalization of a fear may assist the mastectomee in identifying ways of dealing with that fear.	The nurse would observe for: Free verbalization by Ms. R. M. about her fear of an abnormal appearance of her bustline.
	To restore Ms. R. M.'s feminine image.	Direct Ms. R. M. to a surgical appliance firm, an appropriate women's wear department, or an appropriate drugstore.	Mastectomees aware of the appropriate place to obtain a prosthesis will have less anxiety about the availability of the item.	Ms. R. M.'s selection of a prosthesis with which she feels comfortable.
		Provide Ms. R. M. with information about the various types of available prostheses.	A mastectomee aware of the various types of prostheses is better able to select the most appropriate type.	
		Encourage Ms. R. M. to involve Mr. R. M. in taking an active part in choosing the prosthesis.	Involving the sex partner of the mastectomee in the selection of the prosthesis prevents placing the entire responsibility upon the mastectomee.	
		Encourage Ms. R. M. to wait until her wound is healed before being fit with a permanent prosthesis.	Fitting a mastectomee for a permanent prosthesis before the wound is entirely healed may lead to improper fitting since some edema of the wound may still be present.	

	Goals	Nursing Interventions	Rationale	Evaluation
Sexual Impact Unreconciled sexual identity manifested by avoidance of sexual relationship with husband.	To assist Mr. and Ms. R. M. in returning to their premastectomy sexual activities.	Encourage Mr. R. M. and the children to compliment Ms. R. M. on her personal appearance when she begins to wear her permanent prosthesis.	How a mastectomee appears to others is important to the patient.	Ms. R. M.'s demonstration of a sense of pride in her personal appearance.
		Encourage Mr. R. M. to express to his wife his feelings about viewing the mastectomy scar.	Feelings of guilt about one's reaction to the mastectomy scar are difficult to hide and may affect the sex partner's sexual enthusiasm.	The nurse would observe for: Open expression of feelings between Mr. and Ms. R. M. about their sexual activity and whether or not they have returned to their premastectomy level of sexual activity.
	To assist Mr. and Ms. R. M. in dealing with feelings of guilt.	Encourage Mr. R. M. to tell his wife that any hesitant response toward her is not rejection, but rather an expression of empathy.	A mastectomee who is aware of the sex partner's true feelings is less likely to misinterpret the partner's actions.	
		Encourage Ms. R. M. to express to Mr. R. M. her feelings about engaging in sexual relations with him.	Expressing feelings about sexual relations assists the mastectomee and the sex partner in identifying possible reasons for feelings of anxiety and guilt related to the sex act.	
		Encourage Mr. and Ms. R. M. to resume sexual activity as soon as possible.	Early resumption of sexual activity provides recognition of continued affection on the part of the sex partner.	

(cont.)

NURSING CARE PLAN (cont.)

Nursing Diagnoses	Objectives	Nursing Interventions	Principles/Rationale	Evaluations
Occupational Impact Fear of impaired home maintenance management manifested by expressed concern about not being able to carry out usual activities of daily living.	To increase Ms. R. M.'s feelings of self-worth.	Encourage Ms. R. M. to resume usual activities of daily living with the exception of lifting heavy objects. Encourage Ms. R. M. to resume entertaining in her home.	Taking part in premastectomy activities helps reestablish the mastectomee's feelings of self-worth.	The nurse would observe for: Increased resumption of premastectomy activities of daily living.
	To decrease Ms. R. M.'s concern about resuming her activities of daily living.	Reassure Ms. R. M. that activities such as bedmaking, sweeping, typing, washing, and ironing are a few of the activities of daily living that will enhance arm action on her affected side.	Resuming activities done prior to the mastectomy provides physical benefits for arm movement on the affected side.	
Social Impact Withdrawal manifested by refusal to visit friends and associates because of feelings of embarrassment or shame.	To decrease Ms. R. M.'s feelings of embarrassment or shame.	Encourage Ms. R. M. to express her feelings of embarrassment or shame about her altered body structure.	Verbalizing the feelings of embarrassment or shame about altered body structure may assist the mastectomee in identifying ways of dealing with such feelings.	The nurse would observe for: Ms. R. M.'s open verbalization about feelings of embarrassment or shame.
	To increase Ms. R. M.'s contact with friends and associates.	Encourage Mr. R. M. and the children to be firm, yet gentle, in encouraging Ms. R. M. to be with friends and associates.	Reestablishment of social contacts with individuals outside the marital relationship are most vulnerable to decay.	Increased contact with friends and associates by Ms. R. M.

Goal	Nursing Actions	Rationale	Evaluation
To increase Ms. R. M.'s satisfaction with her personal appearance.	Suggest to Ms. R. M. that she resume playing tennis.	Taking part in premastectomy activities that involve individuals outside the marital relationship helps to reestablish these social contacts.	Ms. R. M.'s increased pride and satisfaction with personal appearance.
	Encourage Mr. R. M., the children, and family friends to compliment Ms. R. M. on improvements in tennis.	Positive feedback for accomplishments facilitate feelings of self-worth.	
	Discuss with Ms. R. M. clothing alterations that she feels may be necessary.	Clothing concerns are of vital importance to the mastectomee's social reestablishment.	
	Encourage Ms. R. M. to utilize the assistance of a seamstress in making clothing alterations if she feels it would be helpful.	Assistance in making the necessary alterations in clothing makes the task less burdensome.	
	Encourage Ms. R. M. to stand erect with good posture at all times.	A mastectomee's personal appearance is enhanced by excellent posture.	
	Suggest to Mr. R. M. and the children that they compliment Ms. R. M. on her personal appearance.	Without necessary support and feedback on personal appearance, the mastectomee can easily drift into carelessness.	

PATIENT CARE CARDEX

PATIENT'S NAME: ___Ms. R. M.___   MEDICAL DIAGNOSIS: ___Mastectomy___

AGE: ___49 years___   SEX: ___Female___

MARITAL STATUS: ___Married___   OCCUPATION: ___Housewife___

SIGNIFICANT OTHERS: Husband and three children (20, 18, and 13 years)

Nursing Diagnoses	Nursing Approaches
Psychological: Depression manifested by frequent expressions of hopelessness and despair.	1. Encourage to express feelings to husband and children. 2. Encourage to become involved in mastectomee group sessions. 3. Encourage to become involved in premastectomy activities. 4. Encourage family to take an active part in getting her involved in premastectomy activities. 5. Encourage family to compliment her on accomplishments made in her involvement in premastectomy activities. 6. Encourage family not to reprimand her for behavior during spells of depression. 7. Explain to family the purpose of her crying. 8. Encourage family to sit with her as she cries and to make body contact by holding her hand or touching her arm.

Somatic: Fear of body image alteration manifested by expressed concern that bustline will not have a normal appearance.

1. Encourage family to allow her to verbalize concerns about herself.
2. Direct to surgical appliance firm, an appropriate women's wear department, or an appropriate drugstore.
3. Provide with information about the various types of available prostheses.
4. Encourage to involve husband in taking an active part in the decision regarding the choice of prosthesis.
5. Encourage to wait until wound is healed before being fit with a permanent prosthesis.
6. Encourage family to compliment her on personal appearance when she begins to wear permanent prosthesis.

Sexual: Unreconciled sexual identity manifested by avoidance of sexual relationship with husband.

1. Encourage husband to express to her his feelings about viewing the mastectomy scar.
2. Encourage husband to tell her that any hesitant response toward her is not rejection, but rather an expression of empathy.
3. Encourage to express to husband her feelings about engaging in sexual relations with him.
4. Encourage husband and wife to resume sexual activity as soon as possible.

Occupational: Fear of impaired home maintenance management manifested by expressed concern about not being able to carry out usual activities of daily living.

1. Encourage to resume activities of daily living with the exception of lifting heavy objects.
2. Encourage to resume entertaining in her home.
3. Reassure that activities such as bedmaking, sweeping, typing, washing, and ironing are a few household duties that will enhance arm action on the affected side.

Social: Withdrawal manifested by refusal to visit friends and associates because of feelings of embarrassment or shame.

1. Encourage to express feelings of embarrassment or shame about altered body structure.
2. Encourage family to be firm, yet gentle, in encouraging her to be with friends and associates.
3. Suggest resumption of tennis.
4. Encourage family and friends to compliment her on improvements in tennis.
5. Discuss any clothing alterations that may be necessary.
6. Encourage to utilize the assistance of a dressmaker or friend in making clothing alterations.
7. Encourage to stand erect with good posture at all times.
8. Suggest to family that they compliment her on her personal appearance.

91

REFERENCES

BURDICK, D. Rehabilitation of the breast cancer patient, *Cancer,* 1975, *36* (2), 645-648.

CARROLL, R. The impact of mastectomy on body image, *Oncology Nursing Forum,* 1981, *8* (4), 29-32.

ERIKSON, E. *Childhood and society.* New York: W.W. Norton & Co., Inc., 1963.

GOIN, M., and GOIN, J. Midlife reactions to mastectomy and subsequent breast reconstruction, *Archives of General Psychiatry,* 1981, *38,* 225-227.

GOLEMASTIC, B., DELIKARIS, P., BALARUSTSOS, C., and KARAMONAKOS, P. Lymphedema of the upper limb after surgery for breast cancer, *American Journal of Surgery,* 1975, *129* (3), 286-288.

JAMISON, K., WELLISCH, D., KATZ, R., and PASNAU, R. Phantom breast syndrome, *Archives of Surgery,* 1979, *114,* 93-95.

KAPLAN, H. *The new sex therapy: treatment of sexual dysfunction.* New York: Brunner/Mazel, 1974.

KATZ, J., WEINER, H., GALLAGHER, T., and HALLMAN, L. Stress, distress, and ego defenses, *Archives of General Psychiatry,* 1976, *23,* 131-142.

LONG, B., and MOLBO, D. Problems of the breast. In W. Phipps, B. Long, and N. Woods (Eds.), *Medical-surgical nursing: concepts and clinical practice.* St. Louis: C.V. Mosby, 1983.

MAGUIRE, P. Emotional responses after mastectomy, *Contemporary Obstetrics and Gynecology,* 1975, *8,* 34-38.

MAGUIRE, P. The psychological and social sequelae of mastectomy. In J. Howells (Ed.), *Modern perspectives in the psychiatric aspects of surgery.* New York: Brunner/Mazel, 1976.

MORRIS, T. Psychological adjustment to mastectomy, *Cancer Treatment Reviews,* 1979, *6,* 41-61.

NORTHOUSE, L. Mastectomy patients and the fear of cancer recurrence, *Cancer Nursing,* 1981, *4* (3), 213-220.

NUCKOLLS, K., CASSEL, J., and KAPLAN, B. Psychosocial assets, life crises, and the prognosis of pregnancy, *American Journal of Epidemiology,* 1972, *95,* 431-441.

SAVLOV, E. Breast cancer. In P. Rubin (Ed.), *Clinical oncology.* Rochester, N.Y.: University of Rochester Press, 1978.

SCHMID, W., KISS, M., and HIBERT, L. The team approach to rehabilitation after mastectomy, *AORN Journal,* 1974, *19* (4), 821-836.

SIEMENS, S., and BRANZEL, R. *Sexuality: Nursing assessment and intervention.* Philadelphia: Lippincott, 1982.

SILVERBERG, E. Cancer statistics, 1983, *Cancer Journal for Clinicians,* 1983, *33* (1), 9-25.

WINKLER, W. Choosing the prosthesis and clothing, *American Journal of Nursing,* 1977, *77* (9), 1433-1436.

WITKIN, M. Psychosexual counseling of the mastectomy patient, *Journal of Sex and Marital Therapy,* 1978, *4* (1), 20-28.

Women's attitudes regarding breast cancer, *Occupational Health Nursing,* 1974, *20,* 20-23.

6

VASECTOMY OR HYSTERECTOMY

INTRODUCTION

There is increasing interest in the psychological effects that surgical changes in the reproduction system have upon the individual and his or her family. For some time medical science has been aware of some of the psychosocial effects that a hysterectomy has upon the female. However, the psychosocial effects of surgical alterations in the male's sexual structure, such as a vasectomy, have become an issue of increasing interest in the health care field. With the concern about limiting one's family size, the request for and performance of vasectomies have been on the increase. The economic pressures of living and the increased liberation of the female have added to this increase in demand. Regardless of whether an individual is undergoing a vasectomy or a hysterectomy, a surgical change in sexual structure creates an impact upon one's psychological well-being, somatic identity, sexuality, occupational identity, and social role. This chapter will deal with the impact that the hysterectomy and the vasectomy have upon each of these areas.

VASECTOMY AND HYSTERECTOMY PROFILES

The individual undergoing a vasectomy most often is white, middle class, well educated, in the fourth decade of life, the father of three or four children, of the Protestant religion, and married ten to twelve years to a woman three to five years his junior. The major reason given for obtaining a vasectomy is that it is a safe, effective means of contraception which does not interfere with sexual activity. However, physical illness of either partner or the presence of hereditary disease also are frequently cited reasons.

Certain men are considered poor risks for vasectomies and generally are discouraged from obtaining them. These poor risk individuals include men under twenty-five years of age, with preexisting marital or sexual problems, with psychopathology or whose wives demonstrate psychopathology, and whose wives oppose a vasectomy. If an individual falls into any one of these categories, extensive counseling or even psychotherapy may be required before a vasectomy is performed. The young male (twenty-five and younger) may not be completely cognizant of the impact that a vasectomy could have upon his future. A man, or his sex partner, with preexisting sexual difficulties, marital problems, or psychopathology may be using the vasectomy as an easy solution to more complex problems. Finally, the wife's consent is necessary since the possibilities of legal suits at a later date could occur should she decide that she was not appropriately informed about the procedure (Vaughn, 1979).

Once the man has decided to have a vasectomy, and if he does not fall into any of the above categories, he should be provided with adequate information about the procedure, its desired effects, and the finality of the structural alteration. In addition, he should be encouraged to express his feelings or doubts about the vasectomy. The individual's questions must be answered and any misconceptions must be clarified. Only after such interventions should the man consent to having a vasectomy.

The woman undergoing a hysterectomy presents a different profile from the male consenting to a vasectomy. She generally is married and in the fifth decade of life. It is a time when her financial contributions to the family as a working woman are no longer pressing because children are grown and are ready to leave home. Thus her role within the family structure may be changing.

Unlike the vasectomy, the hysterectomy generally is not performed for the purpose of birth control. Rather, hysterectomies are done as a result of malignant and nonmalignant uterine tumors, menorrhagia, endometriosis, pelvic inflammatory disease, or a ruptured uterus. Regardless of the reason for the hysterectomy, the impact of the loss can affect various facets of the female's life. Just like the male undergoing a vasectomy, the female undergoing a hysterectomy needs to be provided with adequate information about the procedure and the finality of the structural alteration. She must have her questions answered and any misconceptions clarified. Ideally, this should be done before the hysterectomy to allay unnecessary anxiety and fear during the postoperative period.

Whether the individual is male or female, loss is experienced. Regardless of the reasons for the changes in sexual structure, the ability to reproduce has been altered and a number of impacts are sustained by the individual.

IMPACT OF A VASECTOMY OR A HYSTERECTOMY

Psychological Impact

More than 500,000 men a year in the United States undergo vasectomies for the purpose of sterilization (Lipshultz and Benson, 1980). Unlike most surgical interventions, a vasectomy tends to be an operation of choice. Thus, for a short period of time the individual selects to assume the illness role as discussed in Chapter 1.

Men have expressed that one of the most difficult aspects of the vasectomy is deciding to have it done; no doubt this is because of the finality of the alteration. No longer will he be able to father children. Although attempts are being made to develop reversible forms of vasectomy, these surgical procedures are difficult to perform and are not completely effective at this time (Hill, 1980).

If the man is married, it is imperative that the decision to have a vasectomy be a cooperative decision between the man and his wife. Many men feel that it would be more of a health risk for their sex partner to undergo a surgical procedure, such as a tubal ligation, for sterilization than for them to have a vasectomy. Also, more emphasis is being directed toward the male's assumption of equal responsibility in fertility control. Birth control no longer is viewed primarily as the female's task. However, should the man feel pressure from his wife or sex partner to obtain a vasectomy, the psychological impact of the sterilization procedure may produce untoward effects. He may view himself as emasculated and, as a result, become extremely sensitive about comments made to him regarding his sexuality. If the man does not feel pressured to have a vasectomy and if he has chosen to undergo the sterilization process on his own, he is unlikely to exhibit psychological problems as a result of the surgical procedure.

By comparison, the woman undergoing a hysterectomy generally is doing so because of some underlying medical problem. The removal of the uterus thus becomes the surgical procedure of choice to correct or alleviate the pathological alteration. Historically, many individuals in medicine felt that the removal of the uterus would automatically induce emotional problems. Thus, the term hysterectomy was coined to describe the "hysterical" or uncontrollable emotional state that occurred because of the loss of the uterus. This theory has been proven ill-founded and no direct link can be made between emotional disorders and a hysterectomy (Gath, Cooper, and Day, 1982). This is not to say, however, that removal of the uterus cannot create a psychological impact on some women. Since the fantasy of pregnancy can no longer be maintained, some women find this fact difficult to face.

Research findings have suggested that an increase in the severity of psychological responses to a hysterectomy are associated with the persistent desire for children (Kaltreider, Wallace, and Horowitz, 1979). In addition, the removal of the uterus creates a loss, and the woman is faced with the responsibility of dealing with the loss. It is advisable for the reader to refer to Chapter 3 for guidelines on how to assist the hysterectomized woman in dealing with her loss.

The anxiety created by the loss of the uterus tends to be greater in separated and recently divorced women than in married women (Polivy, 1974). No doubt this is because separated and divorced females are faced with not only the loss of a body part but also the loss of a significant other. The compounding effect created by these two major losses cannot help but create coping difficulties. Most likely these difficulties are related to the fact that these women perceive the loss of the uterus as a serious threat to their femininity. If these women do not have the presence of a significant companion, they may question whether they will be capable of attracting a suitable companion now that their female body structure has been altered.

Research has shown that pelvic surgery, such as a hysterectomy, tends to create greater anxiety in the female than does upper abdominal surgery (Janis,1958), such as a cholecystectomy. It is not uncommon for a woman to experience depression or to feel "low" or "weepy" for a few days following her surgical experience. In fact, depression tends to be more common after a hysterectomy than after many other operations (Mathis, 1973).

To deal with this depression, the woman and her family need to be informed and reassured before the hysterectomy that such feelings after surgery are not uncommon. During this period, she needs encouragement to express her feelings, whether it be in the form of crying or verbalization. As the woman begins to deal with her loss, her depression will start to subside. However, the nurse must be aware that some women may experience depression for extended periods of time and thus require professional counseling. In addition, members of her family need to be reminded of the importance of allowing her to express her feelings to them. Family members also may require support from health team members in the form of listening to their feelings about dealing with their loved one's depression after a hysterectomy. During the expression of their feelings, both the woman and her family members should be encouraged to examine: 1) what they are specifically concerned about regarding the hysterectomy and whether the concerns are realistic; 2) whether they feel responsible for the hysterectomy; 3) what they can do to deal with feelings of depression; 4) how they have dealt with feelings of depression in the past; and 5) how they can apply past experiences to the present situation.

For some women, a hysterectomy may be viewed as a welcome relief. They see the removal of the uterus as a new found freedom. No longer will they have to fear the possibility of pregnancy or contend with menstruation. If the hysterectomy resolved underlying pathology, the woman now may be exempt from contending with the concern for an annoying gynecological problem.

Regardless of whether the woman views her hysterectomy as a welcome relief or as a psychological trauma, the nurse must be cognizant of the individual's concept of her newly acquired loss. Only then can appropriate emotional support be provided. If the nurse, however, is unstable in his or her own sexuality then difficulties may be encountered in the provision of emotional support.

Somatic Impact

Alterations in reproductability as with a vasectomized male or hysterectomized female can influence feelings of manliness or womanliness. When a man decides to have a vasectomy, he must explore how he will feel about his manly image once he has lost the ability to reproduce, especially since the surgical procedure generally is irreversible. Some men may postpone, or refuse, a vasectomy because they feel that loss of reproductivity would make them less manly. In addition, a fear that the vasectomy will affect one's masculine appearance, a concern about whether or not voice changes will take place, apprehension about an increase in promiscuity, and anxiety about whether physical weakness will result are potential concerns. The male and his sex partner require reassurance and information that all of these beliefs are ill-founded and do not occur as a result of the sterilization procedure.

The majority of vasectomies occur during young adulthood. This is a time when the individual is ready and willing to merge his identity with that of others. It is during young adulthood that the individual either shares himself with others, both in friendship and in a mutually satisfying sexual relationship, or develops a sense of isolation (Erikson, 1963). Therefore, the male must examine how he believes a vasectomy will affect his ability to merge his identity with others. If he sees himself as "less than a man," he may retreat into isolation and fail to set up both friendships and a mutually satisfying sexual relationship. Since setting up a mutually satisfying sexual relationship is not as likely to occur during the early years of young adulthood, authorities discourage a vasectomy prior to the age of twenty-five years. A man past twenty-five is more likely to have established a sexual relationship and thus may not feel that his ability to procreate is essential in maintaining this relationship.

In the case of the male who is married and over twenty-five years of age, a concern may exist as to how he is perceived by his wife. If he fears that she views him as "less than a man," sexual counseling of both the husband and wife should be done before a vasectomy is performed. If the man believes his masculine image has been altered, he may withdraw from his wife and fail to establish or maintain a healthy sexual relationship.

Just as the male may perceive a vasectomy as an assault on his masculine image, so may the female view a hysterectomy as an assault on her feminine image. The female may describe her hysterectomy as a surgical procedure in which everything was "taken away," whereby she no longer visualizes herself as being physically attractive to others. In fact, some women perceive a hysterectomy as a psychologically mutilating experience. This belief is likely to influence the woman's perception of her bodily appearance and may result in withdrawal from interactions she perceives as oriented toward her feminine appearance (i.e., swim parties). The somatic impact of the hysterectomy is particularly acute in women who feel that it is punishment for past sexually oriented behavior, such as an illicit love affair, masturbation, or the birth of an illegitimate child. Feelings of guilt about such behaviors may be aroused. Thus nursing intervention should include the woman's realistic examination of her guilt feelings and the discussion of the medical reason(s) for her hysterectomy.

Since the majority of hysterectomies occur during the developmental stage of adulthood, alterations may occur in the woman's interest in establishing and guiding future generations, the major focus in life at this time (Erikson, 1963). If the woman feels she is "less than a woman," she may perceive herself as unfit to guide future generations. Instead of becoming generative, the woman may become increasingly concerned over premature aging and may believe that her hysterectomy contributes to the acceleration of her aging process. Preoccupation with every physical change becomes the focus of her life. She becomes engulfed in satisfying personal needs, acquiring self-comforts, and enters a life of self-absorption and stagnation. To aid the woman in dealing with concerns of physical attractiveness she should be encouraged to maintain physical appearance by using make-up appropriately and by wearing an attractive hair style. In addition, the family needs to be encouraged to compliment her about her appearance because not until the woman feels that she is attractive to herself and others will she examine her preoccupation with aging.

Sexual Impact

The sexual impact of surgical alterations in sexual function is one of the greatest concerns of the individual affected. The man undergoing a vasectomy usually does so as a means of birth control. He frequently fears the effects of other methods of contraception on his sex partner's health, especially the birth control pill. Therefore, the man feels that the effects of a vasectomy are minimal compared to the effects encountered by his sex partner when using other means of birth control. Even with these thoughts in mind, prior to a vasectomy the man may be concerned about a possible decrease in sexual desire as a result of the surgical intervention (Vaughn, 1979). Such a concern may be the primary reason for postponing the vasectomy for an extended period of time. However, since the fear of pregnancy is removed from the sexual relationship, many men have noted an increase of enjoyment in their sexual relationships (Lipshultz and Benson, 1980).

The major fear of men preparing to undergo a vasectomy is the fear of castration, the removal of the gonads. Since the surgical incision is located on the scrotum, many men have their fears of castration intensified. Unless thorough preoperative explanation about the procedure is provided, fear of castration may be great at the time of the procedure. However, even with thorough preoperative explanations, some men are not completely convinced that no alterations to their testicles occur. In such situations further examination of the individual's concerns needs to take place. If concerns persist that testicular damage will occur as a result of the vasectomy, it is advisable to encourage the man to reconsider having the surgical procedure carried out.

In addition to the fear of castration is the fear of pain resulting from the surgical intervention. To decrease the fear of pain, thorough preoperative explanation about the surgical procedure and the postoperative course is necessary. Since the male is well aware of the sensitivity of his genital region and thoughts of having a surgical procedure in this region may cultivate intense concern about the pain, information about the use of ice packs to the area and the use of mild analgesics to control the discomfort that can exist in the immediate postoperative period is required. It is advisable to explore with the man what he has done in the past to deal with minor pain. The use of relaxation techniques, such as mouth breathing exercises, may prove helpful as a pain distracting maneuver.

How soon one can resume sexual activity is a question frequently asked by the man undergoing a vasectomy. Since the concerns about sexual desire and castration frequently exist, the need to prove himself sexually to both his sex partner and himself may be important. However, persistent preoccupation with the need to prove himself sexually postvasectomy may be an indication that this surgical procedure is not an advisable means of birth control. In such circumstances the man and his sex partner should reconsider the selection of the vasectomy as their means of controlling the reproduction of offspring.

During the preoperative explanation the man should be instructed that he may resume sexual intercourse as soon as he desires. He and his sex partner must be encouraged to continue previous means of birth control until semen analysis demonstrates the absence of sperm. This time period may extend from six to fifteen ejaculations.

The effect the vasectomy will have upon the marital relationship is important. As pointed out earlier, when the man's wife is adamantly against the procedure, it should not be performed. By the same token, if the man's wife pressures him into having a vasectomy, the impact of the sterilization has a greater chance of creating psychological difficulties.

When the marital relationship is not laden with problems, the performance of a vasectomy that has been selected willingly is unlikely to cause difficulties in the marriage (Lyons, 1978). However, a couple undergoing difficulties may find the vasectomy just one more problem with which to contend. Therefore, during preoperative counseling the husband and wife must be instructed that a vasectomy is not an easy solution to existing marital problems and must not be viewed as such. In some cases, it may be necessary for the husband and wife to seek marital counseling prior to consenting to the performance of a vasectomy.

Just as the male undergoing a vasectomy, the female undergoing a hysterectomy can encounter difficulties in dealing with the sexual impact of a surgical alteration in structure. The hysterectomy is most frequently performed on women during the fifth decade of life, a time when sexual drive tends to be reduced. However, the effects of the surgical procedure on a sexual relationship can be great. The woman involved may question her sexual desirability to her sex partner (Woods, 1979). Such fears are intensified when the woman and her sex partner are of a cultural background in which the presence of the woman's uterus is a way of satisfying *macho* desires. In such instances, the woman may be viewed as being less than perfect now that she is unable to bear children, which is a primary role of her femininity in such a culture. Women affected by such cultural influences may postpone a much needed hysterectomy. Fear of being rejected sexually by the sex partner may become a primary concern. Now that she is unable to bear children she wonders whether her partner will leave her or find another partner.

Since some women are hesitant to express their concerns about the marital ramifications of a hysterectomy, health team members may have to approach the topic for the woman. Even though a woman does not openly express her feelings about the sexual impact of a hysterectomy, it does not mean that concerns do not exist. A leading statement that may encourage the verbalization of feelings about the forthcoming hysterectomy might be, "Many women have expressed anxiety about the effects that a hysterectomy will have upon their femininity. How do you feel your surgery will affect you?" As the woman expresses her concerns she should be guided in examining whether her concerns are realistic; encouraged to explore how she has dealt with similar concerns in the past; assisted in implementing past effective coping strategies; and advised to identify and seek out individuals whom she considers to be her support systems.

It is important that the sex partner be made aware of the woman's potential or actual fears of rejection. He should be encouraged to carry out methods he has used in the past for expressing his affection for her. These methods may include giving her "feminine type" gifts or physically caressing her. Regardless of what means the sex partner uses to express affection, he must be alerted to the fact that the woman may need frequent reminders of his continued affection for her and may respond inconsistently to the affection extended.

To deal adequately with the woman's fear about her sexuality, it is vitally important that both the sex partner and the woman be counseled before the hysterectomy. They must be given explanations about the surgical procedure and what structures are to be removed. If the ovaries are to be removed along with the uterus, and if the woman's age makes reasonable the use of hormonal replacement therapy, such facts must be provided. If the ovaries are not to be removed along with the uterus, the woman and her husband require information that she will not require adjunctive hormone therapy. Above all, the husband and wife need to be guided in recognizing that the woman will not lose her ability to be "female," including her ability to engage in intercourse, even though she will be unable to bear children.

A common concern of the woman in the immediate postoperative period is when she can resume coitus. Women generally are advised not to resume intercourse for approximately six weeks after surgery. The woman should be advised that she may experience some discomfort initially because of the tightening of the vaginal walls and a decrease in natural vaginal lubrication if the ovaries were removed along with the uterus. It should be pointed out that this discomfort will subside and that intercourse actually can help the tissues become supple again. In addition, the use of vaginal creams or lubricants may prove helpful if the discomfort is brought on by the decrease in natural vaginal lubrication. The woman, however, must be told not to use lubricants containing estrogens if she has a history or diagnosis of malignancy since the increased presence of estrogens can cause a growth acceleration of some cancerous tumors. For some women, total enjoyment of sexual intercourse may not occur for three to four months after the surgical intervention since tenderness of the abdomen may persist this long. This is especially true if the hysterectomy was done abdominally. To alleviate this discomfort, the woman may want to try positions for coitus that do not place weight upon the abdomen. Some examples of such positions include a side-to-side position, female superior position, or a male superior "dog-fashion" position (Kaplan, 1975). However, the woman and her sex partner need to determine which positions are most enjoyable for them.

Anxiety that intercourse was the cause of the disease that led to the hysterectomy, that intercourse might reactivate the prehysterectomy pathology, or that intercourse will harm the woman can produce a loss of sex drive for both the woman and her sex partner. These misconceptions must be clarified so unnecessary anxiety is alleviated and the woman and her sex partner can resume prehysterectomy sexual activity.

The frequency of sexual activity after a hysterectomy remains individual. Some women have noted an increase in their sexual activity after a hysterectomy (Humphries, 1980). This is particularly true if the fear of a possible pregnancy existed prior to the surgical intervention. Since the potential threat of pregnancy has been removed, the woman may find the enjoyment of the sex act to be greater.

Occupational Impact

The occupational impact of the vasectomy generally is minimal. Since the procedure is not considered a major surgical intervention by medical standards, it tends to be performed in a clinic or office setting. The vasectomy frequently is performed toward the end of the work week to provide for a rest period of several days over the weekend. If the individual is not able to have a weekend free from job responsibilities, he is encouraged to rest completely for 12 hours following surgery and to take time off the following day if his occupation requires heavy labor. This aids in preventing stress and tension to the suture line, as well as minimizing suture line discomfort. A postvasectomy rest period also facilitates in decreasing anxiety associated with potential job related surgical site injuries following the operative procedure. Once the immediate postvasectomy recovery period has passed (generally two to three days), the male can resume all work related activities.

The occupational impact of a hysterectomy proves to be greater than that of the vasectomy. The hysterectomy, unlike the vasectomy, is performed in a hospital environment as opposed to a clinic or office setting. Thus the surgical procedure is more expensive. In addition to the cost of the procedure, the hysterectomized woman will be required to lose work days. If the female is employed outside the home, she may be required to avoid total resumption of her job responsibilities for a month or two. This, of course, depends upon her job related activities. Job related responsibilities which are prohibited during the immediate postoperative period include driving, lifting anything over five pounds, and/or excessive physical activity.

To deal with the occupational impact of a hysterectomy, the woman employed within the home setting generally is advised to do only light housework for the first two weeks upon her return home and to avoid such activities as vacuuming, lifting, and sports for approximately two months after surgery. It is advisable to suggest to the woman that spacing her job and household responsibilities with rest periods will decrease her chances of excessive fatigue. This practice is especially important during the first two weeks postoperatively when fatigue and weakness are common.

Social Impact

The popularity of a vasectomy stems from the increasing awareness of an improved standard of living resulting from a small-sized family unit. Many individuals request the sterilization procedure because a colleague or friend has undergone the procedure and expressed satisfaction with the outcome. Since today's society discusses sex freely, the topic of vasectomy is dealt with openly. It no longer is exclusively a bedroom topic, but often is an issue dealt with at intimate social gatherings.

Males undergoing a vasectomy are younger, have smaller family units, tend to be from a higher income bracket, and are better educated than the general population. It has been noted that minority groups consistently have been underrepresented in the performance of vasectomies. Reasons cited for this social phenomenon include fear of genocide, concern over an altered masculine gender role, fear of surgery, and feelings of threat to one's masculinity as a result of the inability to father children. In addition to these reasons, some individuals exhibit concerns over societal views about the continuation of tasks that the vasectomized male performs around the house, such as washing dishes or preparing dinner. A fear may exist that others will label him a "sissy." Because of these concerns, the vasectomized male may hesitate to discuss with others the fact that he has undergone a sterilization process or he may hesitate doing household chores that he carried out in the past. Thus, the individual requires information to the effect that vasectomies are being performed as a means of birth control and that vasectomies are more widely accepted and openly discussed by society than in the past. Males who encounter difficulties in dealing with the fact that they have had a vasectomy are likely to retreat from social interactions where their masculine image may be threatened. Not until the male feels secure with his masculine image will he be able to deal with the fact that he has undergone a vasectomy. Thus the individual needs to discuss and examine whether he believes that having a vasectomy will affect his social relationships.

The social effects of a hysterectomy are different from those of a vasectomy, not only in regards to gender roles, but the female also may view her hysterectomy as a social disruption of her previous way of life. Now that the uterus is gone, menstruation, a concrete cyclic symbol of femininity, is absent. No longer can the woman either consciously or unconsciously plan social events around the occurrence of menstruation. For example, in the past, she may have made arrangements for vacations, active sports, or cocktail parties at a time when menstruation did not occur. Now that menstruation is suddenly absent, her cyclic manner of social planning will be altered and she will be forced to adapt.

In addition to the disruption of a cyclic routine of life, women may express concern over their bodily appearance now that their uterus has been excised. Questions frequently asked include whether a swimsuit or other revealing clothing can be worn (if an abdominal hysterectomy was performed) and whether weight gain will be a problem. The woman should be informed that the position of the abdominal scar does vary and is often below bikini level. Thus, if she desires to wear swimwear or other revealing clothing she can do so with relative ease. Weight is a problem only if less exercise is carried out and/or more food is consumed than before the operation. Adequate nutritional intake generally controls this problem. The woman may find that her abdomen bulges initially after surgery, but as the abdominal muscles regain strength the bulging will subside.

The woman who has undergone a hysterectomy may question her feelings of self-worth now that one of her marks of femininity has been lost. This is especially true in women who view their major feminine role as child bearer. To enhance feelings of self-worth, family members should encourage the woman to become involved in activities outside the home, especially if children are grown and have moved away. The woman's interest will affect her choice of activities, and these interests need to be considered as family members assist her in selecting social activities. Possible activities to consider are volunteer work, adult education classes, or learning a new hobby or sport. Since approval from her significant others is so important in reestablishing feelings of self-worth, the woman may require compliments for new accomplishments achieved. Only when feelings of self-worth have been reestablished can the woman resolve the loss of her uterus.

SUMMARY

Surgical changes of the reproductive system are becoming increasingly prevalent in today's society. More men are selecting the vasectomy as a means of controlling family size, and women continue to have a hysterectomy as a necessary treatment for various forms of gynecological pathology. The male undergoing a vasectomy generally is in the fourth decade of life, the father of three or four children, and of the Protestant religion. By contrast, the female undergoing a hysterectomy tends to be in the fifth decade of life and have a grown family.

Unlike most hysterectomies, the vasectomy usually is a surgical procedure of choice. Nonetheless, in both cases, an impact in the life of the individual involved occurs. The presence of surgical sexual alterations can affect one's psychological well-being, somatic identity, sexuality, occupational identity, and social role. The feelings expressed by the spouse or sex partner of the man or woman undergoing a surgical sexual alteration play an important part in how the individual adapts to such loss. Therefore, members of the health care team must prepare both the individual and his or her family for alterations in daily living which may occur as a result of the impact of the vasectomy or hysterectomy and assist them in dealing with each of these changes.

Patient Situation   Mr. V. is a thirty-five-year-old, white, middle-class Methodist with three children. He is a chemical engineer by profession. Mr. V. and his wife do not desire more children and hence have been using birth control. However, Mrs. V. has encountered difficulties and displeasure with the various forms of birth control that she has used. Consequently, she has requested Mr. V. to undergo a vasectomy. Mr. V. has consented to the surgical procedure, but he is experiencing doubts about whether or not he really wants to be sterilized because he has many unanswered questions about the procedure and its effects. Mr. and Mrs. V. are currently being counseled by a nurse in an out-patient clinic. During the initial assessment the nurse identified patient-centered problems related to psychological well-being, somatic identity, sexuality, occupational identity, and social role.

Following are Mr. V's nursing care plan and patient care cardex related to the above mentioned areas of concern.

NURSING CARE PLAN

Nursing Diagnoses	Objectives	Nursing Interventions	Principles/Rationale	Evaluations
Psychological Impact Anxiety manifested by expressed ambivalent feelings about having a vasectomy.	To enhance Mr. V.'s verbalization of his feelings.	Encourage Mr. V. to express to his wife how he feels about having a vasectomy.	Verbalizing feelings can assist the individual in identifying possible solutions to a problem. A sex partner who is aware of the individual's feelings about a surgical sexual alteration is more likely to be able to provide necessary emotional support.	The nurse would observe for: Mr. V.'s expressed feelings about the surgery to his wife.
	To increase Mr. and Mrs. V.'s awareness of the importance of mutual consent about the performance of a vasectomy.	Encourage Mrs. V. to allow Mr. V. to reexamine his feelings about having a vasectomy.	A man who is pressured into making the decision to have a vasectomy is more likely to undergo emotional problems as a result of the surgical intervention.	Mutual reexamination by Mr. and Mrs. V. for the desire for a vasectomy. Definitive plans, by Mr. and Mrs. V., for or against the performance of a vasectomy.
Somatic Impact Fear of body image alteration manifested by expressed concern about being emasculated.	To enhance Mr. V.'s examination of his body image.	Encourage Mr. V. to verbalize how he feels the vasectomy will affect him.	Some men feel that the loss of reproductivity makes them less manly.	The nurse would observe for: Mr. V.'s open verbalization about his masculinity.
		Encourage Mrs. V. to verbalize how she feels the vasectomy will affect Mr. V.	A man who is aware of how his sex partner will view him after a vasectomy is better prepared to make a decision on whether or not he desires it.	

(cont.)

NURSING CARE PLAN (cont.)

Nursing Diagnoses	Objectives	Nursing Interventions	Principles/Rationale	Evaluations
		Inform Mr. and Mrs. V. that a vasectomy does not alter: 1. masculine appearance. 2. voice tone. 3. sexual activity. 4. physical strength.	With a better understanding about the effects of the vasectomy, individuals are more capable of making the decision of whether or not it is their desired means of birth control.	Definitive plans by Mr. and Mrs. V. for or against the performance of a vasectomy.
Sexual Impact Fear of sexual dysfunction manifested by verbalized concern about possible castration.	To decrease Mr. V.'s fear of castration.	Inform Mr. and Mrs. V. that castration (removal of the gonads) does not take place during the surgical procedure.	Fear of castration is compounded when an individual has limited knowledge about the surgical procedure.	The nurse would observe for: A decrease in Mr. V.'s expressed fear of castration.
	To enhance Mr. and Mrs. V.'s knowledge about the vasectomy procedure.	Inform Mr. and Mrs. V. that either a short midline incision is made in the scrotum or a half-inch incision is made on both sides. Both vas deferens (excretory ducts of the testes) are lifted out and a small section is removed. The duct is closed off and placed back into position.		
Occupational Impact Knowledge deficit manifested by the expressed belief that two weeks of work will be missed as a result of the vasectomy.	To increase Mr. V.'s knowledge about the effect which the vasectomy will have upon occupational responsibility.	Explain to Mr. and Mrs. V. that the procedure is performed at the end of the work week (generally on Friday) so that Mr. V. has an opportunity to rest over the weekend before returning to work. If Mr. V. is unable to have a	Increasing an individual's knowledge about the specifics of a surgical procedure can prevent inappropriate postvasectomy behavior.	The nurse would observe for: A decrease in Mr. V.'s expressed belief that numerous work days will be missed as a result of the vasectomy.

Social Impact Potential social isolation manifested by expressed concern about what friends will think and say about him once he has had a vasectomy.	To decrease Mr. V.'s concern about what others think and say about him.	weekend free from his job, he should be informed that he needs to rest completely for twelve hours after the surgery with time off the following day if his work requires heavy labor. Point out to Mr. V. that generally a man undergoing a vasectomy will not be required to lose work days. However, if he has to miss work, the number of days missed is rarely over three. Encourage Mr. V. to verbalize how he feels the vasectomy will affect him.	The male who feels insecure with the masculine image he portrays will be less likely to admit openly and deal with the fact that he has undergone a vasectomy.	The nurse would observe for: Mr. V.'s decreased concern about what others think and say about him.
	To increase Mr. V.'s recognition of the possibility of retreating into isolation.	Inform Mr. and Mrs. V. that: 1. More people are receiving vasectomies as a means of birth control. 2. Vasectomies are more openly discussed by society than in the past. 3. A vasectomy is an acceptable means of birth control. Encourage Mr. V. to discuss how he feels a vasectomy will affect his ability to relate to others.	Increased knowledge and understanding about an issue tend to decrease one's apprehension. A man who views himself as "less of a man" because of the vasectomy may retreat into isolation and fail to set up friendships or a mutually satisfying sexual relationship.	Mr. V.'s discussion and examination of whether he believes that having a vasectomy will affect his social relationships.

PATIENT CARE CARDEX

PATIENT'S NAME: Mr. V.

MEDICAL DIAGNOSIS: Desiring vasectomy for purpose of birth control

AGE: 35 years

SEX: Male

MARITAL STATUS: Married

OCCUPATION: Chemical Engineer

SIGNIFICANT OTHERS: Wife and three children

Nursing Diagnoses	Nursing Approaches
Psychological: Anxiety manifested by expressed ambivalent feelings about having a vasectomy.	1. Encourage to express to wife how he feels about having a vasectomy. 2. Encourage wife to allow him to reexamine his feelings about having a vasectomy.

Somatic: Fear of body image alteration manifested by expressed concern about being emasculated.	1. Encourage to verbalize how he feels a vasectomy will affect him.
	2. Encourage wife to verbalize how she feels the vasectomy will affect husband.
	3. Inform patient and wife that a vasectomy does not alter:
	  (a) masculine appearance.
	  (b) voice tone.
	  (c) sexual activity.
	  (d) physical strength.

Sexual: Fear of sexual dysfunction manifested by verbalized concern about possible castration.

1. Inform patient and wife that castration does not take place during the surgical procedure.
2. Inform patient and wife that either a short midline incision is made in the scrotum or a half-inch incision is made on both sides.
3. Inform patient and wife that both vas deferens are lifted out and a small section is removed. The duct is closed off and placed back into position.

Occupational: Knowledge deficit manifested by the expressed belief that two weeks of work will be missed as a result of the vasectomy.

1. Explain to patient and wife that the procedure is performed at the end of the work week so that there is an opportunity for rest over the weekend before returning to work. If patient is unable to have a weekend free from work, he should be informed that he needs to rest completely for twelve hours after the surgery with time off the following day if work requires heavy labor.
2. Point out that generally a man undergoing a vasectomy will not be required to lose work days, but if days are missed, they rarely number more than three.

Social: Potential social isolation manifested by expressed concern about what friends will think and say about him once he has had a vasectomy.

1. Encourage to verbalize how he believes the vasectomy will affect him.
2. Inform patient and wife that:
   (a) more people are receiving vasectomies as a means of birth control.
   (b) vasectomies are more openly discussed by society than in the past.
   (c) a vasectomy is an acceptable means of birth control.
3. Encourage to discuss how he feels a vasectomy will affect his ability to relate to others.

REFERENCES

ERIKSON, E. *Childhood and society.* New York: W.W. Norton & Co., Inc., 1963.

GATH, D., COOPER, P., and DAY, A. Hysterectomy and psychiatric disorder: levels of psychiatric morbidity before and after hysterectomy, *British Journal of Psychiatry,* 1982, *140,* 335-350.

HILL, G. *Outpatient surgery.* Philadelphia: Saunders, 1980.

HUMPHRIES, P. Sexual adjustment after a hysterectomy, *Issues in Health Care for Women,* 1980, *2* (2), 1-14.

JANIS, I. *Psychological stress.* New York: John Wiley, 1958.

KALTREIDER, N., WALLACE, A., and HOROWITZ, M. A field study of the stress response syndrome, *Journal of the American Medical Association,* 1979, *242* (14), 1499-1503.

KAPLAN, H. *The illustrated manual of sex therapy.* New York: Quadrangle/The New York Times Book Co., 1975.

LIPSHULTZ, L., and BENSON, G. Vasectomy—1980, *Urologic Clinics of North America,* 1980, *7* (1), 89-105.

LYONS, H. Psychological screening for vasectomy, *Ulster Medical Journal,* 1978, *47* (2), 177-185.

MATHIS, J. Psychological aspects of surgery on female reproductive organs, *JOGN Nursing,* 1973, *2,* 50-53.

POLIVY, J. Psychological reactions to hysterectomy: critical review, *American Journal of Obstetrics and Gynecology,* 1974, *118* (3), 319-322.

VAUGHN R. Behavioral response to vasectomy, *Archives of General Psychiatry,* 1979, *36* (6), 815-821.

WOODS, N. *Human sexuality in health and illness.* St. Louis: C.V. Mosby, 1979.

7 |||||||||||||||||||||||||||||||||||||||||||||||||||||||||||||

OBESITY

INTRODUCTION

Excessive weight among members of the population is an ever-increasing concern for health care professionals. Approximately one third of the people in the United States are above their ideal weight and approximately one quarter of a million of them are on some form of diet most of the time to control their weight (Sims, 1979). Undoubtedly, the affluence of Western society contributes greatly to the occurrence of weight related health problems. Food is abundant and accessible for most people. In addition, the standard of living is such that a fair amount of time is available for recreational activities. A large percentage of the population only takes part in sedentary recreational activities such as video games, television, and spectator sports. Thus physical inactivity has become one of the greatest contributing factors to overweight in the American population (Rodin, 1979).

     Some authorities have described overweight as being an excess of weight in comparison to a set standard without consideration for fat deposit, bone structure, or muscle mass (Seltzer and Stare, 1973). Obesity is frequently referred to as a condition in which there is an excess of adipose tissue. The easiest and most direct means of determining the presence of obesity is by measuring the thickness of the individual's skinfold because large quantities of adipose tissue are located under the skin. Detailed studies of skinfolds on many sites of the body show that the amount of fat at the upper arm site, over the triceps and at the subscapular site, correlates highly with total body fat (Renold, 1981). An upper arm skinfold measurement of 3.0 centimeters and above for a woman and a measurement of 2.3 centimeters and above for a man are considered standard measurements of obesity by many authorities (Seltzer and Stare, 1973).

Regardless of whether the individual is excessively overweight or is actually obese, similar problems are encountered by both. For clarity of the topic related to an individual experiencing a weight problem, this chapter will refer to these individuals as obese.

OBESITY PROFILE

Obesity generally is recognized by health care professionals as a major health hazard both physically and emotionally. Research has shown that individuals who are obese are more prone to additional health care problems such as diabetes mellitus, cardiovascular disorders, and renal disease (Cavallo-Perin, Sorbo, Morra, Pagani, Tagliaferro, and Lenti, 1981; Kalisch, 1972; Kannel and Gordon, 1979). Nevertheless, few individuals in the general population view obesity as ill health. For many it has become a way of life, since historically obesity has been viewed as a weakness, a sin, or inadequate self-control rather than as a medical condition.

Obesity is one of the most common chronic illnesses in American women. Obese men outnumber obese women in the early adult years, but women increasingly outnumber men after age thirty-five. Nearly two and one half times more obese women than nonobese women were overweight as children (Rimm and Rimm, 1976). Obese children and adolescents are a major reservoir for obesity in adults since over three quarters of them go on to become obese adults (Feig, 1980).

A familial tendency has been found to exist since children who have one obese parent have a 40 percent chance of being obese themselves and children who have two obese parents have an 80 percent chance of being obese themselves. Generally, only 7 percent of the children with nonobese parents become obese (Fisch, Bilek, and Ulstrom, 1975).

Socioeconomic factors play an important part in the prevalence of obesity. Studies have shown that obesity is six times more common in women of lower socioeconomic class than in women of higher socioeconomic class (Salans, 1979). For men, social class also has a significant relationship to obesity, but the relationship is less pronounced than in women (Bray, 1976).

In addition to socioeconomic factors, cultural background contributes to the development of obesity. Bray (1976) and Stunkard (1976) note that individuals originating in Eastern Europe and living in the United States have a higher incidence of obesity than individuals from Western Europe. The incidence of obesity increases steadily as one moves eastward across Europe, starting with Great Britain and continuing with Ireland, Germany, Italy, Czechoslovakia, Hungary, and a Polish-Russian group. Stunkard (1976), however, notes that one ethnic group, the Czechoslovakians, does not fit this pattern. The Czechoslovakians demonstrate the highest rate of obesity among any of the groups, with 34 percent of them being obese. Research also has shown that the time spent in the United States has an effect upon the frequency of obesity since the lowest incidence of obesity has been found among individuals whose families have been in the United States for a long period of time (Stunkard, 1976). Consequently, recent immigrants to the United States demonstrate a higher incidence of obesity than fourth-generation Americans of the same cultural heritage.

Religion has a decided relationship to the frequency of obesity. Obesity has been found to be most common among Jews, followed by Catholics, and then Protestants. When the Protestant religion is further examined with respect to some of its denominations, the occurrence of obesity mirrors the social class stereotyping conventionally ascribed to each of these divisions. Baptists have the highest incidence of obesity, followed by Methodists, Presbyterians, and finally Episcopalians (Stunkard, 1976).

Although various interpretations can be placed upon these findings, major contributing factors to the prevalence of obesity are, most likely, increased standard of living, abundance of food, decreased physical activity, and basic food habits. Food of high carbohydrate and caloric content may frequently comprise the diet of individuals of lower socioeconomic status. One-dish meals designed to stretch meat allowances for a family often contain high carbohydrate foods, such as noodles or macaroni. Thus, caloric consumption increases. In addition, increased use of "junk foods" has affected the additional caloric intake of many individuals, regardless of social class. Cultural food patterns in which potatoes, pastas, and sweet pastries are important constituents also can contribute to increased weight. If the main meal of the day is high in calories and if physical activity becomes increasingly less, obesity is likely to ensue.

Regardless of the factors that contribute to obesity, its presence can create problems that affect psychological well-being, somatic identity, sexuality, occupational identity, and social role. The remainder of the chapter will discuss how obesity can affect each of these areas.

IMPACT OF OBESITY

Psychological Impact

The presence of obesity has many psychological ramifications. A question frequently asked by members of the health care team is, "Which came first, the psychological difficulties or the obesity?" Advocates for both sides exist. Regardless of which occurred first, both facets greatly contribute to the survival of the other.

Individuals who are obese frequently are seen by others as stubborn, defiant, and wary, characteristics that form the basis for a passive-aggressive personality organization. They may intentionally miss clinic appointments or they may take their daily prescribed vitamins and minerals haphazardly, even though the importance of adhering to both regimens has been explained.

When asked to describe themselves, the obese individuals are ambivalent. Obese individuals are unaware of the esthetic drawbacks of obesity, yet they are very embarrassed about viewing themselves in a mirror or in photographs (Castelnuovo-Tedesco and Schiebel, 1975). Some obese individuals refuse to shop for clothing because they dislike having to view themselves in a mirror when trying on garments. In addition, the clothing store environment (small dressing rooms and narrow passageways) frequently reminds them of their size.

Obese individuals usually view food as a self-administered gratification to decrease emotional upheavals. Although such individuals are aware that the food they eat is not good for them (Plutnick, 1976), they have an intense desire to eat. Thus, a strong sense of denial is manifested. External stimuli such as the smell of food, the sight of food, and the discussion of food play a vital role in encouraging obese individuals to eat. Unlike the case for non-obese individuals, internal stimuli, such as gastric contractions and changes in blood sugar levels, play a minor role in initiating the obese individual's drive to consume food. Rodin (1975) found that obese individuals perceive time as passing more slowly than nonobese individuals and thus eat sooner. Consequently, obese individuals are greatly affected by the stimuli from the environment and, because of these stimuli, increase their food consumption. Such findings lend themselves to the belief that eating disorders are learned behaviors that have become reflexive in the obese individual's pattern of daily living.

Obesity, like alcoholism, drug abuse, and gambling, is a complex problem. Individuals exhibiting any one of these disorders frequently demonstrate an obsessive-compulsive syndrome which is manifested by rigid behavior, especially in those areas of their emotional life which are not completely under voluntary control. Since they are unable to be in absolute control, they often attempt to control by totally avoiding any kind of control. They are either totally organized or totally unorganized, meticulously clean or very sloppy. The obsessive-compulsive individual tends to be concerned about being in control either through extreme active attempts at control or complete abandonment of all efforts to control. This behavior is manifested by the obese individual's obsession to eat and the compulsion to eat. ''What difference does it make how much I eat? Everything turns to fat anyway!'' These are common statements made by the obese person demonstrating an obsessive-compulsive syndrome.

Research has shown that adults who were obese as children encounter more difficulties in the treatment of their weight problem than adults who were not obese as children (Gold, 1976). The prognosis and psychological aspects of obesity are different in individuals who have become obese in their middle adult years from those who have been obese since early life. Individuals who were obese as children are more likely to be obsessively concerned about their self-image than persons who have middle-age, adult-onset obesity. The child-onset obese individual tends to view his or her obesity as a badge of shame rather than a medical problem. In addition, the individual usually demonstrates a long history of repeated failures to control weight.

By contrast, middle-age, adult-onset obesity is less inundated with diffuse psychological factors. The adult-onset obese individual generally views his or her condition as reversible, provided he or she obtains appropriate medical guidance. In addition, the individual tends to realize the health hazards of obesity, thus creating a more cooperative and conducive climate with the health care team and their approach to the obesity problem. This is not necessarily true of the person with child-onset obesity who does not view the excessive weight as harmful to physical health and thus demonstrates less cooperation in the institution of therapy. Consequently, one can see the importance of knowing the age of the individual's obesity onset in developing and implementing an appropriate plan of care.

Since treatment of obesity is complex, a multidimensional approach is necessary for successful treatment. Simply placing the individual on a weight reduction diet and encouraging more physical activity often are not enough to accomplish the goal of taking off pounds.

To deal with the psychological aspects of the individual's weight problem, one of the first goals in therapy is to establish sound rapport with the individual. Acceptance of the individual must occur before weight reduction therapy is instituted. Since the obese individual harbors feelings of shame and guilt about his or her condition, the individual may find it difficult to express these feelings if he or she feels that the therapist or family members are not accepting of him or her; consequently, treatment efforts are doomed before they start.

A family member or health care provider who holds unwarranted prejudices about obesity must identify and work through these prejudices before attempting to become involved in therapy with the individual manifesting a weight problem. If the family member or the health team member views obesity as incurable or only slightly amenable to therapy, these feelings may be transmitted to the obese individual. Such prejudices may have contributed to the low success rate experienced by the individual in past attempts at weight reduction.

The obese individual and his or her family need to be told that feelings of depression during the first twelve months of weight reduction (with the first six months being the most difficult) are not uncommon (Kalucy and Crisp, 1974) and that such feelings will subside as weight reduction is stabilized at the lower desired weight. Since feelings of discouragement are evident, frequent strong, positive encouragement to continue therapy may be necessary. Encouraging the dieting individual to verbalize his or her feelings to significant others and the therapist is vital. By the same token, the significant others and the therapist must provide positive reinforcement for the accomplishment in weight loss that has been made.

Throughout the obese individual's life, he or she most likely has been reminded of the negative effects of eating to excess. The use of negative reinforcement of the problem may often intensify the existence of that problem (Pierre and Warren, 1975). Instead of using negative feedback, positive reinforcement on the part of those in the environment of the obese individual may prove more beneficial. For example, health team members and family members should comment in a positive way about the individual's decrease in food consumption instead of commenting that he or she still is eating too much even though the individual has attempted to reduce caloric intake. Comments indicating positive feedback can include such statements as: "I've noticed that you are eating less at each meal. It must be difficult and I'm proud of your attempts."

As previously mentioned, environmental factors play a major role in contributing to the obese individual's compulsion to eat. Therefore, one of the first acts that health care providers must carry out is an assessment of the individual's eating *behaviors* (Hagenbuch, 1982). The obese person and his or her family require instructions on how to keep a record of the obese individual's eating patterns for approximately one week. This record must include: when eating takes place, what is eaten, where eating takes place, what is being done while eating, and how the obese individual feels prior to eating. To assist the obese person and his or her family in controlling the effects that environmental factors have upon the obese person's eating patterns, attempts must be made to decrease such stimuli. Based upon the assessment of the obese individual's eating behavior the following interventions are recommended to facilitate the reduction of these stimuli:

1. Eat meals slowly so that they last at least twenty minutes.
2. Chew each mouthful of food ten times.
3. Place the utensils on the plate between mouthfuls.
4. Decrease the size of food portions.
5. Serve the meals restaurant style.
6. Discard leftover food immediately after the meal is completed.
7. Avoid keeping prepared snack food in the house.
8. Leave small portions of food on the plate at each meal.
9. Alter the composition of foods (if possible) high in caloric content. For example, over a period of days or weeks decrease the amount of bread used to make a sandwich until no bread is used at all.
10. Use low-calorie substitutes with meals, such as low-calorie sodas.
11. Shop for groceries after eating a full meal.

12. Shop from a prepared grocery list.
13. Turn off the bulb in the refrigerator.
14. Keep all foods in covered containers.
15. Eat only in one room and in one chair.
16. Avoid carrying out household and personal activities, such as telephone calls or letter writing, in the kitchen.
17. Reward appropriate dietary behavior by engaging in a pleasurable "non-food" oriented activity.

As the obese individual attempts the above suggested measures to decrease environmental stimuli to eat, he or she may identify other helpful maneuvers. Using a small dinner plate to eat from, placing a picture of a slender person on the door of the refrigerator as a reminder to decrease food consumption, or chewing "sugar free" gum each time the urge to eat occurs are but a few possible maneuvers to consider. Regardless of which measures an individual uses, those that are helpful in decreasing environmental stimuli are the ones of importance.

Family members and friends can play a vital role in assisting the obese individual in carrying out diet therapy. They can help by facilitating the reduction of environmental stimuli and by providing reinforcement for accomplishments made. Thus, the obese individual does not feel alone in the effort for weight reduction.

In addition to the support provided by family and friends, the use of group interaction can be helpful to some obese individuals. Group interaction can take several forms, including group therapy sessions with a psychiatric clinical nurse specialist or the use of organized societal groups such as Weight Watchers or TOPS (Take Off Pounds Sensibly). These sessions provide a means for obese individuals to share similar problems and possible solutions to their problems. Since the obese person has a great need to be liked, peers in group interaction provide a realistic means for such acceptance. In addition, group interactions serve as another available source of positive reinforcement for continuation with weight-reduction therapy and for accomplishments achieved.

Somatic Impact

Three components have been identified as major contributing factors to the development of a disturbed body image in an obese individual: age of onset, presence of emotional problems, and negative appraisal of obesity by other individuals during the formative years (Noppa and Hallstrom, 1981). Disturbances in body image related to age of obesity onset occur primarily among individuals who became obese during childhood and adolescence. Generally, an individual who is obese in childhood also tends to be obese in adolescence (Feig,

1980). As pointed out in Chapter 2, it is during adolescence that the individual becomes concerned about his or her body contour. The female adolescent takes on a rounded feminine form and the male assumes a muscular masculine appearance. However, both the male and the female adolescent see the body as something useful to them that allows engagement in activities valued by their peers. The success with which the adolescent utilizes the body is important because the body contributes to the value placed upon oneself. If the adolescent views the body as "less than desirable" because of obesity, he or she will encounter difficulties in establishing a healthy view of personal capabilities and, in turn, will have a distorted body image.

According to Stunkard (1976), the basic feature of the obese individual's disturbed body image is a constant preoccupation with obesity. This preoccupation actually may lead to the exclusion of other personal characteristics such as intelligence, wealth, or theatrical talent. The obese person often views the entire world in terms of body weight and divides society into classifications of differing weight and responds to them accordingly. The thinner individual is viewed with envy, while someone fatter is looked upon with contempt. The obese person appraises his or her body as grotesque and feels that others view his or her body with horror. These feelings are exemplified in such statements as, "Who would want to marry an elephant?"

Long-term results for weight reduction in the juvenile-onset obese individual are poor. Studies have found that when undergoing weight reduction a variety of behavioral changes such as distortions of time, inaccuracies of body size estimation, and depressive symptoms occur in juvenile-onset individuals. Adult-onset individuals do not experience any of these alterations (Grinker, 1973; Grinker and Hirsch, 1972). Thus, it is apparent that the age at which obesity occurs has profound effects on both the individual's body image and the success encountered in dealing with weight loss.

The second contributing factor in the alteration of the obese individual's body image is the presence of emotional disturbances. The juvenile-onset obese individual frequently manifests emotional disorders (Stunkard and Mendelson, 1967). By contrast, the adult-onset obese individual tends to demonstrate a variety of emotional disorders with few, if any, related to his or her obesity (Stunkard and Mendelson, 1967). Emotional disturbances can contribute to a disruption in body image, but they are not necessarily a primary constituent of its development.

Negative evaluation of obesity by significant others comprises the third predisposing factor to a disturbed body image in the obese individual. Today's society has an almost universal devaluation of obesity. The obese individual frequently is ostracized by others during social functions, becomes the target of jokes, and often is viewed with hostility and contempt. How others view the obese person is important not only to the obese adult, but to the obese child as well. Fat children are known to encounter more difficulties with interpersonal relationships and are discriminated against by peers. Richardson and Goodman (1961) investigated children's reactions to the physical attributes of other children. Their findings indicate that almost unanimously the nonobese child was the most preferred and the obese child was the least desired.

The occasional existence of juveniles who do not face censorship because of their size reinforces the importance this factor can play in the formation of a disturbed body image. Stunkard and Mendelson (1967) found that men coming from families in which large body size was valued and overweight was viewed as a sign of strength and health escaped body image disturbances. Such individuals frequently are in demand as football players.

One reason given for society's negative attitudes toward obesity is that often success depends upon physical attractiveness. Another justification offered is that excess weight is detrimental to health, and health is an important measure of status and security. Regardless of the justifications offered by society, the views society holds and the feelings society expresses play a vital role in the individual's development of his or her body image in childhood and in adolescence. Without a doubt, the most devastating result of the stigmatizing attitude displayed by society is that the afflicted individuals come to accept the negative evaluation placed upon them.

The negative feelings the obese individual harbors because of his obesity can have an effect upon the stage of development that he or she is currently experiencing. If the obese individual is in the stage of young adulthood (eighteen to forty-five), the individual is in the period in which merging his or her identity with others is vital to maturation. Since the obese individual feels grotesque and believes that others view him or her with contempt, the individual will undoubtedly experience difficulty in sharing himself or herself with others, both in friendships and in a mutually satisfying sexual relationship. In fact, a study has shown that obese women encounter more difficulty in establishing a satisfying sexual relationship with members of the opposite sex than nonobese women (Stunkard and Mendelson, 1967). Because of the fear of negative evaluation by significant others, the obese young adult may retreat into isolation instead of establishing a sense of intimacy with other individuals. The existing state of isolation leads to boredom whereby a need to eat may develop in an attempt to cope with the feelings of loneliness. Thus, a vicious cycle develops and obesity ends up generating obesity.

The developmental stage of adulthood (forty-five to sixty-five years) may create problems of stagnation for the obese individual. The middle years, as pointed out in Chapter 2, are a time when vital interests outside the home are founded and a concern for guiding future generations evolves. If an obese individual views himself or herself with contempt and becomes preoccupied with obesity, he or she devalues other personal attributes. Regardless of the positive characteristics that may exist, only the negativeness of obesity is seen. The individual becomes self-absorbed, stagnates, and feels that he or she has nothing of value to offer forthcoming generations. Chronic defeatism results and the individual isolates himself or herself in self-pity.

As pointed out in Chapter 2, the stage of maturity (sixty-five and over) is when the individual derives satisfaction from life's experience and accomplishment. Obese individuals may not be satisfied with past accomplishments and may develop an altered sense of self-worth. In addition to the impact of obesity upon body structure, the obese person must contend with the frequent body changes brought about by aging. Ego integrity is weak and it is not uncommon for a state of despair to exist for an obese individual experiencing the final developmental stage of life. Obesity can have an adverse effect upon successful accomplishment of each developmental stage of adulthood since it does alter one's mental picture of oneself.

The nurse's role in dealing with an obese individual's altered body image revolves around assisting him or her in reestablishing a new body image. It has been found that a formerly obese person who has not reestablished his or her self-image will most likely be unable to retain weight loss (Kalisch, 1972). This is often the result of harbored feelings of self-hate and inadequacy. Encouraging the obese person to verbalize feelings may assist him or her in recognizing possible ways of dealing with his or her feelings. It also provides a means of releasing pent-up emotions so that these internalized emotions do not further intensify feelings of self-hate and inadequacy.

The obese individual needs encouragement to express how he or she believes members of society view him or her. The individual requires assistance in awareness of and resistance to stigmatizing attitudes that the community may express. Instead of retreating into isolation and further compounding these feelings of inadequacy, the obese individual must be assisted in understanding why people react the way they do. The obese individual needs help in realizing that ostracizing and stigmatizing someone who is different is often the way people deal with their own insecurities. If the obese person can understand and accept this, he or she may encounter fewer difficulties in relating to members of society.

In addition to verbalizing personal feelings and attempting to understand other individuals' reactions, the obese individual requires positive feedback for attempts and accomplishments made in weight reduction. The feedback may be encouragement about the use of willpower at a party serving many high-caloric foods or compliments about weight lost. Since the obese person has frequent moments of discouragement and depression, positive feedback is necessary both from significant others and members of the health care team. Not until the obese individual reevaluates and restructures his or her body image will the individual consistently be able to lose the necessary amount of weight and maintain the desired level of weight (Cozens, 1982; Jordan, Levitz, and Kimbrell, 1977).

Sexual Impact

Sexual behavior is affected by the way an individual perceives his or her body and the obese individual certainly is no exception. The obese individual finds his or her body ugly and loathesome and continually avoids mirrors and scales. He or she tends to think of himself or herself as fat, and awareness of body size rarely is far from conscious thoughts. Thus it is not surprising that homogamy or assortive mating (interbreeding of individuals of like characteristics) occurs with obese persons (Garn, 1976).

Displeasure at looking at one's nude body is not uncommon. The obese individual dislikes being seen in the nude and even avoids being seen in a bathing suit. Therefore, it is not unusual for the obese person to carry out sexual intercourse in the dark or while partially clothed (Castelnuovo-Tedesco and Schiebel, 1975). In addition, sexual activity is significantly diminished which is related to the fact that the obese individual encounters serious difficulties in relationships with members of the opposite sex.

Some individuals have used obesity as a protective means of lessening heterosexual opportunities. Such a maneuver is related to fears about one's sexual potential. When weight loss occurs the individual may be confronted with feelings of frigidity and/or increased anger toward potential sex partners who "come too close."

In addition to the psychological effects that obesity may have upon one's sexual activity, physical difficulties in carrying out intercourse also may be encountered. Because of the excessive body fat, the ability to assume various coital positions may be difficult. Vaginal penetration may become complicated because there is an excess of adipose tissue in the pelvic region. Such distribution of excessive body fat does not lend itself to close body positioning. The obese individual may find it necessary to experiment with various coital positions before deciding which one(s) provides the greatest comfort and enjoyment. For example, the male superior position may create breathing difficulties for the female because of either her own obese state or the weight of her sex partner. The "doggy-fashion" position may be impossible because of the excessive fat on the female buttocks. The inability to carry out the sex act satisfactorily can create anxieties in the sexual relationship and/or intensify existing difficulties.

Proper feminine hygiene after intercourse may pose problems for the obese female. Because of the excessive body fat the woman may encounter difficulties in adequately cleansing the perineal area. She may be unable to see or to reach her perineum so that she can clean herself properly. As a result, the woman may hesitate to engage in intercourse. The outcome may be the creation of difficulties or intensification of existing problems within the sexual relationship. If the obese female has difficulty in cleansing the perineal area, the nurse should instruct her on how to use a small hand mirror to assist in the visualization of the perineum. Assuming a sitting position on the toilet may facilitate the ability to reach the area. The use of a bidet or a squeeze bottle with a spray tip for external cleansing may also prove helpful.

The nurse needs to encourage the obese individual to express feelings about his or her sexual relationship. Unless feelings are expressed, the identification of problems is difficult and the internalization of ill feelings can only add to the creation of tension in the sexual relationship. The obese individual should be guided by the nurse in examining: what his or her expectations are in regards to the sexual relationship; what a sexual experience means to him or her; whether he or she desires sexual intercourse; and what alternatives exist, other than intercourse, for sexual expression. It may be necessary for the nurse to direct the obese individual to appropriate members of the health team who are prepared in counseling individuals with sexual difficulties. If the nurse is a prepared sex therapist, then he or she can carry out the necessary interventions.

Occupational Impact

The obese individual often finds his or her condition a barrier to obtaining privileges, opportunities, and status granted to others. He or she may encounter difficulties in acquiring the necessary preparations for certain jobs or in securing employment. It has been noted that applicants who are obese are less likely to be admitted to college than non-obese applicants even when there is no measurable difference in academic achievement, social class, and motivation (Canning and Mayer, 1966). In addition, many companies have regulations for acceptable body weight that hinder the obese individual from securing a job. Such occupational restrictions only add to the obese person's already altered self-concept.

Even if the individual is not discriminated against because of weight, job requirements may make it difficult, if not impossible, for the individual to function. Body fat may actually get in the way if the obese individual is required to operate certain machinery or if he or she is expected to maneuver down small passageways or sit on small stools. In addition to increased body size, the obese individual may demonstrate a decrease in physical capabilities manifested by the inability to tolerate the same amount of physical strain as a non-obese person.

Aside from the fact that certain occupations are unsafe and/or impossible for the obese person, certain jobs actually foster the potential occurrence of obesity. Consider the businessman or woman who frequently is expected to "wine and dine" clients as part of his or her job responsibilities. The owner of a delicatessen or a bakery easily may become a "nibbler" since pieces of food often are left over. The factory worker who is required by union law to take coffee breaks may munch on "goodies" from the ever-present vending machine during these breaks. Excess weight may be put on by the housewife because food is always available. She may find herself eating the leftovers from the family meals or eating what the children have left on their plates because she cannot tolerate seeing food wasted. It is evident that the obese individual may not only encounter problems in obtaining employment but also in losing and maintaining weight because he or she may be constantly bombarded by food-related stimuli in conjunction with job responsibilities.

To assist the obese individual in dealing with the occupational issues of obesity, the nurse needs to guide the individual in recognizing ways in which obesity is affecting his or her occupation. The obese person needs to: verbalize how excessive weight is affecting work performance and occupational advancements; identify how he or she feels about the influence obesity has upon work performance; and explore whether he or she desires to alter weight because of the effect it has upon occupational pursuits. Unless the individual is aware that the obese state has an impact upon employment, he or she may not be ready to deal with its control.

If the work situation fosters obesity, means of dealing with the situation should be explored. The individual who frequently is required to "wine and dine" clients, as part of the job, needs assistance in learning how to select low-caloric foods from a menu. Encouragement to set limits prior to the meal on how much one intends to eat and drink is advisable. The individual then must function within these self-imposed limits. If one usually eats high-caloric "goodies" from the vending machine during cofee breaks, it may be helpful to take breaks where the vending machines are not accessible. If this is not possible or if the obese individual has a great need to eat during the coffee break, encouragement to bring low-caloric beverages or low-caloric foods, such as celery and carrot sticks, from home may prove beneficial. For the housewife or the delicatessen owner, possible ways of decreasing the availability of leftover food are to dispose of it immediately in the garbage or to package and put it in the freezer for future use. Such an act decreases or eliminates food-related stimuli that foster overconsumption.

Social Impact

The meaning of food in the social structure has greatly contributed to the occurrence of obesity. For centuries food has been the symbol of many religious and secular rituals such as weddings, baptisms, confirmations, bar mitzvahs, fund-raising banquets, cocktail parties, and graduation galas. People cannot escape the existence of food even when relaxing in front of the television set since commercials for hamburgers, sodas, candy, and ice cream continually are being aired. Even though society believes that fatness is unacceptable, it does little to assist the individual in achieving the goal of weight reduction.

Obesity presents a greater social disadvantage for women than it does for men. Physical attractiveness becomes a major factor in a woman's social success, with obese females finding it difficult to progress up the social ladder, relate to others, and find a suitable marriage partner (Kalisch, 1972). Since physical desirability is not one of her outstanding features, she finds herself often taking second best. For men, educational achievement, occupation, and financial status are the valued social traits. Hence, physical attractiveness plays less of a role in their social achievements.

Clothing plays a part in the social impact of obesity. Men's clothes often are designed to conceal body form and thus hide bulges. Women's clothes, however, frequently are fashioned to reveal body configurations and hence expose fat bulges. When extra weight is gained clothing may not be purchased. However, should the obese female purchase new clothing because of her weight gain she may look at her new wardrobe with feelings of despair. After all, she may feel that "one can't be choosy when Omar the tentmaker is your dressmaker!" Because of this, some women hesitate to be seen at social functions.

The obese individual is extremely concerned about being liked by others, yet worries about being too agreeable lest he or she be "used" or "put down." The obese person often appears awkward, tense, withdrawn, and seclusive during social contacts. One of the most frequent complaints related to the social impact of obesity is the feeling of humiliation at parties. The obese person often is found sitting along the sidelines at a dance or standing alone at a cocktail party. "Who wants to dance with a blimp!" is a statement frequently made by the obese person in reference to social functions. Thus, the comment that an obese individual is inherently jolly and the life of the party is a fallacy. Diminished social contact may further intensify the tendency to overeat, one of the obese individual's few remaining gratifications. The obese person bemoans the fact that he or she is fat and frequently uses it as an alibi for other handicaps. Yet the obese individual feels helpless, trapped, and incapable of altering his or her situation.

The nurse, when assisting the obese individual to cope with the social impact of obesity, needs to facilitate the individual's ability to develop adaptive responses to unavoidable social situations, such as banquets and weddings. The obese individual must be taught strategies for dealing with the presence of attractive and abundant foods to prevent unnecessary and excessive food consumption. However, realistic expectations of his or her behavior at such functions must be considered when planning these strategies. Setting extremely high goals that are unachievable and unrealistic can only lead to discouragement and failure.

Preplanning eating behavior, standing away from the serving table at a cocktail party, leaving small amounts of each kind of food on the dinner plate at a banquet, and constantly "thinking thin" are a few possible strategies the obese person can use. The primary goal is to enjoy the food at the social function while eating less.

The obese individual should not avoid social functions because isolation and loneliness often encourage the tendency to overeat. Some obese persons have found group interaction with other obese persons (e.g., Weight Watchers and Overeaters Anonymous) helpful in identifying and sharing ways of coping with social difficulties. Such groups may not be helpful for everyone; therefore, the nurse and other members of the health team must identify which obese individuals would benefit from such interactions.

Above all, the obese person needs encouragement from the nurse and significant others not to use obesity as an excuse to avoid social interactions. In addition, the result of social isolation should be made known to the individual. Since the obese person has frequent feelings of helplessness and hopelessness, constant positive feedback and support from significant others is a must. Unless the obese person's attitude toward social interaction is altered, he or she will continue to be socially isolated and to indulge in self-pity.

SUMMARY

Obesity is a prevalent and ever-increasing health care problem. It affects individuals of all ages and is a hazard both physically and emotionally. Research has shown that obesity tends to be more common in women of lower socioeconomic class, individuals originating from Eastern Europe, persons of recent immigration to the United States, and individuals of the Jewish faith. However, regardless of the factors that contribute to a person's obesity, its presence can create difficulties in the individual's psychological well-being, somatic identity, sexuality, occupational identity, and social role.

The obese person often is forced to deal with his or her health care problem alone. Society frowns on obesity, but it does little to assist the obese person in losing weight or maintaining weight already lost. Therefore, the role of the health care team is to assist the obese person in identifying how obesity affects his or her everyday life and guide the person in dealing with each of these alterations.

Patient Situation   Mrs. O. is a twenty-eight-year-old married woman with children ages two and four. Mrs. O's parents were immigrants from Hungary, but Mrs. O. was born in the United States. Her husband is currently employed as a gas station attendant. Mrs. O. has had a weight problem since the birth of her second child. She has come into the free clinic requesting assistance in dealing with her obesity. During the initial assessment the nurse identifies patient-centered problems related to psychological well-being, somatic identity, sexuality, occupational identity, and social role.

Following are Mrs. O's nursing care plan and patient care cardex related to the above mentioned areas of concern.

NURSING CARE PLAN

Nursing Diagnoses	Objectives	Nursing Interventions	Principles/Rationale	Evaluations
Psychological Impact Dysfunctional eating patterns manifested by inability to control eating habits.	To assist Mrs. O. in identifying uncontrollable eating behavior.	Instruct Mrs. O. and her family on how to keep a record of Mrs. O.'s eating habits. The record must include: 1. when she eats. 2. what she eats. 3. where she eats. 4. what she is doing while she eats. 5. how she feels prior to eating.	Identifying eating patterns assists the individual in recognizing her eating behavior.	The nurse would observe for: Recognition by Mrs. O. that her eating habits are uncontrollable.
	To identify means of controlling Mrs. O.'s eating behavior.	Involve Mrs. O. in group interactions in weight control programs.	Interacting with individuals with similar problems can provide emotional support and may facilitate in the solution of individual problems.	A change in Mrs. O.'s eating habits.
		Instruct Mrs. O. and her family on ways to decrease environmental stimuli that may be affecting Mrs. O.'s eating patterns. Include the following maneuvers: 1. Eat meals slowly so that they last at least twenty minutes. 2. Chew each mouthful of food ten times. 3. Place the utensils on the plate between mouthfuls.	Increasing understanding about factors that contribute to obesity can enhance the desire to control eating habits. Prolonging the meal can aid in the prevention of rapidly consuming excessive amounts of food.	

4. Decrease the size of food portions.	Decreasing the amount of readily available food for consumption can decrease food intake.
5. Serve the meals restaurant style on small plates.	
6. Discard leftover food immediately after the meal is completed.	
7. Avoid keeping prepared snack food in the house.	
8. Leave a small portion of food on the plate at each meal.	Decreasing the amount of calories consumed can lead to a loss in weight.
9. Alter the composition of foods high in caloric content (if possible).	
10. Use low-calorie substitutes with meals.	
11. Shop for groceries after eating a full meal.	Shopping from a prepared list while not hungry can prevent the purchase of unnecessary food items.
12. Shop from a prepared grocery list.	
13. Turn off the bulb in the refrigerator.	Decreasing the visibility of food can decrease the urge to eat.
14. Keep all foods covered in containers.	
15. Eat only in one room and in one chair.	Increasing the difficulty to eat can decrease the desire to eat.
16. Avoid carrying out household and personal activities in the kitchen.	
17. Reward appropriate dietary behavior by engaging in a pleasurable "non-food oriented" activity.	Positive feedback for accomplishments facilitates the feelings of self-worth.

(cont.)

NURSING CARE PLAN (cont.)

Nursing Diagnoses	Objectives	Nursing Interventions	Principles/Rationale	Evaluations
Somatic Impact Body image alteration manifested by devaluation of self.	To assist Mrs. O. in establishing a new body image.	Encourage Mrs. O. to verbalize the feelings she has about herself.	Verbalization of feelings can assist the individual in recognizing possible ways of dealing with feelings.	The nurse would observe for: A decrease in Mrs. O.'s verbalization that she is of little importance.
		Encourage Mrs. O. to express how she feels members of society view her.	Verbalizing feelings provides a release of pent-up emotions.	An increase in Mrs. O.'s pride about herself.
		Assist Mrs. O. in understanding that individuals who may ostracize and stigmatize her often do so because of their own insecurities.	Understanding the reasons for others' actions can aid the obese person in relating to other members of society.	
		Encourage Mr. O. to provide positive feedback to Mrs. O. for attempts and accomplishments made in weight reduction.	Positive feedback for accomplishments facilitates feelings of self-worth.	

Sexual Impact Sexual dysfunction manifested by expressed concern about increased avoidance of sexual relationship with husband.	To facilitate a healthy and satisfying sexual relationship between Mr. and Mrs. O.	Encourage Mrs. O. to verbalize her feelings about her sexuality.	Verbalization of feelings about one's sexuality may assist the individual in identifying a specific problem.	The nurse would observe for: Open expression of feelings between Mr. and Mrs. O. about an increased satisfaction with their sexual relationship.
		Encourage Mr. and Mrs. O. to discuss openly with each other their feelings about their sexual relationship.	Discussion of feelings between sex partners assists in their identifying specific sexual problems and aids in the prevention of internalized feelings that can create tension in the sexual relationship.	
		Inform Mrs. O. that her expressed concern about avoiding sexual contact with her husband is not abnormal.	Providing information can decrease anxiety that can interfere with sexual activity. Diminished sexual activity is not uncommon for obese persons. In addition, they often encounter difficulties in relationships with members of the opposite sex because they are self-conscious about how others view them.	

(cont.)

NURSING CARE PLAN (cont.)

Nursing Diagnoses	Objectives	Nursing Interventions	Principles/Rationale	Evaluations
Occupational Impact Deficit in health management activities manifested by increased tendency to eat excessive amounts of food at home.	To assist Mrs. O. in recognizing how obesity may be affecting her occupation as a housewife.	Encourage Mrs. O. to verbalize how her excessive weight is affecting her ability to perform her household duties.	Being aware of the impact that obesity has upon occupational performance facilitates the individual's readiness to deal with its control.	The nurse would observe for: Recognition by Mrs. O. that her obesity is affecting her performance as a housewife.
	To decrease external stimuli in the occupational situation that foster food consumption.	Encourage Mrs. O. to discard leftover foods immediately after the meal by disposing of them in the garbage or freezing them for future use. Encourage Mrs. O. not to eat the food her children leave on their plates and to dispose of it instead. Encourage Mrs. O. not to purchase snack foods high in calories, such as potato chips and cookies.	Decreasing the amount of available food for consumption can decrease food intake.	

Social Impact				
Social isolation manifested by avoidance of social contacts.	To enhance Mrs. O.'s social interaction.	Encourage Mrs. O. to take part in social functions because avoidance of social contact can be detrimental to the obese person.	Isolation and loneliness often encourage the tendency to overeat.	The nurse would observe for: Mrs. O.'s increased involvement in social functions.
	To facilitate Mrs. O.'s feelings of comfort when at social functions.	Instruct Mrs. O. on various strategies to use in social situations for dealing with the presence of attractive and abundant food (e.g., preplanning of eating behavior, standing away from the serving table at a cocktail party, and constantly thinking thin).	Developing adaptive responses to eating for social situations that are unavoidable and unchangeable can facilitate the obese person's comfort in taking part in social contacts.	Mrs. O.'s verbalization about increased comfort and enjoyment at social functions.
		Encourage Mrs. O. to maintain an attractive appearance by wearing makeup and clothing that deemphasize her size (i.e., dark colors and slenderizing lines).	Feeling attractive to oneself and others facilitates feelings of self-worth.	

PATIENT CARE CARDEX

PATIENT'S NAME: _____ Mrs. O. _____   MEDICAL DIAGNOSIS: _____ Obesity

AGE: _____ 28 years _____   SEX: _____ Female

MARITAL STATUS: _____ Married _____   OCCUPATION: _____ Housewife

SIGNIFICANT OTHERS: Husband and two children (2 and 4 years)

Nursing Diagnoses	Nursing Approaches
Psychological: Dysfunctional eating patterns manifested by inability to control eating habits.	1. Instruct Mrs. O. and her family on how to keep a record of Mrs. O.'s eating habits. The record must include: (a) when she eats. (b) what she eats. (c) where she eats. (d) what she is doing while she eats. (e) how she feels prior to eating. 2. Involve in group interactions in weight control programs. 3. Instruct Mrs. O. and her family on ways to decrease environmental stimuli that may be affecting Mrs. O.'s eating patterns. Include the following: (a) Eat meals slowly so that they last at least twenty minutes. (b) Chew each mouthful of food ten times. (c) Place the utensils on the plate between mouthfuls. (d) Decrease the size of food portions. (e) Serve the meals restaurant style on small plates. (f) Discard leftover food immediately after the meal is completed. (g) Avoid keeping prepared snack food in the house. (h) Leave a small portion of food on the plate at each meal.

(i) Alter the composition of foods high in caloric content (if possible).
(j) Use low-calorie substitutes with meals.
(k) Shop for groceries after eating a full meal.
(l) Shop from a prepared grocery list.
(m) Turn off the bulb in the refrigerator.
(n) Keep all foods in covered containers.
(o) Eat only in one room and in one chair.
(p) Avoid carrying out household and personal activities in the kitchen.
(q) Reward appropriate dietary behavior by engaging in pleasurable "non-food oriented" activity.

Somatic: Body image alteration manifested by devaluation of self.

1. Encourage to verbalize the feelings she has about herself.
2. Encourage to express how she feels members of society view her.
3. Assist in understanding that individuals who may ostracize and stigmatize her often do so because of their own insecurities.
4. Encourage husband to provide positive feedback to patient for attempts and accomplishments made in weight reduction.

Sexual: Sexual dysfunction manifested by expressed concern about increased avoidance of sexual relationship with husband.

1. Encourage to verbalize feelings about sexuality.
2. Encourage husband and patient to discuss openly with each other their feelings about their sexual relationship.
3. Inform that her expressed concern about avoiding sexual contact with husband is not abnormal.

Occupational: Deficit in health management activities manifested by increased tendency to eat excessive amounts of food at home.

1. Encourage to verbalize how excessive weight is affecting ability to perform household duties.
2. Encourage to discard leftover foods immediately after the meal by disposing of them in the garbage or freezing them for future use.
3. Encourage not to eat food her children leave on the plates and to dispose of it instead.
4. Encourage not to purchase snack foods high in calories, such as potato chips and cookies.

Social: Social isolation manifested by avoidance of social contacts.

1. Encourage to take part in social functions because avoidance of social contact can be detrimental to the obese person.
2. Instruct on various strategies to use in social situations for dealing with the presence of attractive and abundant food (e.g., preplan eating habits).
3. Encourage to maintain an attractive appearance by wearing makeup and clothing that deemphasizes her size (e.g., dark colors).

REFERENCES

BRAY, G. The overweight patient, *Advances in Internal Medicine,* 1976, *21,* 267–308.

CANNING, H., and MAYER, J. Obesity—its possible effect on college acceptance, *New England Journal of Medicine,* 1966, *275* (21), 1172–1174.

CASTELNUOVO-TEDESCO, P., and SCHIEBEL, D. Studies of superobesity: I—psychological characteristics of superobese patients, *International Journal of Psychiatry in Medicine,* 1975, *6* (4), 465–480.

CAVALLO-PERIN, P., SORBO, R., MORRA, G., PAGANI, A., TAGLIAFERRO, V., and LENTI, G. Correlation between obesity and other risk factors for coronary heart disease in a group of 4124 volunteers. In G. Enzi, C. Crepaldi, G. Pozza, and A. Renold (Eds.), *Obesity: Pathogenesis and treatment.* New York: Academic Press, 1981.

COZENS, R. Obesity in the aged: not just a case of overeating, *Nursing Clinics of North America,* 1982, *17* (2), 227–232.

FEIG, B. *The patient's guide to weight control for children ages 5–13 years.* Springfield: Charles C. Thomas, 1980.

FISCH, R., BILEK, M., and ULSTROM, R. Obesity and leanness at birth and their relationship to body habits in later childhood, *Pediatrics,* 1975, *56,* 521–528.

GARN, S. The origins of obesity, *American Journal of Diseases of Children,* 1976, *130,* (5), 465–467.

GOLD, D. Psychologic factors associated with obesity, *American Family Physician,* 1976, *13* (6), 87–91.

GRINKER, J. Behavioral and metabolic consequences of weight reduction, *Journal of the American Dietetic Association,* 1973, *62* (1), 30–34.

GRINKER, J., and HIRSCH, J. Metabolic and behavioral correlates of obesity, *Ciba Foundation Symposium,* 1972, *8,* 349–374.

HAGENBUCH, V. Obesity and the school-age child, *Nursing Clinics of North America,* 1982, *17* (2), 207–216.

JORDAN, H., LEVITZ, L., and KIMBRELL, G. Psychological factors in obesity. In E. Wittkower and H. Warnes (Eds.), *Psychosomatic medicine: its clinical applications.* New York: Harper & Row Pub., 1977.

KALISCH, B. The stigma of obesity, *American Journal of Nursing,* 1972, *72* (6), 1124–1127.

KALUCY, R., and CRISP, A. Some psychological and social implications of obesity, *Journal of Psychosomatic Research,* 1974, *18* (6), 465–473.

KANNEL, W., and GORDON, T. Psychological and medical concomitants of obesity: the Framingham study. In G. Bray (Ed.), *Obesity in America* (NIH Publication No. 79-359). Washington, D.C.: U.S. Government Printing Office, 1979.

NOPPA, H., and HALLSTROM, R. Weight gain in relation to socioeconomic factors, mental illness and personality traits: a prospective study of middle-aged women, *Journal of Psychosomatic Research,* 1981, *25* (2), 83–89.

PIERRE, R., and WARREN, C. Smoking and obesity: the behavioral ramifications, *Journal of School Health,* 1975, *45* (7), 406–408.

PLUTNICK, P. Emotions and attitudes related to being overweight, *Journal of Clinical Psychology,* 1976, *32* (1), 21–24.

RENOLD, A. Epidemiologic considerations of overweight and of obesity. In G. Enzi, C. Crepaldi, G. Pozza, and A. Renold (Eds.), *Obesity: Pathogenesis and treatment.* New York: Academic Press, 1981.

RICHARDSON, S., and GOODMAN, N. Cultural uniformity and reaction to physical disability, *American Sociological Review,* 1961, *26,* 241–247.

RIMM, I., and RIMM, A. Association between juvenile onset obesity and severe adult obesity in 73,532 women, *American Journal of Public Health,* 1976, *66* (5), 479–481.

RODIN, J. Causes and consequences of time perception differences in overweight and normal weight people, *Journal of Personality and Social Psychology,* 1975, *31* (5), 898–904.

RODIN, J. Pathogeneses of obesity: energy intake and expenditure. In G. Bray (Ed.), *Obesity in America* (NIH Publication No. 79-359). Washington, D.C.: U.S. Government Printing Office, 1979.

SALANS, L. Natural history of obesity. In G. Bray (Ed). *Obesity in America* (NIH Publication No. 79-359). Washington, D.C.: U.S. Government Printing Office, 1979.

SELTZER, C., and STARE, F. Obesity, *Medical Insight,* 1973, *5* (4), 10–22.

SIMS, E. Definitions, criteria, and prevalence. In A. Bray (Ed.), *Obesity in America* (NIH Publication No. 79-359). Washington, D.C.: U.S. Government Printing Office, 1979.

STUNKARD, A. *The pain of obesity.* Palo Alto: Bull Publishing Co., 1976.

STUNKARD, A., and MENDELSON, M. Obesity and the body image: I—characteristics of disturbances in the body image of some obese persons, *American Journal of Psychiatry,* 1967, *123* (10), 1296–1300.

8 |||||||||||||||||||||||||||||||||||||||||||||||||||||||||

BURN INJURY

INTRODUCTION

Being burned is one of the most devastating, dehumanizing experiences known. Not only is the injury frightening, but the individual involved may be faced with pain, helplessness, dependency, prolonged illness role assumption, possible disfigurement, and death. Between 2½ and 3 million people are burned yearly with approximately 3 percent of these individuals requiring hospitalization and less than four tenths of a percent dying. Involvement in an uncontrolled fire or explosion and contact with a hot object constitute the most common causes of burns that lead to death, while nonfatal injuries caused by burns are more likely a result of hot liquids, acids, or flames (Hummel, 1982).

The individual sustaining a burn is most often a nonwhite female living in a low-income area (Crawford, 1981; MacArthur and Moore, 1975). The individual's home is usually the site of the burn incident, with hair or clothing, a mattress, bedclothes, or an overstuffed chair being the items of initial ignition. Certain predisposing factors such as alcoholism, senility, psychiatric disorders, and neurological disease tend to contribute to the likelihood of a burn, with alcoholism being the most frequent contributing factor.

TYPES OF BURNS

The classification of a burn is determined by the depth of tissue injury. Based on this fact, burns are categorized in the following manner:

First-degree burn: a burn caused by brief contact with hot liquids or prolonged exposure to sunlight. The burn area is painful and appears red and dry. Blister formation generally is absent.

Second-degree burn: a burn caused by short periods of exposure to intense flash heat or contact with hot liquids. The burn area is very painful, is moist, and has a mottled red or pink appearance. Blister formation is a characteristic feature.

Third-degree burn: a burn caused by flames or contact with hot objects. Electrical burns are generally third-degree. The burn area is dry and pearly white or charred in appearance. The area is not very painful since terminal nerve endings are destroyed by the deep injury.

The depth of a burn depends upon the intensity and duration of the heat. Below forty-five degrees centigrade injury from heat does not occur, while above sixty-five degrees centigrade cell death takes place. Between forty-five and sixty-five degrees centigrade, the amount of injury that occurs depends upon the duration of exposure. For example, in a hot water burn, the body temperature cools the heat from the hot water with the result generally being a superficial second-degree burn. The heat from a flame burn, however, cannot be rapidly cooled by the body and the result is usually a deep second-degree or third-degree burn.

As mentioned previously, the majority of burn victims do not require hospitalization. Most burn victims sustain either superficial second-degree burns of less than 15 percent of the body, deep second-degree burns of less than 6 percent of the body, or third-degree burns that cover small areas of the body. Most other burns, however, do require hospitalization.

Once the individual is admitted to the hospital, maintenance of the burned individual's life becomes the primary goal and concern of the health care team. The outcome of the burn therapy depends upon the extent and degree of the burn, with the very young and the elderly having the lowest survival rate. In addition, supporting nutrition, antibiotic resistance, and the individual's will to live become major factors contributing to a successful recovery.

Once the acute phase has passed and death no longer is the major concern, the health care team turns its focus toward cosmetic reconstruction and rehabilitation. At this time many burned individuals also change their focus of concern from the strangeness of the hospital and the fear of impending death to the total impact of their experience. Thoughts of what effects the burn will have upon their future are common.

A burn experience creates an impact upon one's psychological well-being, somatic identity, sexuality, occupational identity, and social role. The remainder of this chapter will discuss how a burn experience can affect each of these areas of concern.

IMPACT OF BURNS

Psychological Impact

The individual undergoing a burn experience not only is faced with physiologic shock resulting from hypovolemia, but also emotional shock resulting from the burn experience. According to Andreasen, Noyes, Hartford, Brodland, and Proctor (1972), the initial emotional shock of burns can take one of two forms: a calm dream-like state or an acute traumatic response. If the burned individual enters a calm dream-like state, he or she manifests little awareness of the immediate surroundings. During this time the individual may talk lucidly. However, as recovery progresses the individual has limited or no recollection of these conversations.

The other, and more common, initial emotional reaction to a burn experience is an acute traumatic response. Such a reaction is characterized by insomnia, an exaggerated startle response, anorexia, emotional liability, and nightmares about the burn incident (Andreasen, Noyes, Hartford, Brodland, and Proctor, 1972; Davidson, 1973).

During the initial emotional shock of a burn experience the individual is rarely troubled about deformity (Andreasen, Noyes, Hartford, Brodland, and Proctor, 1972). Some individuals manifest confusion about the burn experience and express fears of impending death. However, their major concerns deal with the strangeness of the hospital, the cost of hospital care, and who is caring for their affairs and family.

In dealing with the initial shock reaction to a burn experience, an important nursing intervention is to provide the individual with reassurance that he or she will not be abandoned by members of the health care team. A trusting relationship between the individual and the staff is crucial and should be established at the time of admission and continued through discharge. Explaining procedures, responding promptly to individual needs, being available to listen and talk to the individual and the family, and providing explanations about the body's reaction to thermal injury are interventions that enhance a trust relationship. Often the use of a psychiatric nurse consultant to help the individual, the staff, and the family deal with the impact of a burn injury can be valuable (Tringali, 1982).

If the nurse notices that the burned individual is extremely restless during sleep, it is likely that a nightmare is occurring. Gently awakening and encouraging the individual to verbalize feelings and fears decreases anxiety caused by nightmares and provides positive reinforcement that someone is close by. Verbalization can assist in alleviating fears of what sleep may bring and hence prevent insomnia.

If nightmares are experienced, informing the individual that this reaction is normal, but temporary, may 'assist in decreasing anxiety elicited by such dreams. Encouraging the individual to describe the dream can provide an additional outlet for anxiety; however, the individual should be told that description of the dream can cease at anytime he or she desires. At the termination of the dream description the person should be encouraged to examine the reality of the present situation and to recognize the personal significance of the dream.

After going through the initial period of shock, burned individuals frequently become acutely aware of their environment. Every minute noise or movement in their surroundings is noticed. This initial lucidity, however, usually is short-lived and periods of delirium soon follow (Davidson, 1973).

Delirium is characterized by impaired orientation, restlessness, agitation, altered cognitive abilities, fluctuating levels of awareness and consciousness, visual hallucinations, and insomnia (Andreasen, Noyes, Hartford, Brodland, and Proctor, 1972). The manifestations of delirium tend to worsen at night when the individual is deprived of familiar, orienting environmental cues, such as the face of a staff or family member. The degree and duration of delirium are variable. However, the frequency tends to increase with age and the severity of the burn.

A burned individual who is delirious requires orientation to time, place, and person. Examples of statements providing such orientation are: "Good morning, Mr. B., today is Monday, January 13th. You are in your room at University Health Sciences Center. It is 8:00 a.m. and I have your breakfast." Repetitive orientation may be necessary because the burned individual frequently may fade in and out of periods of disorientation. A clock, a calendar, or a radio often prove helpful in assisting the individual in orientation. The attendance of a familiar individual, such as a family member or friend, often is beneficial. To prevent unnecessary disorientation at night, a light should be kept on in the individual's room to prevent misinterpretation of the surroundings. Placement of the light should avoid the creation of shadows which can increase the incidence of illusions.

Physical restraint of the delirious individual should be avoided, if possible, since it frequently arouses additional fears and anxieties. The restrained individual may feel that he or she is unable to protect himself or herself against illusions such as snakes and bugs which are believed to be harmful. Restraint may be perceived by the individual as a threat to sexuality since during the illusions the burned individual may interpret restraint as a preliminary to castration or rape. Medication to control the individual's restlessness and agitation can prove beneficial, but barbiturates should be avoided because they further decrease cerebral function and enhance confusion.

Above all, the burned individual and the family require reassurance that the manifestations of delirium are frequent in individuals sustaining severe burns. They must be informed that such manifestations do not imply the existence of a severe emotional disorder and that as the individual's physical condition improves, generally, so will the level of orientation (Andreasen, Noyes, Hartford, Brodland, and Proctor, 1972).

Because of the overwhelming stress of the situation, burned individuals often utilize the mechanism of regression which appears to be the psyche's attempt to conserve energy. Regression, as discussed in Chapter 1, is the act of returning to an earlier level of adaptation. In other words, the individual reverts to childlike ways of dealing with illness role assumption which is manifested by a low tolerance for frustration, hypochondriasis, dependency, temper tantrums, poor cooperation, and demanding infantile behavior. This behavior is demonstrated by such acts as complaining about mistreatment, threatening to strike someone, and using foul and abusive language that contains sexual overtones. Mild regression is common and benign, but marked regression, unfortunately, becomes difficult for family and health team members to handle.

Since the family and health care team members are closest to the burned individual, they frequently become the object of regressive acts. This is especially true of the nurse because of the frequent interactions with the individual. Unless each member of the family and health care team recognizes and understands the basis for the burned individual's behavior, a vicious cycle of attack and counterattack is likely to occur.

To deal with regressive behavior, the family and the nurse and other members of the health team must realize that the individual requires acceptance at his or her own regressed level. The burned individual needs assurance that when he or she is unable to control his or her behavior, limits and controls will be provided. The individual must be dealt with in a firm, kind, and nonrejecting manner. For example, if the burned individual refuses to eat, he or she should be informed of the importance of nutrition in a nonpunitive manner and be offered a choice between nasogastric feedings and eating self-selected food (Andreasen, Noyes, Hartford, Brodland, and Proctor, 1972). In other words, the family and health care team basically assume a parental role.

Conversation with the burned individual during periods of regression should be simple and concrete. Short frequent visits throughout each shift by a variety of family and health team members who utilize a consistent, supportive approach are beneficial in reassuring the individual of support. Prolonged visits by a few select persons can result in a vicious cycle of hostility when the burned individual's regressive acts no longer can be tolerated.

As the burned individual becomes less regressed, positive feedback on his or her behavior is necessary for acknowledging progress achieved. Providing the individual with additional choices about his or her care can be helpful in preserving the individual's autonomy and in enhancing cooperation.

Concerned and embarrassed family members require reassurance that the regressive acts of their loved one are not unusual. As the individual's physical condition improves his or her behavior tends to become more appropriate. Allowing the family the opportunity to ventilate their feelings about the burned individual's actions is important because they too may become intolerant of these regressive acts. In addition, the family should be informed about the approach to be used when the burned individual demonstrates regressive behavior; otherwise inconsistency in care can develop. If the family does not understand the rationale for a prescribed approach to care, feelings of hostility may arise between the family and the health team, resulting in the emanation of undue anxiety in the burned individual's environment.

If the burned individual is hospitalized more than a month, depression is likely to occur (Andreasen, Noyes, Hartford, Brodland, and Proctor, 1972). Although the onset frequently is during the middle of hospitalization, the time of occurrence does vary. Depression in its mildest form is manifested by loss of interest in one's self and surroundings, anorexia, frequent crying spells, insomnia, and helplessness about the future. In its severest form, depression is demonstrated by refusal to eat, lethargy, severe insomnia, loss of the desire to cooperate with the health team members, and a desire to be left alone to die in peace. Severe depression can hinder the effects of the health team to carry out necessary treatments such as nutritional and physical therapy. In such cases, it is imperative that appropriate psychotherapy be instituted. Research has shown, however, that generally the burned individual can and does make a positive adjustment to the injury despite age, sex, or severity of the burn (Knudson-Cooper, 1981).

Often the existence of depression has been precipitated by a specific problem that possibly can be relieved. For example, some burned individuals experience depression secondary to their silent frightening fantasies, such as fear of impotence when a burn has occurred in the genital region. If the depression is precipitated by such a problem, clarification of the situation may relieve the burned individual's anxiety and hence lessen his or her depression. If the problem is a realistic one, such as depression precipitated by viewing one's scarred face in the mirror, the individual requires assistance in identifying ways of approaching the problem. Gradually building up time spent viewing the face and discussing specifically what about the scarred face bothers the individual are two possible approaches. As the individual identifies what about his or her appearance is bothersome, the reality of these concerns needs to be examined.

In summary, the individual sustaining a burn is likely to experience a variety of emotional reactions. Initially, the victim may undergo an acute traumatic reaction followed by a keen awareness of the environment. This initial lucidity may be followed by a state of delirium that varies in degrees and duration. Next, in order to cope with the overwhelming stress of the burn, the individual also may manifest behaviors of regression ranging from mild to severe. Finally, a state of depression can develop, especially when the burned individual is hospitalized more than a month. The nurse's primary role in dealing with the psychological impact of burns is to be cognizant of the manifestations of each behavioral reaction and initiate the appropriate intervention.

Somatic Impact

An alteration in body image is undoubtedly one of the most devastating impacts of a burn. The burn injury and the necessary treatments that follow often disrupt the body boundary concept due to alterations in bodily appearance, in sensation, and in perception of the body surface. Dressing changes, whirlpool baths, and pain tend to alter the limits of one's body boundary. Dressing changes and whirlpool baths may produce a loss of body boundaries, while dressing application may represent the reestablishment of an intact body surface. Pain can distort the body boundaries to the point of producing a sense of swelling or enlargement. Thus, the burned individual undergoes contractions and expansions of the body boundaries at various times during illness role assumption.

Pain varies in character and severity among burned individuals. However, pain suffering tends to be most intense during debridement and/or dressing changes. It has been noticed that pain threshold and the ability to withstand pain decrease the longer a burned individual is hospitalized. No doubt, the anxiety caused by the expectation of pain related to anticipated dressing changes or forthcoming surgery contributes to this reduction in pain tolerance. Pain also reminds the individual of the initial injury which, in turn, incites additional anxiety and possibly leads to a reduction in pain tolerance.

The burned individual may find it difficult to control his or her emotions during pain and, as a result, lash out at family members and health team members. The emotionally controlled individuals may fear the consequences of exhibiting anger toward family and health care members who directly care for them and instead vent their feelings of anger and frustration on individuals indirectly responsible for their care, such as housekeeping personnel, dietary staff, or visitors.

During treatment some degree of moaning and yelling is acceptable, but if such a practice is continued for a long period of time, it can have a demoralizing effect upon other burned individuals in the immediate area. The burned individual finds that he or she must develop various ways of controlling pain expression during pain provoking therapies. Such maneuvers can include placing something in the mouth to bite on; using self-hypnosis by loudly saying, "It doesn't hurt. It doesn't hurt"; or distracting oneself by turning up the volume on radio earphones. Simply knowing that a great deal of pain will subside once grafting has occurred gives many burn victims a feeling of hope. Reinforcement of this fact by a grafted burn victim to a newly burned individual may prove beneficial. "Just knowing that someone else has made it through a similar experience is comforting" may be a typical statement expressed by a newly burned individual after conversing with a burned individual in a more advanced stage of therapy.

The burned individual often views the availability of pain medications as a sign of the health care team's interest in his or her welfare. The individual's requests for analgesics, however, may become a means of expressing fears and seeking much needed reassurance. Andreasen and associates (1972) suggest that some form of pain medication be available to the burned individual at all times, even if it is a mild analgesic or if the burned individual does not believe that it is helpful. The lack of available pain medication can be interpreted by the burned individual as evidence of little or no concern for his or her welfare by health team members. The administration of pain medication prior to painful debridement and dressing changes does seem to assist in alleviating a fair amount of pain and in decreasing anxiety for the burned individual.

When pain becomes inevitable and irreducible, often health team members tend to direct their interest to other concerns. For example, concern over the complexities of dressing changes may become their primary focus, with pain management and its psychosocial implications receiving minimal attention. To avoid this situation, the nurse must directly approach the individual's reactions to pain by encouraging free ventilation of feelings about the anticipation and sensation of pain being experienced. During the expression of feelings the burned individual needs to be directed in examining what specifically about the anticipation of pain concerns him or her. Is it the fear of the unknown or does the pain conjure up thoughts about the initial burn incident? As the individual describes the specifics of his or her concerns, he or she should be encouraged to identify how pain has been dealt with in the past. Maneuvers for dealing with past pain experience may prove helpful for the present.

Pain not only exists during debridement and dressing changes, but many burned individuals have described its presence in donor sites once grafting has occurred. Some individuals believe that the pain experienced in the donor site is more intense than the pain experienced in the burn site. This will vary among individuals and depends upon such factors as the severity and depth of the burn, the individual's anxiety level, and the individual's pain tolerance at the time of grafting. Nonetheless, pain in the donor site can exist and the previously mentioned interventions for dealing with pain should be instituted.

When an individual sustains a burn, body boundaries are altered. Touching of the dressing and affected parts is necessary to aid in redefining one's body boundaries after a burn. Tactile stimulation of the body surface not only assists in reidentifying one's body surface, but it also enhances one's awareness of true body boundaries. Encouraging the burned individual to touch the dressings and body parts can facilitate the necessary relinquishment of dressings (a temporary body boundary) with little or no anxiety. Thus, the new body surface will more readily be accepted as the new body boundary. If the burned individual is not allowed to carry out necessary tactile stimulation, difficulties in establishing a new body image, as discussed in Chapter 2, may ensue.

Fears of deformity and mutilation start to develop once the acute phase of injury passes. The burned individual has become familiar with the hospital surroundings and routines and begins to focus attention upon the future. The two most commonly voiced fears deal with loss of function (especially the hands) and cosmetic deformities as indicated by such questions as, "Will I ever be able to use my hands again?" and "How can anyone love someone that looks like me?"

Research has shown that men usually are more concerned about loss of function, whereas women have a greater fear of cosmetic deformity following a burn experience (Noyes, Andreasen, and Hartford, 1971). This results from the man's concern about being able to function in order to continue his job. A woman, however, may feel greater pressure than a man to appear physically attractive in order to achieve in the occupational and social world. With the changing roles among men and women, these concerns may be undergoing alterations. Regardless, during the early phases of the illness role, burned individuals usually require assistance in dealing with their concern about possible deformities.

The initial reaction to viewing a deformity may be repudiation (as discussed in Chapter 3) of the existence of the deformity or a severe state of depression (as discussed in Chapter 1). Most burned individuals will be reticent to view their deformity and will avoid looking in a mirror until they are ready. This is particularly true when the deformity involves facial disfigurement. When the burned individual is ready to view his or her deformity, a supportive individual needs to be present to provide an outlet for the expression of feelings. The burned individual's response to the disfigurement must be dealt with in an honest and hopeful manner. Statements commenting on the improvement of the wounds are important because such statements supply both honesty and optimism.

The fear of rejection may arise when the burned individual realizes the full impact of his or her deformity. This rejection may be demonstrated by a strong tendency to increase personal space. The burned individual may avoid intimate and personal distances, function in a zone of social distance but prefer a public distance of twelve feet or more (Bernstein, 1976). Unless health team members and family members are aware of these maneuvers, they unconsciously may allow the burned individual to distance himself or herself from others. Standing close and touching in an accepting manner can aid in preventing the burned individual's loneliness and withdrawal. Pointing out what the individual is doing and encouraging him or her to identify ways in which to avoid distancing may prove beneficial. Frequent reminders of the individual's importance to others such as the presence of family pictures and get well cards also are helpful in preventing withdrawal and loneliness.

As discussed in Chapter 2, the stage of development being experienced by an individual is influenced by a trauma such as the burn experience. For example, the young adult (eighteen to forty-five years) is in the stage of intimacy versus isolation (Erikson, 1963). It is during this developmental stage that the individual is ready to merge his or her identity with others, both in friendship and in a mutually satisfying sexual relationship. The body becomes a major factor in relating to others. If the individual experiences disfigurement when a burn is sustained, he or she may view his or her physical appearance as unacceptable, since Western society places a great deal of emphasis upon physical attractiveness. If the burned individual feels less than acceptable because of physical appearance, he or she may retreat into isolation instead of establishing a state of intimacy with other individuals.

The impact of a burn is somewhat different in the developmental stage of adulthood (forty-five to sixty-five years). The middle years are a time when the individual directs energies toward establishing and guiding future generations with the hope of improving society (Erikson, 1963). The presence of a burn may alter this goal and instead of being generative, the adult may become self-absorbed and stagnate. The middle-aged burned individual may feel that he or she has nothing of value to offer other generations. Chronic defeatism may result and the individual may become isolated in self-pity.

The burned individual in the final stage of life, maturity (sixty-five years and over), may view the presence of a burn as a prelude to the end of life since thoughts of death frequently occur during this stage. Hence, the mature adult may enter a stage of despair (Erikson, 1963) and have the feeling of having little to offer others. Whatever the individual's stage of development, body boundaries have changed at the time of the burn and the individual's personal mental picture is altered.

The nurse's role in assisting the burn individual in establishing a new body image should involve encouraging the burn individual to examine personal feelings about himself or herself. If the individual believes that he or she is "a freak" or "a monster," or if he or she encounters problems in dealing with questions that society poses about the burn incident, the individual will experience difficulties relating and interacting with others. Group sessions with burn victims and their families may be helpful, for they afford the opportunity of sharing ideas on ways to cope with society (Bailey and Moore, 1980). Instead of retreating into isolation and further compounding the sense of rejection, burned individuals require assistance in understanding why society may react the way it does. Burned individuals need to realize that other people may view them with a sense of curiosity, sympathy, and fear. They are curious about how the incident occurred, they sympathize with them about how they live with the disability, and they fear that a burn incident could easily happen to them.

Sexual Impact

The sexual impact of burns frequently is overlooked by members of the health care team. Often it is a topic not openly approached by the burned individual and his or her family. This does not mean, however, that the burned individual or the family members are unconcerned about the effect that the burn injury has upon their sexual relationships.

The fear of personal rejection becomes a grave fear for many burned individuals. They believe that their disability threatens their capacity to be loved by others; this is especially true if the burn occurs on the face or genital region. A minor burn of the genitalia may evoke more emotional distress than more serious burns elsewhere on the body. Females are likely to be concerned about their fertility, especially if the menses are interrupted as a result of the physical or emotional stress of the burn experience. By the same token, castration anxiety can occur in the male when perineal burns are present (Bernstein, 1976). The male may become convinced that he is sterile and may feel embarrassed and ashamed about his imagined inadequacy. Such beliefs make the burned individual hypersensitive to the reactions of others, with the slightest indication of possible rejection being blown out of proportion.

Since the sexual impact of burn trauma usually is not approached by the individual involved, the family, the nurse, or other members of the health team may have to initiate discussion on the topic. Leading statements such as, "Individuals sustaining burns similar to yours have indicated a concern about being rejected by others. How do you feel about this?" may initiate a much needed discussion about the sexual impact of burns. The burned individual's significant others must be informed that the fear of rejection is common. They may need encouragement to show outward signs of acceptance for the burned individual by using such maneuvers as physical caressing, gift giving, or including the burned individual in family decision making. Whatever means were used to demonstrate affection prior to the burn incident would be appropriate for use at this time.

The sex partner must be aware that the burned individual may encounter difficulties in the sexual relationship because of fear of infertility or impotence. Open discussion about these fears must be encouraged between the burned individual and sex partner. As with any physical disability, if the sex partner is repulsed by the appearance of the burn, personal sexual satisfaction may be threatened. Unless the sex partner is assisted in expressing these feelings, extreme guilt may be aroused as a result of thoughts which are uncontrollable. In an attempt to hide these feelings, the sexual enthusiasm displayed by the sex partner probably will decrease. This decrease in sexual enthusiasm can be interpreted by the burned individual as rejection. Thus, it is advisable that the burned individual and sex partner share their fears and emotions with each other and avoid the pretense of being unaffected by the presence of the burn. The sex partner needs to make it clear to the burned individual that any hesitant response does not imply rejection, but rather an expression of empathy. If the sexual impact of the burn becomes too difficult for the burned individual and sex partner to resolve, they should be directed to a member of the health team experienced in sex counseling.

Occupational Impact

Recovery of the burned individual is never totally dependent upon one person; it is dependent upon every member of the health care team. But since the professional nurse spends more time in direct contact with the burned individual than anyone else, the nurse has the greatest potential influence on the success of the rehabilitation program.

Total rehabilitation is accomplished when the burned individual returns to society as a contributing member and is living to his or her fullest capacity. In order for the individual to achieve a successful rehabilitation, the process must begin at the time of admission to the burn-care facility. Everything that is done for the burned individual from the time of admission contributes in some way to a successful return to society.

During the acute phase of treatment the burned individual is dependent upon members of the family and the health care team for his or her total care. As therapy progresses, however, the individual should become more responsible for his or her own care. An activity that the burned individual should be carrying out as soon as possible is personal hygiene, which includes bathing, shaving, combing the hair, and brushing the teeth. The nurse and/or family members are responsible for supervising these activities and providing assistance when needed. In addition to providing the individual with a sense of self-pride and independence, these activities require muscle movements needed to prevent contracture formation.

As the burned individual assumes more responsibility for self-care, fears of neglect and abandonment by the family and health care team may be elicited. The burned individual may feel physically and emotionally unprepared to deal with increased independence. Reassurance by way of verbal interactions is required regarding the fact that such fears are not unnatural and that many other individuals sustaining burns have encountered the same fears.

Physical therapy continues throughout the rehabilitation period. It includes hydrotherapy (to assist in exercise and with the removal of wound crusts), active and passive range of motion, and ambulation (Braddom, Boe, Flowers, and Johnson-Vann, 1982). In addition, splints or functional devices may be necessary to control contracture formation. It should be pointed out that all physical therapy activities are as important to a successful recovery as are medications and grafting procedures. To aid in facilitating compliance with physical therapy activities it is advisable to verbally encourage and to allow the burned individual to express how he or she feels about going through the therapy sessions.

Since the burned individual may require a lengthy rehabilitation program, family members must be incorporated into the program early in its development. During periods of physical therapy, family members must be taught how to carry out needed exercise programs, dressing applications, and splint applications. Before sending the burned individual home, the health care team must be sure that written instructions for care are ready and that the family is capable of carrying out necessary therapies. Having a family member demonstrate to a health team member the necessary therapies proves very beneficial. If home follow-up is necessary, a community health nurse should be notified so that appropriate exchange of information can take place before the burned individual is discharged. If possible, the community health nurse should visit the burned individual and the family in the burn-care facility to help allay unnecessary fears and concerns of being left alone to deal with their problems.

Before the burned individual is discharged he or she requires a realistic appraisal of what to expect at home. Once the initial excitement of returning home subsides, the individual is likely to experience feelings of depression. A sense of being overwhelmed is not unusual since therapies that seemed simple in the hospital setting may seem burdensome upon returning home. If the burned individual and family members feel unable to cope with the home situation, they should be instructed to contact the community health nurse or the burn-care facility. If adequate preparation is given prior to discharge, the burned individual and family members are not likely to encounter extreme difficulties in the home situation.

Occupational retraining may be necessary for some burned individuals since the effect that the burn has upon one's future plans is a common concern. If the burned individual's former occupation depended upon the use of his or her hands, and if the hands were badly burned, retraining may be in order. By the same token, nonvocational activities such as recreational sports are affected by the presence of a burn. If an individual derives great satisfaction from basketball or cycling, leg burns may prove extremely threatening and the burned individual may require introduction to and training in some other form of activity.

Andreasen, Norris, and Hartford (1971) found that the burned individual's capacity and desire to work are not significantly influenced by the severity of the burn. Adults who encounter exaggerated feelings of inadequacy and are disturbed by their dependency upon others because of their physical helplessness are, most likely, individuals who had difficulty coping with adult responsibility prior to their burn incident. Often disabled individuals, such as severely burned people, thrust ahead vocationally and become obsessed with achieving and reaching a goal. Many burned individuals emerge with a new identity because they have been able to triumph over external limitations.

The financial impact of a burn may be overwhelming, particularly if lengthy health care treatment, reconstructive surgery, and extensive rehabilitation are required. If the burned individual is employed, he or she will be unable to work during the duration of the hospitalization. Should the hospital stay be lengthy, accumulated sick leave will be used up, resulting in possible dismissal from the work setting. Lack of income plus loss of job can place an additional financial burden on the family which can result in a lowered standard of living. If the family is unable to deal with the financial impact of the burn incident, the economic aspects of a burn trauma become the responsibility of society. Thus, it can be seen that a burn incident not only affects the individual involved, but it may influence family members and members of society at large.

Social Impact

How well the burned individual will be received by society is a common concern of both the burned individual and his or her family. If scarring and contractures are readily visible, the burned individual may fear what others think about his or her appearance and as a result hesitate to be seen socially. In an attempt to deal with social encounters, the burn individual often finds it necessary to provide others with a socially acceptable justification for the burn incident. This justification may carry religious overtones which speak of punishment for wrongdoings or allude to a test of faith. However, the individual's religious justification for the burn need not reflect any specific religious doctrine.

During this justification period, it is the nurse's responsibility to convey acceptance of the burned individual's religious frame of reference. This is done by providing nonjudgmental feedback during the individual's verbalization of his or her religious beliefs. When the health team conveys acceptance instead of judgment of the burned individual, reconciliation of the burn experience can be reinforced in the individual's own frame of reference. A hospital chaplain may prove helpful for interpreting and meeting the burned individual's specific religious needs.

As the burned individual extends social contacts, he or she generally finds most people supportive. Those who appear tactless, curious, and hostile tend to be strangers or casual acquaintances (Andreasen, Norris, and Hartford, 1971). The burned individual may require assistance in how to contend with these people. Encouraging the burned individual to verbalize how he or she may deal with such a situation is beneficial because it prepares the individual for the situation before it occurs. Burned individuals and their families often share ideas in group sessions on how they personally have contended with awkward situations involving tactless and curious people. Some suggestions have included directly approaching the curious and tactless person and introducing oneself or walking away from the situation and ignoring the individual.

Many burned individuals resolve their crisis concerning others' response toward them by reformulating their sense of identity. Instead of developing an identity based upon physical appearance, they construct an identity emphasizing inner self-worth. By means of reassurance of continued affection, the burned individual shifts his or her orientation toward the internal "good-self" which has not been damaged by the burn. Often the burned individual believes that the burn experience has made him or her a better person and feels more resourceful and compassionate. Concern for others, solidarity of family relationships, and a renewed religious faith may become important components of the burned individual's life.

SUMMARY

Almost 3 million people are burned each year. Such an experience can be devastating and dehumanizing. The individual sustaining a burn is most often a nonwhite female living in a low-income area. The home is the usual site of the burn incident, with the hair, clothing, a mattress, or an overstuffed chair being the items of initial ignition. Predisposing factors such as alcoholism, senility, psychiatric disorders, or neurological disease may contribute to the likelihood of the burn.

If the burn is severe and/or extensive, hospitalization may be required, but most burns are not treated in a hospital setting. If hospital care is required, the treatment most likely will be lengthy and expensive. Thus, the burned individual often is forced to assume the illness role for an extended period of time and is faced with pain, helplessness, dependency, possible disfigurement, or death.

Regardless of the extent or the degree of the burn, each burned individual undergoes an impact to his or her psychological well-being, somatic identity, sexuality, occupational identity, and social role. Members of the health care team must assist the burned individual in identifying how the presence of the burn affects his or her everyday life and must assist the burned individual and his or her family in dealing with each of these alterations.

Patient Situation   Miss B. is a twenty-two-year-old single, engaged, black salesgirl who sustained burns over 20 percent of her body. She fell asleep one evening in an overstuffed chair while smoking a cigarette. The lit cigarette caused the chair and her clothing to ignite. As a result, she suffered burns of the perineum, thighs, and abdomen. The fire was extinguished by the fire squad and Miss B. was admitted to the burn-care facility at the University Health Sciences Center.

Miss B. is currently ten days postburn. The nurse caring for her has identified patient-centered problems related to Miss B.'s psychological well-being, somatic identity, sexuality, occupational identity, and social role.

Following are Miss B.'s nursing care plan and patient care cardex dealing with each of these areas of concern.

NURSING CARE PLAN

Nursing Diagnoses	Objectives	Nursing Interventions	Principles/Rationale	Evaluations
Psychological Impact Regression manifested by refusal to eat.	To avoid fostering Miss B.'s regressive behavior.	Have family and health team members approach Miss B. in a firm, kind, and nonrejecting manner (e.g., "I'll position your breakfast tray to facilitate your eating").	Demonstrating acceptance can decrease the need for using regressive behavior as a means of relieving anxiety.	The nurse would observe for: A decrease in Miss B.'s regressive behavior.
		Inform Miss B. that when she is unable to control her behavior, limits and controls will be provided by family and health team members.	Providing limits creates a consistent and stable environment. Providing limits shows the out-of-control individual that he or she will not be allowed to harm himself/herself or others.	
	To increase Miss B.'s food consumption.	Inform Miss B. of the importance of nutrition in a nonpunitive manner (e.g., give her a choice between nasogastric feedings and eating self-selected foods).	Allowing the patient the right to control one's environment implies respect as an adult. Decision making fosters autonomy and can enhance cooperation.	An increase in Miss B.'s food consumption.
		Keep conversation simple and concrete during periods of regressive behavior.	Preventing sensory overload can decrease the need for regressive behavior as a means to deal with anxiety.	
		Utilize a variety of family and health team members who maintain a consistent supportive approach with Miss B.'s behavior.	Prolonged visits by a few select members of the family and health team can result in a vicious cycle of hostility and counterhostility when family and health team members no longer can tolerate the burned individual's regressive behavior. Conflicting approaches toward an individual can foster regressive behavior.	

NURSING CARE PLAN (cont.)

Nursing Diagnoses	Objectives	Nursing Interventions	Principles/Rationale	Evaluations
Somatic Impact Inappropriate verbal communication manifested by excessive and prolonged screaming during and after painful dressing changes.	To decrease Miss B.'s pain during dressing changes.	Encourage Miss B. to verbalize her feelings about the anticipation of and sensation of pain.	Ventilating feelings about pain can assist in decreasing anxiety related to the pain experience.	The nurse would observe for: A change in Miss B.'s expression of pain.
	To assist Miss B. in venting her expression of pain in a more acceptable manner.	Administer analgesics *prior* to the dressing change.	Administering analgesics prior to a dressing change assists in alleviating pain and decreasing anxiety associated with the dressing change.	Miss B.'s increased use of less demoralizing means of pain expression.
	To prevent demoralizing effects that Miss B.'s screaming may have upon other burned individuals in the immediate area.	Encourage the discussion of pain and ways of dealing with it between Miss B. and an individual in a more advanced stage of burn therapy.	Knowing that someone else has made it through a similar experience can be comforting.	
		Suggest various maneuvers to be used to control the expression of pain during painful dressing changes, for example: Placing something in the mouth to bite on. Using self-hypnosis by loudly saying, "It doesn't hurt."	Sharing and developing ways of distracting one's attention during a painful dressing change can decrease the patient's need to express pain inappropriately for extended periods of time.	

Sexual Impact Potential sexual dysfunction manifested by expressed fear of being rejected by her fiancé because of perineal burns.		Reassure Miss B. that a great deal of the pain will subside once grafting takes place.	Knowing that pain will decrease with grafting leaves a feeling of hope for many burned individuals.	
		Encourage Miss B. to identify how pain has been dealt with within the past.	Utilizing maneuvers which were helpful for dealing with past pain experiences may prove helpful for dealing with the present pain experience.	
	To decrease Miss B.'s fear of rejection.	Encourage Miss B. to express her fear of possible rejection by her fiancé.	Expressing feelings of rejection may assist the patient in developing ways of dealing with such feelings.	The nurse would observe for: A decrease in Miss B.'s expressed fear of rejection by her fiancé.
	To assist Miss B. in dealing with her fears of rejection.	Encourage Miss B. and her fiancé to discuss with each other her fears of rejection.	Knowing how an individual reacts to a crisis situation can assist significant others in understanding and dealing with the individual's behavior.	An increase in discussion between Miss B. and her fiancé about her fears of rejection.
		Encourage Miss B.'s fiancé to express to her his feelings about her perineal burn.	Feelings of guilt about one's reaction to a perineal burn are difficult to hide and may affect the fiancé's sexual enthusiasm.	
		Encourage Miss B.'s fiancé to tell her that any hesitant response toward her is not rejection, but rather an expression of empathy.	An individual with perineal burns who is aware of his or her sex partner's true feelings is less likely to misinterpret the sex partner's actions.	

(cont.)

NURSING CARE PLAN (cont.)

Nursing Diagnoses	Objectives	Nursing Interventions	Principles/Rationale	Evaluations
	To increase Miss B.'s feminine self-concept.	Encourage Miss B.'s fiancé to demonstrate affection toward her by carrying out maneuvers used prior to the burn to express such feelings. Such acts may include physical caressing or the giving of gifts.	Expression of acceptance by significant others can aid the individual with perineal burns in decreasing fears of rejection.	An increase in Miss B.'s expressed feelings of feminine self-worth.
Occupational Impact Potential impaired job management manifested by expressed fear of being unable to resume the duties of a salesgirl.	To decrease Miss B.'s fear of physical incapacity.	Encourage Miss B. to take an active part in daily personal hygiene. Encourage Miss B. to carry out her required physical therapy each day.	Taking an active part in one's own therapy program assists in the achievement of physical function and fosters independence.	The nurse would observe for: Miss B.'s increased participation in her burn therapy program.
		Explain to Miss B. and her family the importance of carrying out all components of her burn therapy.	Understanding that all components of burn therapy are vital for a successful recovery facilitates the individual's likelihood of adhering to prescribed therapies.	Miss B.'s decreased verbalization about her fear of not being able to resume occupational activities.

	To increase Miss B.'s feelings of self-worth.	Have family and health care members compliment Miss B. on each improvement and accomplishment made during her rehabilitation program.	Positive feedback for accomplishment fosters a feeling of self-worth and a feeling of achievement.	Miss B.'s expression of the fact that she is still a worthwhile human being.
Social Impact Unreconciled loss manifested by expressed belief that the burn incident was a punishment from God.	To assist Miss B. in dealing with her thoughts about justification for the burn incident.	Convey acceptance of Miss B.'s religious frame of reference by providing nonjudgmental feedback during verbalization of religious beliefs.	Demonstration of acceptance of the burn individual reinforces concepts of forgiveness and reconciliation within the individual's religious frame of reference.	The nurse would observe for: Miss B.'s decreased expression about the belief that her burn incident was a punishment from God.
		Notify the hospital chaplain of Miss B.'s feelings.	A member of the health team prepared in religious thought may prove helpful for interpreting and meeting the burn individual's religious need.	Miss B.'s verbalization of the fact that the burn was an accident.

PATIENT CARE CARDEX

PATIENT'S NAME: ___Miss B.___   MEDICAL DIAGNOSIS: ___Burns___

AGE: ___22 years___   SEX: ___Female___

MARITAL STATUS: ___Single___   OCCUPATION: ___Salesgirl___

SIGNIFICANT OTHERS: ___Fiancé___

Nursing Diagnoses	Nursing Approaches
Psychological: Regression manifested by refusal to eat.	1. Have family and health team members approach in a firm, kind, and nonrejecting manner (e.g., "I'll position your breakfast tray to facilitate your eating"). 2. Inform that when she is unable to control her behavior, limits and controls will be provided by family and health team members. 3. In a nonpunitive manner inform of the importance of nutrition (e.g., give her a choice between nasogastric feedings and eating self-selected foods). 4. Keep conversation simple and concrete during periods of regressive behavior. 5. Utilize a variety of family and health team members who maintain a consistent supportive approach with the patient's behavior.

Somatic: Inappropriate verbal communication manifested by excessive and prolonged screaming during and after painful dressing changes.	1. Encourage to verbalize feelings about the anticipation and sensation of pain.
	2. Administer analgesics prior to the dressing change.
	3. Encourage the discussion of pain and ways of dealing with it between the patient and an individual in a more advanced stage of burn therapy.
	4. Suggest various maneuvers to be used to control the expression of pain during painful dressing changes, such as:
	  (a) placing something in the mouth to bite on.
	  (b) using self-hypnosis by loudly saying, "It doesn't hurt."
	5. Reassure that a great deal of pain will subside once grafting takes place.
	6. Encourage to identify how pain has been dealt with in the past.

Sexual: Potential sexual dysfunction manifested by expressed fear of being rejected by fiancé because of perineal burns.	1. Encourage to express fear of possible rejection by fiancé. 2. Encourage patient and fiancé to discuss with each other patient's fears of rejection. 3. Encourage fiancé to express to patient his feelings about her perineal burns. 4. Encourage fiancé to tell patient that any hesitant response toward her is not rejection, but rather an expression of empathy. 5. Encourage fiancé to demonstrate affection toward her by carrying out maneuvers used prior to the burn.
Occupational: Impaired job management manifested by expressed fear of being unable to resume the duties of a salesgirl.	1. Encourage to take an active part in daily personal hygiene. 2. Encourage to carry out required physical therapy each day. 3. Explain importance of carrying out all components of burn therapy. 4. Have family and health care members compliment on each improvement and accomplishment made during rehabilitation program.
Social: Unreconciled loss manifested by expressed belief that the burn was a punishment from God.	1. Convey acceptance of religious frame of reference by providing nonjudgmental feedback during verbalization of religious beliefs. 2. Notify hospital chaplain of patient's feelings.

REFERENCES

ANDREASEN, N., NORRIS, A., and HARTFORD, C. Incidence of long-term psychiatric complications in severely burned adults, *Annals of Surgery,* 1971, *174* (5), 785–793.

ANDREASEN, N., NOYES, R., HARTFORD, C., BRODLAND, G., and PROCTOR, S. Management of emotional reactions in seriously burned adults, *New England Journal of Medicine,* 1972, *286* (2), 65–69.

BAILEY, E., and MOORE, D. Group meetings for families of burn victims, *Topics in Clinical Nursing,* 1980, *2* (2), 67–75.

BERNSTEIN, N. *Emotional care of the facially burned and disfigured.* Boston: Little, Brown, 1976.

BRADDOM, R., BOE, L., FLOWERS, L., and JOHNSON-VANN, T. The physical treatment and rehabilitation of burn patients. In R. Hummel (Ed.), *Clinical burn therapy: a management and prevention guide.* Boston: John Wright. PSG Pub., 1982.

CRAWFORD, J. Incidence and prevention of burn injuries. In M. Wagner (Ed.), *Care of the burn-injured patient: a multidisciplinary involvement.* Littleton: PSG Pub., 1981.

DAVIDSON, S. Nursing management of emotional reactions of severely burned patients during the acute phase, *Heart and Lung,* 1973, *2* (3), 370–375.

ERIKSON, E. *Childhood and society.* New York: W.W. Norton and Co., Inc., 1963.

HUMMEL, R. Introduction. In R. Hummel (Ed.), *Clinical burn therapy: a management and prevention guide.* Boston: John Wright. PSG Pub., 1982.

KNUDSON-COOPER, M. Adjustment to visible stigma: the case of the severely burned, *Social Science and Medicine,* 1981, *15B* (1), 31–44.

MACARTHUR, J., and MOORE, F. Epidemiology of burns, *Journal of the American Medical Association,* 1975, *231* (3), 259–263.

NOYES, R., ANDREASEN, N., and HARTFORD, C. The psychological reaction to severe burns, *Psychosomatics,* 1971, *12* (6), 416–422.

TRINGALI, R. The role of the psychiatric nurse consultant on a burn unit, *Issues in Mental Health Nursing,* 1982, *4* (1), 17–24.

9 ‖‖

SENSORY
ALTERATIONS

INTRODUCTION

Humans are continually exposed to sensory experiences which are constantly changing. Sleep exposes an individual's senses to a low degree of activity, while taking part in an active sports event subjects an individual's senses to a high degree of activity. How one interprets and deals with a specific sensory experience will vary among individuals. A sensory experience described as pleasant by one individual may be described as unpleasant by another. Rock concerts may be pleasant to the young adult but unpleasant to the elderly individual. Regardless of whether a sensory experience is pleasant or unpleasant, it must be remembered that sensory experiences provide data about the environment.

The nurse often is required to deal with persons who are undergoing alterations in sensory function. Patients in protective isolation, individuals with visual impairments, people with progressively decreasing hearing ability, patients in pain, and individuals with altered smell and/or taste because of the common cold are but a few examples of individuals undergoing an alteration in a sensory function. How an afflicted individual deals with an altered sensory experience varies, but an altered sensory experience, regardless of its type, is likely to create an impact upon the afflicted individual's psychological well-being, somatic identity, sexuality, occupational identity, and social role.

SENSORY PROCESS

In order for the nurse and other health care professionals to deal effectively with alterations in sensory function, they must be cognizant of the sensory process. The sensory process consists of two components: (1) the ability to receive mental impressions by way of the body organs and (2) the ability to *perceive* or organize the stimuli received.

Reception is the biological component of the sensory process and includes such functions as hearing, seeing, smelling, and touching. Perception is the psychological component of the sensory process and involves the individual's ability to select and organize the impressions received by the body organs. Without selection and organization of the mental impressions received, the stimuli remain meaningless to the individual involved.

The selection of an impression received is affected by the intensity, size, change, and repetition of the stimulus. The more intense the sound, the more likely it is to be heard. The larger the visual stimuli, the more likely they are to attract attention. A change in stimuli, such as a pink dot in a field of black dots, demands attention because there is a break in the monotony. Finally, frequently repeated stimuli are more likely to be remembered than are infrequently repeated stimuli. It must be remembered, however, that there is a limit to the effectiveness of repetition and, with time, change may become more effective than repetition.

By the same token, the organization of mental experiences received is influenced by certain factors. These factors include past experiences, knowledge, and attitudes. If an individual has encountered a prior experience with a stimulus, how the individual has dealt with the stimulus will have an affect upon the way in which the individual will deal with it now. Knowledge about the stimulus influences how the person will assimilate his or her interpretation of the stimulus into his or her cognitive process. Finally, attitudes about the stimulus will affect the individual's acceptance or rejection of his or her interpretation of the stimulus. If the individual likes the stimulus, no doubt he or she will accept it. If the individual finds the stimulus displeasing, he or she probably will reject it. In other words, the receptive component of the sensory process is an involved experience that depends upon many environmental and personal factors.

SENSORY RESTRICTION VERSUS SENSORY OVERLOAD

An individual's sensory experiences can be perceived as existing on a continuum. Sensory balance lies in the center of the continuum with sensory deprivation and sensory overload lying on opposite ends (see Figure 9.1). Since

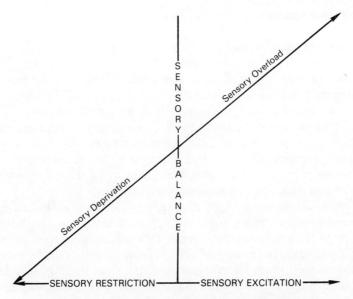

Figure 9.1   An individual's sensory experience continuum

sensory experiences constantly are changing, an individual will be in a constant state of flux on this continuum. When an individual is confronted with a decrease in sensory balance, he or she falls in the area of sensory restriction (to the left of the sensory experience continuum). When a person is bombarded and becomes overtaxed with a sensory experience, he or she falls in the area of sensory overload (to the right of the sensory experience continuum).

Health team members frequently are confronted with clinical situations in which sensory restriction or sensory overload occurs. For example, sensory restriction can occur with the eye-patched cataract patient, with the individual who is in isolation because of a contagious disease, with the individual who is suffering from loss of sight because of glaucoma, with the person who is losing his or her sense of hearing because he or she is aging, and even with the individual who is living in an isolated region of the country. By comparison, sensory overload is not uncommon for the individual requiring care in the intensive care unit, for the newly diagnosed diabetic being taught all of his or her necessary health care measures, for the individual admitted to an acute care setting for the first time, or for the recently discharged patient returning home to curious and inquisitive relatives and neighbors.

The manner by which an individual perceives and deals with each sensory experience makes him or her unique. Therefore, the nurse and other health team members must be cognizant of the individuality of each person when planning and instituting health care related to sensory function.

IMPACT OF SENSORY ALTERATIONS

Psychological Impact

Since humans rely upon sensory experiences in order to function, it is no wonder that when alterations in sensory experiences occur the afflicted person manifests certain psychological responses. Research shows that persons subjected to both sensory restriction and sensory overload manifest boredom, impaired concentration, lack of coherent thinking, anxiety, fear, depression, rapid mood changes, and even the extreme of auditory and visual hallucinations (Bolin, 1974: Lindsley, 1961). The intensity of these responses is very individual and may range from mild to severe.

The major responsibility of the nurse when dealing with an individual with an alteration in sensory function involves manipulation, clarification, and validation of the environmental stimuli. This is done in an attempt to prevent and/or decrease the occurrence of psychological responses that may result due to the altered sensorium. The manipulation, clarification, and validation of the environmental stimuli involve stimulus substitution or stimulus modification.

To facilitate the provision of appropriate health care for an individual who is subjected to alterations in sensory function, it is essential for the nurse to first obtain a data base from both the individual and the family about past activities in which the sensory impaired person has taken part. This prepares the nurse to identify activities and situations that will provide meaning for the individual's sensory experiences. Boredom, one of the responses to an altered sensory experience, can be best dealt with by providing the afflicted person with a variety of ways to explore his or her environment. For example, the individual in protective isolation can be given puzzles to put together, books to read, television to watch, a radio to listen to, or handicrafts with which to work. Before providing any of these activities, it is best for the nurse to discuss with the patient his or her interests and then to determine the feasibility of each activity. By involving the afflicted person and his or her family in the identification of activities of interest, provisions are made for the selection of endeavors that are personally meaningful.

Impaired concentration and lack of coherent thinking can be best dealt with by engaging the sensory afflicted person in conversation on topics that he or she finds meaningful and by providing him or her with time orientation. If the family, the nurse, or other members of the health team have identified an individual's interest as sports, involving the person in conversation with others who share a similar interest can provide a meaningful sensory experience, facilitate appropriate reality testing, and enhance a meaningful relationship. If an individual afflicted with a hearing impairment has a problem with verbal communication, written communication or sign language may have to be utilized. Time orientation can be facilitated by the use of clocks, calendars, and verbal input regarding the correct month and date. The following statements are beneficial in facilitating time orientation: "This certainly is a cold October morning!" or "Mr. J., how are you this fine Thursday afternoon?"

To deal with the responses of anxiety, fear, and depression in the individual afflicted with sensory alteration, the nurse will find it helpful to provide the individual with experiences which activate the unaltered senses and/or with meaningful reference points that indicate progress toward a goal. To activate the unaltered senses of the visually impaired individual, increased sensory input by way of auditory communication is in order. This can include announcing one's presence to the afflicted individual and describing activities that are occurring in the environment. For the hearing-impaired individual, utilizing communication through sight, as in the written form, is beneficial. Human touch also can transmit a great deal of sensory input, since it provides not only comfort but an additional means of nonverbal communication. Simply holding an individual's hand gives the feeling of caring and emphasizes the existence of another's presence.

Provision of meaningful reference points can be achieved through indicating to the individual experiencing sensory overload, while learning necessary health care regimens, what therapies he or she has mastered to date. Pointing out to the hearing-impaired individual how his or her observational skills have improved is another possible means of suggesting progress toward a goal. Above all, the individual should be encouraged to express feelings related to the alteration in sensory function. During the expression of feelings, the individual needs to be encouraged to look at the reality of these feelings, to examine how he or she has dealt with past feelings of anxiety, fear, or depression, and to identify and activate the use of his or her social support systems.

A sudden change in mood constitutes another response experienced by the individual afflicted with an alteration in sensory function. Before the nurse concludes that an individual's mood change is a result of an alteration in sensory function, it is necessary for a complete physical and psychosocial assessment to be made. Since there are many physical conditions and psychosocial situations that can contribute to sudden mood changes, it is best that these contributing factors be ruled out. Once an alteration in sensory experience has been identified as the contributing factor in the person's sudden mood change, the nurse must determine whether the alteration in sensory function is a result of sensory restriction or sensory overload and respond accordingly.

Experiencing hallucinations (auditory and visual) is one of the most devastating responses to an alteration in sensory function. To deal with such a response, the nurse needs to provide the afflicted individual with reality validation so that he or she does not have to read nonexistent stimuli into the environment. In other words, the nurse must not feed into or challenge the individual's hallucinatory experiences. If the afflicted person says that he or she hears the androids calling, an appropriate response from the nurse would be, "I'm sure the androids seem real to you, but I do not hear them. It must be very frightening for you to have these experiences." When the nurse encounters a hallucinating person, it is highly advisable to have the psychiatric clinical nurse specialist evaluate the individual so that appropriate referrals can be initiated. In some circumstances, psychotherapy and psychotropic drugs may be required.

Somatic Impact

The impact that an alteration in sensory function has upon a person's body image varies among individuals. Both the specific sensory alteration and how the afflicted person perceives the alteration play vital roles in the resulting changes in body image. A visual impairment may be perceived by the afflicted person as impinging upon the ability to communicate effectively since he or she cannot see the eye movements or facial expressions of others. An auditory alteration often is perceived as a "nonvisible" handicap, since others cannot see the deficit. Unfortunately the person with a hearing deficit tends to be labeled slow or dull because his or her sensory alteration causes a response delay. By the same token, the individual placed in protective isolation may perceive his or her body image as dirty and undesirable since everyone coming near wears protective clothing.

As discussed in Chapter 2, the stage of development being experienced by an individual will have an influence upon how the individual will adapt to an alteration in sensory function. The afflicted person in the stage of young adulthood (eighteen to forty-five years) may encounter difficulties in sharing himself or herself with others both in friendship and in a mutually satisfying relationship. It is during this developmental stage that the young adult is ready and willing to merge his or her identity with that of others (Erikson, 1963). Since the individual is suffering from an alteration in a sensory experience, the individual may view the body as less than perfect or desirable and withdraw from others. If an individual in the stage of adulthood (forty-five to sixty-five years) encounters an alteration in sensory function, he or she may feel ill-equipped to guide future generations, the major focus of this developmental phase (Erikson, 1963). The individual may view his or her altered sensory function as a premature sign of old age, become engulfed in personal needs and self-comforts, and enter a state of self-absorbtion and stagnation. When an alteration in sensory function occurs in the mature adult (sixty-five years and over), he or she may develop feelings of despair with frequent thoughts of death. These feelings are prematurely intensified when the mature adult has not derived satisfaction from life experiences and accomplishments (Erikson, 1963). As a result, the sensory alteration may be interpreted as a prelude to death.

The nurse's first task in dealing with the individual who has sustained an alteration in sensory function involves providing the individual with correct data about himself or herself in regard to the environment. For example, does the individual feel less than perfect because he or she cannot see? Does the individual feel that others think him or her dull or slow because he or she cannot hear? Does the individual think that he or she is repulsive to others because he or she requires protective isolation? Finally, does the individual feel emotionally incompetent because he or she finds it impossible to tolerate the noises in the intensive care unit? As the individual discloses his or her body image perceptions, the nurse must assist the individual and family members in developing adaptive modes for dealing with alterations.

Since a visually impaired person cannot see the intricacies of body lesions he or she may have, the nurse must make a concerted effort to describe the appearance of these lesions and to allow for touching of the area to prevent misinterpretation and distortion about the individual's body image. The auditory impaired person who encounters difficulties in verbally communicating with others may perceive himself or herself as less than perfect and withdraw from others. To prevent withdrawal, alternate means of communication must be explored and pursued. If the auditory impaired person feels ostracized by others during conversation, the individual and his or her family need to be encouraged to verbalize to others ways to include the impaired person in the conversation (i.e., use of sign language, written communication, or measures to facilitate lip reading). The individual placed in protective isolation may feel that others are avoiding him or her because of feelings of disgust. Stopping in to visit with the person in protective isolation and making body contact, by touching, are two basic and helpful measures that can prevent misinterpretation of the environment as a result of altered sensory experiences. If the person is suffering from an overload of sensory experiences, the nurse needs to encourage the person to aid others in helping him or her identify those environmental factors which are overwhelming (e.g., the presence of constant, bright lights or the continual beeping of the cardiac monitor). Once overwhelming stimuli are identified, such maneuvers as dimming the lights or providing soft relaxing radio music through earphones can be provided.

Sexual Impact

The specific impact that an alteration in sensory experience may have upon one's sexuality often depends upon the specific alteration in sensory function. For example, the individual suffering from visual impairment cannot rely solely upon sight for sexual stimulation and may need to resort to sound and touch for achieving a satisfying sexual experience. The auditory impaired person may be unable to hear whether his or her sex partner is enjoying the maneuvers of sex play. As a result the other senses may need to be utilized for creating a mutually satisfying sexual encounter. If the sense of touch or smell is impaired, the afflicted person may be unable to utilize these senses for enhancing erotic feelings. Caressing sensory impaired body areas or using colognes when olfaction is altered may fail to arouse sexual feelings. This ultimately can lead to a sense of frustration for both the afflicted person and the sex partner.

The individual placed in protective isolation may find that sexual needs cannot be met in a physical manner because of bodily removal from others. He or she may attempt to meet sexual needs through delusional means (i.e., dreaming about sexual fulfillment or imagining the effect his or her sexual prowess has upon members of the opposite sex) or through acting out inappropriate sexual behavior (i.e., a male patient patting a female nurse's buttocks). The individual suffering from an overload of sensory stimulation finds that dealing with a constant bombardment of stimuli from the environment may render him or her totally incapable of dealing with sexual needs. Since part of one's sexuality is psychic, the sensory overloaded person may be unable to relax enough to enjoy a sexual experience. In any case, the person afflicted with an alteration in sensory function will need to identify sensory experiences that will aid in providing the fulfillment of a sexual relationship for both the afflicted person and the sex partner.

The nurse's role in dealing with the sexual impact of an alteration in sensory function involves assisting the afflicted person and the sex partner in identifying and utilizing alternate sensory experiences that can enhance a fulfilling sexual relationship. To accomplish this goal, the nurse needs to encourage the afflicted person and his or her sex partner to verbalize feelings to each other about the effect the alteration in sensory function is having upon their sexual relationship. By sharing their feelings, the couple can more easily identify possible and existing areas of concern. For example, the sex partner may be caressing a sensory-deprived body part of the afflicted person and becoming totally frustrated because no sexual arousal results.

Once areas of concern are identified, methods of dealing with each of the areas of concern need to be developed. If an individual suffers from auditory impairment, the sex partner and afflicted person may have to develop some means of communicating during their sexual experience. To communicate to the hearing-impaired individual that certain sexual activities are pleasurable, the sex partner could gently stroke the arm of the hearing-impaired person to transmit the message of pleasure. For the person placed in protective isolation, the nurse may find it advisable to encourage uninterrupted sessions for the individual and his or her sex partner so that private conversation and caressing may take place. In the case of sensory overload, the afflicted person and his or her sex partner may have to be encouraged to discuss and to identify ways of assisting the afflicted person to relax so that he or she can have a fulfilling sexual experience. Taking warm baths or showers, listening to relaxing music, or discussing pleasant topics prior to sexual activity are but a few possible maneuvers to use in aiding relaxation.

Whether the afflicted person suffers from sensory restriction or sensory overload, the nurse needs to encourage the individual to maintain a high standard of personal appearance. An appealing appearance not only increases one's feelings of self-worth, but it also makes one appealing to others.

Occupational Impact

The impact that an alteration in sensory function has upon one's occupational pursuits depends upon the specific requirements of the job, the type of sensory alteration, and the intensity of the sensory dysfunction being experienced. For example, moderate difficulties in visual acuity, color blindness, and total blindness are all visual alterations, but each imposes a different impact upon the person's occupational situation. Before an individual can be labeled as ill-suited for an occupation, the precise effect that the alteration in sensory function imposes upon the work situation must be identified.

Alterations in visual experiences can create a variety of problems for an afflicted person. If the job entails reading fine print, visual acuity is essential. If one's visual acuity is less than desirable, but can be improved by corrective lenses, the problem may be solved. Should wearing corrective lenses in an attempt to deal with an impairment in visual function become a hazard in the work situation, the individual may find it necessary to make alterations in his or her job. Color blindness, another alteration in visual function, can create difficulties in the work situation when identifying colors is essential, as in the case of an air traffic controller or an interior decorator. The person afflicted with severe hearing deficiencies may find it difficult to carry out a job that involves identifying and recording various sounds. Occupations involving use of the telephone, such as that of a receptionist, might be out of the question for the auditory impaired person. If, however, the hearing deficit is manageable by amplification of the sound, as with a hearing aid or by using a printout of the spoken word, jobs involving phone usage would be feasible. In some occupations being able to identify sounds may not be crucial, but the hearing impairment itself may be a safety hazard for the afflicted person. A heavy machine operator may not need excellent hearing to operate machinery but must be able to hear verbal commands from others to stop or start the machinery so that the safety of self and others is not jeopardized.

Alterations in smell, taste, and touch can create an impact upon one's occupational pursuits. Someone involved in the culinary arts may find it difficult to judge the quality of fine foods and drink if taste and/or smell are hindered. An altered sense of touch could create an occupational hazard for someone who works with very hot and very cold items; the sensory loss may impede also the ability of the individual, such as a musician, who relies upon sensitive hands and fingers to carry out occupational endeavors.

Sensory overload is just as likely as sensory restriction to have an impact upon one's occupational pursuits. Undoubtedly, the greatest occupational impacts created by sensory overload deal with safety and high-quality performance in the work setting. The person encountering sensory overload is less likely to focus total attention on his or her work. If the individual is bombarded by sensory experience, chances for an accident will increase and the quality of work will decrease. The bookkeeper afflicted with sensory overload is more likely to make errors than the bookkeeper not afflicted with sensory overload. The assembly line worker suffering from sensory overload is more likely to be involved in an accident caused by lack of attention than is the worker who is not sensory overloaded.

The nurse's responsibilities related to the occupational impact of alterations in sensory function involve identifying whether the altered sensory experience will affect the afflicted person's ability to perform job responsibilities. If necessary the nurse should help the person to seek assistance in obtaining alternate occupational pursuits. If the alteration in sensory function creates difficulties in the occupational setting, the family, the nurse, and other health team members need to identify ways in which changes can be made in the work environment to deal with the afflicted person's altered sensory experience. Should an individual suffer from auditory alterations and his or her job involves using the telephone, possibly a sound amplifier could be installed or the telephone responsibilities could be delegated to someone else in the work setting. If sensory overload creates problems in the job environment, an alteration of the stimulus or its removal from the environment should be considered. However, should adjustments in the environment be impossible, the afflicted person may have to consider job retraining. The nurse will find it helpful and beneficial to call upon the expertise of the social worker, the occupational therapist, or the rehabilitation counselor for assistance in identifying alternate occupational endeavors for the sensory impaired individual.

Social Impact

The social impact created by an alteration in sensory function will depend upon the specific sensory experience that has undergone change. In cases of sensory restriction, such as auditory, visual, olfactory, and gustatory impairment, the effect that each change imposes will depend upon the specific social encounter.

Social events that deal exclusively with visual interaction may not be enjoyable for the visually impaired person. For example, movies are enjoyable only when they do not depend greatly on visual detail for their impact. When attending a movie, the visually impaired person may find it beneficial to have a family member along to describe what is occurring visually. Unfortunately, this often creates difficulties because it annoys other people in the theater. Attending concerts, lectures, or conversational social engagements may be desirable alternatives. Many visually impaired people find enjoyment in touring historical sections of cities and walking through arboretums and gardens where braille signs and recorded speeches describe the site and/or the foliage. To access social functions, the visually impaired individual will need to rely upon others for transportation. In rural areas transportation will have to be provided by family and friends since public transportation modes are not readily available. In metropolitan areas, however, the visually impaired person can be instructed on how to use a variety of public transportation systems. In any event, the visually impaired person requires assistance in exploring how he or she can safely get to and from social events.

The individual afflicted with an alteration in auditory function is faced with social setting problems of a different nature. At social gatherings where conversation is the primary entertainment, the person with an auditory impairment may feel isolated if he or she cannot read lips or communicate with others by sign language or the written word. Even if the person with an auditory impairment can read lips, he or she may find lip reading difficult if eye-straining fluorescent lights are present or the lighting creates shadows on the face of the individual who is speaking. In addition, lip reading for extended periods of time has proven to be tiring. Activities that a hearing-impaired person might find enjoyable include observing a sports event, visiting museums and art centers, or attending a movie that has subtitles. Television also has proven enjoyable since a number of programs now provide the verbal message by way of "signing."

The individual with an alteration in olfaction and gustation may not find it enjoyable to attend social events centered around the consumption of tasty food and drink. Thus, it would be advisable for the individual to engage in entertainment that does not focus primarily on the partaking of culinary delights.

Individuals undergoing sensory overload also encounter difficulties in the social setting. If a person is overwhelmed by sensory stimuli, he or she may find it difficult to enjoy the social engagement. The person from a rural area who has come to a metropolitan area for the sole purpose of entertainment may feel overwhelmed and stressed by the large number of people and the congested traffic. The individual's inability to relax and enjoy the social encounter because of an overloaded sensorium may make him or her unpleasant company.

The nurse's role in dealing with the social impact of an alteration in sensory function involves assisting the individual and his or her family in identifying social encounters that are enjoyable for the sensory impaired person and/or assisting in making necessary adaptations in the social setting to facilitate the afflicted person's comfort. If the visually impaired person enjoys movies or plays but is uncomfortable in public because someone has to verbalize the visual data of the production, an alternative may be to watch television at home or attend drive-in movies. If a visually impaired person enjoys playing cards, braille playing cards can be used so that the individual can play both with sighted and nonsighted friends. Reading braille or being read to, either by way of a recorded message or with the assistance of a reader, are other forms of entertainment that the visually impaired individual may enjoy.

If sensory overload is a problem in the social setting, the nurse needs to aid the person and family members in identifying those social settings that may add to sensory overload. For example, a sports event in a large arena where there is a large crowd may overwhelm the individual who comes from a small, noncongested community. Placing this person in such a social setting will undoubtedly decrease the chances for enjoying the event. It may be advisable to encourage the selection of a social event that is not so crowded. By comparison, when a person from a large metropolitan area moves to an isolated rural town, sensory restriction may result. In such a situation the nurse will find it necessary to identify events and activities that the person can attend for a stimulating sensory experience.

SUMMARY

Humans are continually exposed to a variety of sensory experiences. How each person deals with each sensory experience makes him or her unique. An experience seen as pleasant by one individual may be seen as unpleasant by another.

The nurse often is required to deal with individuals who are undergoing alterations in sensory function. These alterations may include a restriction or an overload in sensory function. Whether the person is afflicted with a restriction or an overload in sensory function, the alteration is likely to create an impact upon his or her psychological well-being, somatic identity, sexuality, occupational identity, and social role.

Patient Situation   Miss S. A. is a forty-nine-year-old, single, American Sioux Indian who is suffering from progressive loss of vision due to glaucoma. For the past twenty-five years she has been living in a small housing project on an Indian reservation. For economic support, Miss S. A. beads Indian jewelry which she sends to jewelry stores in surrounding cities.

Miss S. A. is currently being treated for glaucoma at the health clinic on the reservation. During her last clinic visit the nurse in charge of her care identified problems related to Miss S. A.'s psychological well-being, somatic identity, sexuality, occupational identity, and social role.

Following are Miss S. A.'s nursing care plan and patient care cardex dealing with each of these areas of concern.

NURSING CARE PLAN

Nursing Diagnoses	Objectives	Nursing Interventions	Principles/Rationale	Evaluations
Psychological Impact Anxiety manifested by expressed "uneasy" feelings about the presence of visual impairment.	To decrease Miss S. A.'s anxiety.	Provide Miss S. A. with meaningful reference points indicating progress toward a goal (e.g., explain and point out to Miss S. A. that by adhering to her prescribed therapies, the incidence of her progressive visual impairment will be greatly reduced).	Having a meaningful reference point with which to relate aids in decreasing anxiety.	The nurse would observe for: Miss S. A.'s verbalization about how her anxiety concerning her visual impairment has decreased.
Somatic Impact Fear of body image alteration manifested by expressed concern about appearing distorted.	To decrease Miss S. A.'s misconception about her body image. To provide Miss S. A. with correct data about her body image.	Provide Miss S. A. with accurate verbal data about her personal appearance (e.g., describe to her how she appears).	Visually impaired individuals must rely upon touch to obtain data about their body image. As a result, distortions in their interpretation of their body image may occur. Providing a visually impaired person with verbal feedback about the actual appearance of the body can aid in decreasing misconceptions about body image.	The nurse would observe for: Miss S. A.'s accurate description of her body image.
		Encourage Miss S. A. to verbalize how she feels about herself (e.g., does she view her body as less than perfect since she has a visual impairment?).	Verbalization of feelings aids the individual in exploring ways of dealing with an alteration.	

(cont.)

NURSING CARE PLAN (cont.)

Nursing Diagnoses	Objectives	Nursing Interventions	Principles/Rationale	Evaluations
Sexual Impact Unreconciled sexual identity manifested by verbalized fear of appearing unfeminine.	To enhance Miss S. A.'s feelings of self-worth.	Encourage Miss S. A. to maintain an appealing personal appearance (e.g., dress neatly, keep hair clean and arranged in an orderly fashion, and wear garments that are becoming to her).	Maintaining a high standard of personal appearance aids in increasing one's feelings of self-worth and makes one appealing to others.	The nurse would observe for: Miss S. A.'s verbalization about feeling attractive to herself and others.
Occupational Impact Potential deficit in job management activities manifested by expressed concern about being unable to continue beading Indian jewelry.	To enhance Miss S. A.'s ability to maintain her occupational pursuits.	Encourage Miss S. A. to use visual aids (e.g., her prescribed glasses and/or a magnifying glass).	Providing appropriate alterations in the work environment can facilitate the visually impaired individual's chances of maintaining occupational endeavors.	The nurse would observe for: Miss S. A.'s verbalization that she is able to carry out her Indian beading.
		Encourage Miss S. A. to use good lighting when she works with her beads.	Lighting that does not cause shadows or eyestrain facilitates the individual's ability to carry out activities that involve vision.	

172

Social Impact Potential social isolation manifested by withdrawal from social events that take place on the reservation.	To prevent Miss S. A. from becoming socially isolated.	Encourage Miss S. A. to take periodic breaks during her beading sessions.	Resting the eyes periodically aids in preventing eyestrain and, in turn, facilitates the ability to carry out activities that involve vision.	The nurse would observe for: Miss S. A.'s increased involvement in social activities.
		Encourage Miss S. A. to attend social activities on the reservation.	Engaging in social activities prevents withdrawal and social isolation.	
	To involve Miss S. A. in social activities.	Encourage Miss S. A. to contact friends for transportation to and from the social activities.	Lack of public transportation in rural areas may hinder the visually impaired person's ability to get to and from social activities.	

PATIENT CARE CARDEX

| PATIENT'S NAME: | Miss S. A. | MEDICAL DIAGNOSIS: | Glaucoma and progressive visual impairment |

PATIENT'S NAME: Miss S. A.

MEDICAL DIAGNOSIS: Glaucoma and progressive visual impairment

AGE: 49 years

SEX: Female

MARITAL STATUS: Single

OCCUPATION: Beader of Indian jewelry

SIGNIFICANT OTHERS: Fellow tribal members

Nursing Diagnoses	Nursing Approaches
Psychological: Anxiety manifested by expressed "uneasy" feelings about the presence of visual impairment.	1. Provide meaningful reference points indicating progress toward a goal (e.g., explain and point out how adherence to prescribed therapies will reduce the incidence of progressive visual impairment).
Somatic: Fear of body image alteration manifested by expressed concern about appearing distorted.	1. Provide accurate verbal data about her personal appearance (e.g., describe to her how she appears). 2. Encourage verbalization of how she feels about herself. (Does she view her body as less than perfect because she has a visual impairment?)
Sexual: Unreconciled sexual identity manifested by verbalized fear of appearing unfeminine.	1. Encourage maintenance of an appealing personal appearance (dress neatly, keep hair clean, and wear becoming clothing).
Occupational: Potential deficit in job management activities manifested by expressed concern about being unable to continue beading Indian jewelry.	1. Encourage use of visual aids (e.g., prescribed glasses and/or a magnifying glass). 2. Encourage use of good lighting when working with beads. 3. Encourage taking periodic breaks during beading sessions.
Social: Potential social isolation manifested by withdrawal from social events that take place on the reservation.	1. Encourage to attend social activities on the reservation. 2. Encourage contacting friends for transportation to and from social activities.

REFERENCES

BOLIN, R. Sensory deprivation: an overview, *Nursing Forum,* 1974, *13* (3), 241–258.

ERIKSON, E. *Childhood and society.* New York: W.W. Norton and Co., Inc., 1963.

LINDSLEY, D. Common factors in sensory deprivation, sensory distortion, and sensory overload. In P. Solomon, P. Kutzansky, P. Leiderman, J. Mandelson, R. Trumbull, and D. Wexler (Eds.), *Sensory deprivation.* Cambridge: Harvard University Press, 1961.

10

MYOCARDIAL INFARCTION

INTRODUCTION

Western society's standard of living offers many luxuries and comforts. People no longer have to fight for survival from the elements but are able to partake of many of the "finer" things in life. Sedentary activities have become prevalent and life spans have grown longer. However, with an increase in luxuries and comforts come disadvantages such as the increased incidence of coronary heart disease. At the present, coronary heart disease constitutes the leading cause of incapacitation and death in both Europe and the United States (Fishman, 1982).

Historically, the heart has been identified as the maintainer of life, since it pumps life-giving blood throughout the body. The heart's continual beating provides people with an ever present reminder of its value. Early medical observers held romantic notions about the pathology of the heart manifested by the belief that the presence of fibrinous pericarditis was an indication of a heroic death. As a result, the heart has been credited with the expression of such emotions as fear, courage, sadness, desire, and love. Religiously, the heart has been designated as a substitute for both the body and the spirit as demonstrated by the heart burials of the ancient rulers of the Holy Roman Empire. Thus, the importance of the heart has been acknowledged throughout history.

PATIENT PROFILE

Research has shown that the presence of various factors increases the incidence of coronary heart disease. Such predisposing factors include obesity, cigarette smoking, consumption of a high-caloric and high-fat diet, a sedentary life-style, hypertension, stress, and the presence of specific personality traits (Jenkins, 1979; Protos, Caracta, and Gross, 1971).

Physiological factors such as cigarette smoking, hypertension, consumption of a high-caloric and high-fat diet, and obesity create vasoconstriction, myocardial damage, lipid abnormalities, and an increased cardiac workload. Psychosocial factors such as a sedentary life-style, the presence of stressful situations, and the existence of certain personality traits often lead to overeating, smoking, and hypertension, all of which produce deleterious effects upon cardiac function. The exact effect, however, that psychosocial factors have upon the occurrence of coronary heart disease is not known and all theories at present are speculative.

Some authorities (Friedman, 1969; Haynes and Feinleib, 1981) advocate that individuals who display a certain behavior pattern are more prone to succumb to coronary heart disease when physiological predisposing factors are present. Friedman (1969) has defined the coronary-prone behavior pattern as "type A personality."

According to Jenkins (1979) if one were to examine the behavior of the individual manifesting the type A personality, the following traits could be identified:

Values

1. Sets high standards for self.
2. Critical of self and others when self-established standards are not met.
3. Is intense and inflexible.
4. Prefers respect for achievements made rather than for who he or she is.
5. Feels a need to maintain productivity in order to maintain a feeling of self-worth.
6. Craves recognition and power.
7. Is competitive with self and others.
8. Is gratified primarily by occupation and aggressive avocational pursuits (e.g., political and community affairs).

Style of thought

1. Simultaneously pursues several lines of thought and action (e.g., eats while working).
2. Anticipates the future and begins to react prematurely.
3. Appears alert and ready to move.
4. Is compulsive about completing tasks.
5. Demonstrates poor observation skills.

Interpersonal relationships

1. Is self-centered.
2. Feelings of anger easily aroused.

3. Is easily frustrated in a work situation.
4. Is aggressive sexually, but enjoys the chase more than the consummation.
5. Emits a certainty about his or her own correctness.
6. Becomes a victim of his or her own behavior pattern (e.g., pushes beyond his or her limits).

Style of response

1. Reacts rapidly.
2. Speaks with certainty and emphasis.
3. Does not waste words.
4. Gives nods and "ahems" while listening to another speaker.
5. Becomes emotionally and physically involved when describing a situation that characteristically frustrates him or her.
6. Finds it uncomfortable to slow down the speed of his or her speech or writing when requested to do so.

Gestures and movements

1. Uses tense, energetic movements.
2. Clenches fists when tense.
3. Shakes hands with a firm grip and uses active motion.
4. Finds it difficult to remain still when sitting or standing.

Facial expression

1. Uses momentary tense smiles with a tight horizontal lip line.
2. Uses brief smiles to emphasize comments or reveal impatience.
3. Tenses jaw muscles or grits teeth when emphasizing comments.

Breathing

1. Has frequent breaks in breathing rhythm.
2. Inhales more air than necessary when speaking.

Being characterized as a type A personality depends upon the number of characteristics possessed and their intensity. It is possible for an individual to be classified as having a type A personality without demonstrating all of the aforementioned characteristics. When examining the relationship between the presence of a type A personality and the incidence of coronary heart disease, one must realize that most research has been limited to male members of industrialized societies. A limited number of studies suggest that females who manifest a type A personality also are subject to an increased incidence of coronary heart disease (Kenigsberg, Zyzanski, Jenkins, Wardwell, and Licciardello, 1974; Rosenman and Friedman, 1961). According to Jenkins (1979), the incidence of type A personality tends to be highest among young males and decreases with age. It is important to note, however, that not *all* individuals afflicted with coronary heart disease manifest a type A personality pattern.

The importance of the identification of type A behavior patterns among individuals who are physiologically prone to cardiovascular disease is multidimensional. Understanding its foundation in personality structure, realizing how it is reinforced by our society, knowing what effect it has upon cardiac medical therapy, and identifying possible approaches to modifying it are all part of a long-term rehabilitation program for the individual sustaining coronary heart disease. Just as the individual is instructed in ways to alter the predisposing physiologic factors to coronary heart disease, so must he or she learn about altering predisposing psychosocial factors.

As long as coronary heart disease remains a major health care problem, nursing must be cognizant of the effects that it has upon the individual's life. The remainder of this chapter will deal with the impact that coronary heart disease—namely, myocardial infarction (M.I.)—has upon an individual's psychological well-being, somatic identity, sexuality, occupational identity, and social role.

IMPACT OF MYOCARDIAL INFARCTION

Psychological Impact

The use of denial to protect oneself from facing the full impact of impending death, impaired function, and disability is a phenomenon that has been noted clinically in every type of disease and disability. The individual sustaining an M.I. is no exception and the use of denial can be identified as early as the preadmission period. A typical response of actual or potential coronary patients, just prior to hospital admission, is to delay seeking medical advice or treatment. This delay can range from less than one hour up to several days. However, the average time for hospital arrival is between two and one-half to four hours after the onset of symptoms. This time period often is referred to as the individual's *decision time,* the period of time starting from the onset of symptoms until the individual obtains medical assistance. The prolongation of the decision time concerns medical authorities since approximately 50 to 70 percent of the individuals experiencing a myocardial infarction die within one hour after the onset of acute symptoms and prior to obtaining medical treatment (Gentry, 1979).

Demographic characteristics, perception of the illness, and the social context at the onset of symptoms are three factors which have been identified as determinants of an individual's preadmission behavior (Gentry, 1979). Demographic characteristics include the individual's age, sex, educational background, occupation, socioeconomic class, ethnic background, and history of coronary heart disease. Research suggests that older individuals tend to take longer to seek medical attention than younger individuals (Moss and Goldstein, 1970). Men demonstrate a shorter decision time than women. Education, occupation, and socioeconomic class appear to have no relation to preadmission behavior (Gentry, 1979). Ethnic background, however, appears to have a decided effect upon preadmission behavior, with individuals of Jewish and Italian origins demonstrating a higher proportion of denial than individuals from the Irish and British old American groups (Croog, Shapiro, and Levine, 1971). Individuals with a past history of myocardial infarction generally are better able to diagnose their initial symptoms as a cardiac problem than are individuals without such a history. However, a history of coronary heart disease either has no effect on or actually increases the individual's decision time (Alonzo, 1973; Goldstein, Moss, and Green, 1972), hence prolonging the seeking of medical attention.

How the individual perceives the illness is the second factor determining preadmission behavior. An individual's ability to seek medical attention following the occurrence of symptoms requires three cognitive functions: perception of the symptoms, recognition of their meaning, and realization that medical attention is necessary. If the individual follows this cognitive sequence (perception-recognition-realization), he or she will seek medical attention in a reasonably short period of time. Should the individual not follow the sequence, delay in obtaining medical care will occur. Although the symptoms are perceived, they may be attributed to other causes or assessed as being less severe than they actually are. Denial of the seriousness of the symptoms may serve as a temporary means of reducing anxiety about the immediate situation; however, it also serves to decrease the acquisition of appropriate health care.

The social context at the onset of symptoms is the third factor determining preadmission behavior. When symptoms occur in the presence of others (especially the spouse), the afflicted individual decreases his or her decision time in seeking medical assistance (Alonzo, 1973; Goldstein, Moss, and Green, 1972). Decision time tends to increase, however, when the symptoms occur in the absence of others or when the afflicted person is enjoying a weekend away from work responsibilities (Tjoe and Luria, 1972).

No *single* factor determines whether or when an individual seeks medical attention. Gentry (1979) believes that the most important factor is the social context at the time of symptom onset. If others are around, if the individual is not involved in an activity that is difficult to terminate, and if the symptoms occur at a time when they appear more serious (the middle of the night), the individual is likely to respond with greater speed in seeking medical attention. Without a doubt, educating the public concerning the symptoms of a myocardial infarction and the necessity of seeking appropriate medical attention is one important intervention for decreasing the incidence of death caused by a prolonged decision time.

Once the individual is diagnosed as having sustained an M.I., he or she is faced with a loss, as discussed in Chapter 3. Since the individual sustaining an M.I. generally loses wellness suddenly, he or she is thrust into illness role assumption, as discussed in Chapter 1, with little time for role assimilation.

Repudiation is the first reaction to a myocardial infarction. This response occurs immediately and generally lasts twenty-four to forty-eight hours. It is during this time that the individual refuses to believe what has occurred and demonstrates a stunned numbness about the experience (Bigos, 1981). Manifestations of repudiation may include avoidance of discussing the M.I. and its significance, minimizing the seriousness of the condition and its consequences, engaging in social humorous interactions with health members, and asking different staff members the same questions in an attempt to find the desired answer.

During repudiation the individual afflicted with an M.I. must be allowed to deny the loss of wellness. Encouraging free verbalization about his or her feelings is important, but at no time should the family, the nurse, or other members of the health team join the individual in denial. Should the individual verbalize that increased activity has no effect upon the heart, others must not agree. Such a comment is the individual's way of telling health team members that he or she is not ready to accept the M.I. or its imposed restrictions.

The nurse's response to such a comment should be an open-ended statement which allows for additional verbalization. The nurse could say, "You don't believe that increasing your activities affects your heart. Why don't you feel that you need restricted activity?" As the individual begins to delineate his or her reasons as to why restricted activity is *not* necessary, the nurse needs to guide the individual in examining the reality of the rationale. *Forcing* the individual to accept the fact that an M.I. has been sustained should be avoided since the individual is not ready to cope with such a realization.

In addition to allowing the individual the right to deny the loss of wellness, the nurse must assess whether the denial is interfering with medical and nursing regimens. Accurately assessing the consequence of the individual's noncompliance to prescribed therapies is necessary. Monitoring vital signs and observing for fatigue and shortness of breath when restricted activities are carried out by the individual are means of assessment. Sharing with the individual afflicted with an M.I. the data obtained from monitoring vital signs can assist in providing reality testing concerning noncompliant behavior. However, the data must be shared in a nonpunitive manner since punitive behavior on the part of the nurse will intensify repudiation.

Conveying concern and allowing the individual more control over the environment is beneficial in modifying behavior. Providing the cardiac patient the opportunity to be involved in deciding the sequence and manner in which morning care is carried out is a possible approach. By compromising and allowing involvement in care, the nurse assists the individual in altering or modifying his or her behavior to an acceptable therapeutic level.

Recognition, the second behavioral reaction to an M.I., generally begins forty-eight hours after hospitalization and extends into the discharge period. During this time the individual's physiologic condition becomes more stable and the fear of impending death decreases. The individual begins to wonder how the illness will affect his or her job, whether he or she will become dependent upon others, and whether this illness is a prelude to premature aging. Denial becomes difficult to maintain, the reality of the situation begins, and depression, overt anger, and/or negotiation emerge.

Depression results when the individual is unable to express feelings outwardly and is manifested by a sense of listlessness, expressions of hopelessness, loss of appetite, crying, and slowness in movement and speech. If these manifestations are not dealt with successfully, they hinder the individual's recovery by preventing the institution of various medical and nursing regimens. Essential nursing interventions for dealing with depression caused by myocardial infarction include reflecting upon observations made, informing the individual that these feelings are typical and that many people feel depressed about their hospital situation, and soliciting and listening to the individual's feelings about the illness. As the individual begins to verbalize his or her feelings, positive comments concerning progress made in health care status are important. Such comments may allude to improvements in cardiac function, to decreased fatigue and shortness of breath, or to improved facial color.

Instead of internalizing feelings in the form of depression, some individuals overtly express feelings in the form of anger, such as striking out at family and health team members or at circumstances in the environment. Overt anger may be expressed by refusing to remain in bed, failing to take prescribed medications, or accusing others of not caring about his or her well-being. If the individual expresses anger toward family or health team members, the anger should not be taken personally. It must not be forgotten that the angry individual experiencing loss is not necessarily angry at those nearby but at others' attributes, such as wellness, freedom, vitality, mobility, and the ability to control one's life.

To deal with the individual's anger, the family, the nurse, and other members of the health care team need to remain matter-of-fact about the anger, to listen to the individual's expression of anger, and to show neither approval nor disapproval of this behavior. Being matter-of-fact aids in preventing the individual's guilt about the expression of feelings. Listening to the individual's expression of anger provides the nurse with the opportunity for examining what it is that is anger provoking. Once the anger provoking issues are identified then the individual requires assistance in examining how best to deal with each of these issues. For example, if the anger-provoking issue is the individual's perception that he or she has lost the ability to control the surroundings, actively involving the person in planning and instituting daily health care would be advisable. Such an activity provides for involvement in the very issue that incited the person's anger. In addition, allowing the individual to express anger without repercussion aids in preventing the internalization of feelings which ultimately may lead to depression.

Negotiation also may be used by the individual with myocardial infarction. Common negotiating statements include: "If I hadn't been in such a hurry to catch that train, I wouldn't be in the hospital now" or "If *only* I had lost weight as the doctor told me." Negotiation is an attempt to deal with feelings of guilt. The individual afflicted with an M.I. may believe that his or her actions had an effect upon the present dilemma and has a need to purge such beliefs. Not until the individual with an M.I. is ready to face directly the loss of wellness will the individual be capable of relinquishing the need for negotiation.

During negotiation the nurse's primary role is to guide the individual in looking at the *reasons* for using such a maneuver. Encouraging the verbalization of guilt feelings for the purpose of purging is vital. As the individual begins to express feelings of guilt, the *reality* of these feelings needs to be examined. For example, is it realistic to believe that if one had not hurried to catch the train or if one actually had lost weight, a myocardial infarction would not have occurred? Above all, the nurse must avoid such statements as, "Oh, I'm sure everything will work out and you will be out of the coronary care unit in no time." Such a response is an abortive attempt on the part of the nurse to pacify the individual and to direct the conversation to a topic that may be more comfortable.

Reconciliation, the third behavioral response to the M.I., tends to take place after the individual is discharged from the acute care setting. It is at this time that the individual reorganizes his or her feelings about the loss of wellness and the need for anger, depression, and negotiation no longer exists.

During reconciliation the individual becomes less preoccupied with the illness and starts to develop a more factual approach to the myocardial infarction. The person begins to deal with the consequences of the M.I. by giving up some of his or her dependency upon others and by assuming responsibilities in identifying realistic goals to health care and ways of achieving these goals. For example, the individual accepts the effects that smoking has upon the heart condition and decreases the number of cigarettes smoked or stops smoking altogether. Weight reduction is taken more seriously and attempts are made to follow a reducing diet. Stress provoking situations are identified and ways of dealing with these situations are examined and instituted. In other words, the cardiac patient in reconciliation demonstrates the assumption of new ways for dealing with health care needs.

The nurse's role involves encouraging the cardiac patient in the stage of reconciliation to verbalize how he or she feels now that reconciliation of the occurrence of the myocardial infarction has taken place. Does the individual see himself or herself as being different from before the myocardial infarction? In what way has the individual assimilated the current state of health into his or her life-style? How does the individual view the effects of his or her state of health upon occupation, social life, or sexuality? These may be but a few of the individual's concerns and feelings that should be expressed verbally.

Reconciliation of the myocardial infarction is accomplished when the individual accepts his or her state of health and, with no hesitation, is able to verbalize freely to family, friends, and health team members about his or her condition. The nurse must be cognizant of the fact, however, that an individual experiencing a loss, such as an M.I., may undergo the entire process of loss (repudiation, recognition, and reconciliation) each time a new loss is encountered. Such a loss may be another myocardial infarction, a new health care problem, or a loss situation unrelated to health status.

In addition to the cardiac patient's psychological response to the M.I. itself, an emotional reaction to the coronary care unit (C.C.U.) also may be experienced. Since the unit may be viewed as a threat by the individual, it is not uncommon for anxiety to be exhibited (Cay, 1982). The anxious individual will manifest such behaviors as increased verbalization, inability to concentrate, restlessness, insomnia, tachycardia, and palmar sweating. For the individual who has sustained an M.I., three situations can be identified as producing unusually high levels of anxiety: admission to the C.C.U.; transfer from the C.C.U. to the step-down unit; and discharge from the hospital.

Upon admission and during the individual's stay in the C.C.U., orientation to the unit's routines, explanation about procedures to be performed, and description of the equipment being utilized are helpful maneuvers for allaying anxiety about environmental activities. In addition, encouraging the expression of feelings, concerns, and questions is imperative because it enables the nurse to identify situations which the individual with an M.I. finds anxiety producing. Not understanding why bedrest is necessary may provoke unnecessary anxiety in some people. Concerns about one's sexuality may prove extremely upsetting for another individual. Each person's perception of a situation is different and what one individual finds anxiety producing another individual may not. Therefore, clarifying areas of concern and misunderstanding is necessary to aid in decreasing a cardiac patient's anxiety.

Consistent and continuous nurse-patient contact must be maintained during periods of severe anxiety to establish a trust relationship. If possible, the cardiac patient should be assigned to the same nurse each shift so that a therapeutic relationship can be formed. Above all, the nurse must convey a feeling of competence in both performance and ability to foster a feeling of security. Feeling insecure about the manner in which he or she is cared for can provoke additional and unnecessary anxiety for the individual who has sustained a myocardial infarction.

Transfer from the C.C.U. and discharge from the hospital are periods when increased anxiety are experienced because of changes in the environmental milieu. Preparation for these changes should begin shortly after admission with the individual and his or her family being told that the stay in the C.C.U. is temporary and that the transfer out of the unit and eventually home is a positive step toward recovery. It is helpful for the nurses from the step-down unit to visit the individual in the C.C.U. prior to the individual's transfer. During their visit, the nurses from the cardiac step-down unit can explain how the environment and routines in their unit differ from those in the coronary care unit. This interaction not only provides the cardiac patient and the family with information about the environment, but also aids in preparing the patient psychologically for the transfer. It is helpful to have significant others present during the transfer to provide additional support and comfort. If possible, it is advisable to avoid transferring the cardiac patient at night since such a maneuver tends to increase anxiety and disorientation.

If the cardiac patient does not require cardiac monitoring upon leaving the C.C.U., the monitor should be removed one to two hours before the transfer. Some patients and their families develop a great attachment to the monitor and feel that the heart's function is dependent upon the machine, even after explanations to the contrary. Removal of the monitor several hours before the transfer provides the individual and the family time to adjust to the fact that he or she can survive without it.

Many cardiac patients transferred out of the C.C.U. find it comforting to be visited occasionally by the nursing staff from the unit since an emotional attachment for those working in the C.C.U. often has been fostered. The individual may find it easier to relate to the staff on the cardiac step-down unit when he or she does not feel abandoned by the staff of the coronary care unit. Knowing that communications exist between the nurses in both units creates a sense of security in the cardiac patient since he or she feels that there is continuity of care.

Somatic Impact

A major source of stress for the cardiac patient is the alteration of his or her life-style caused by the illness. Such alterations may include losing weight, changing dietary habits, abstaining from smoking, or changing occupations. The cardiac patient is confronted with these alterations while in the hospital, but their total impact is not realized until after he or she is discharged.

How well an individual accepts his or her altered life-style affects the ability to formulate a new body image. The individual who was well-adjusted and stable before the myocardial infarction probably will accept his or her new body image without extreme difficulty, but the individual who is less able to deal with crisis situations may encounter problems in accepting his or her changed body image caused by the illness.

The person who encounters problems in accepting himself or herself after the myocardial infarction may manifest regressive behavior and become passive and dependent. Such a person allows and expects others to take charge and tell him or her what should and should not be done. In the early course of illness such behavior is acceptable, but as the recovery period progresses this dependency should begin to subside. When passive-dependent behavior continues, difficulties in accepting one's new body image most likely have occurred.

The individual who does not want to relinquish the illness role and who continues to be dependent often enjoys the secondary gains offered by the existence of the M.I. The cardiac status becomes a central part of his or her way of life and the individual uses this physical condition as a means of exploiting interpersonal relationships. The individual not only expects to be cared for, but demands and enjoys it. Such a person may view himself or herself as being weak, as less than a man or woman, and as requiring constant care and attention. Thus, the individual truly becomes a "cardiac invalid."

In such a situation, the cardiac patient must be provided with limits in which to function and not be allowed to exploit interpersonal relationships by refusing to relinquish the illness role. Expectations need to be well-defined and this information should be relayed to both the patient and the family. For example, if the patient manifests passive-dependent behavior by expecting to be fed when capable of such a task, the food should be prepared, placed in front of the individual, and removed at the end of an allotted time. During the meal the cardiac patient may require encouragement to the effect that he or she is physically capable of feeding himself or herself and that each additional activity assumed is a step closer to recovery.

How the cardiac patient feels about himself or herself as a result of the myocardial infarction also is affected, as pointed out in Chapter 2, by the stage of development that the individual is currently experiencing. If the individual is in the stage of young adulthood (eighteen to forty-five years), difficulties may be encountered in developing a mutually satisfying friendship and/or sexual relationship (Erikson, 1963). As a result of the M.I., the individual may feel less than perfect in interactions with others and hence retreat into isolation and avoid developing or maintaining interpersonal relationships. The individual in the stage of adulthood (forty-five to sixty-five years) focuses upon establishing and guiding future generations (Erikson, 1963). If the cardiac patient believes that the myocardial infarction has made him or her an unfit person to guide others, engulfment in meeting personal needs and acquiring self-comforts may occur with the ultimate result of stagnation. Since the illness may require alterations in life-style, the cardiac patient may see the future less optimistically and may view the M.I. as a deterrent to future aspirations and successes. The stage of maturity (sixty-five years and over) is a time when the individual focuses upon his or her accomplishments, as well as having frequent thoughts of death. Physiological changes have occurred throughout life, but the occurrence of the myocardial infarction may be seen as the "final blow" of old age. Hence, the mature adult sustaining a myocardial infarction may feel despair (Erikson, 1963) and question the value of his or her achievements in life.

The nurse's role in dealing with the cardiac patient's altered body image involves assistance in integrating the changed image into the patient's life-style.

It is important to encourage the individual, regardless of developmental stage, to verbalize feelings about self. Does the individual feel incapacitated and less than acceptable to others? How does the individual feel the illness affects relationships with others? As the cardiac patient verbalizes these feelings, the nurse can assess the individual's reactions to the illness. Once it is determined how the individual feels, family and health team members can assist the individual in identifying ways of dealing with these feelings.

If the individual describes himself or herself as weak, worthless, or less than a man or woman because of the cardiac condition, the positive aspects of the individual's life should be pointed out in a realistic manner. For example, if the individual is in business, book work and business calls may be carried out at home. The individual who enjoys walks can still engage in walking, but instead of taking long walks, the individual should take short but frequent strolls because they are less tiring and less physically demanding. If the individual finds luncheon engagements a necessary part of life, a dietician should instruct him or her on ways to select low-sodium, low-caloric, and low-cholesterol foods. The major goal, when emphasizing to the cardiac patient the positive aspects of life, is to demonstrate that with alterations many of the premyocardial infarction activities can still be carried out. It is important to stress this fact since an individual who is capable of developing the ability to focus attention from somatic concerns to other objectives more readily demonstrates the ability to effectively deal with his or her new body image.

Sexual Impact

The effect that myocardial infarction has upon one's sexuality is an area that all too often is avoided by members of the health care team. The sexual ramifications of an M.I. generally begin early in the hospitalization period. Once the threat of death is no longer the major concern, the cardiac patient's behavior may shift from concern for life to concern for the quality of remaining life. As a result, the cardiac patient's behavior may manifest sexual overtones. Since limited research exists on the sexual impact of an M.I. on the female patient, the remainder of this section will deal exclusively with the *male* patient who has sustained a myocardial infarction.

Anxiety resulting from threats to one's self-image as an adult and from fear of sexual inadequacy are possible reasons for the male cardiac patient's sexually oriented behavior. Postmyocardial infarction patients usually question their sexual identity and thus find a need to test their feelings of sexuality. The male cardiac patient may respond to some members of the health care team with sexually aggressive behavior such as grabbing and touching body parts of health care providers. This behavior demonstrates a maladaptive effort on the part of the individual to test virility, autonomy, and external achievement.

Often the nurse's initial response to such behavior is embarrassment, fright, discomfort, and finally withdrawal from the individual. Such reactions feed into flirtatious behavior by demonstrating to the sexually oriented individual that the nurse is being manipulated and/or demoted as an authority figure. If the sexually aggressive male patient does not elicit such a response, he probably will alter his behavior.

Instead of supporting such behavior by reacting to it or withdrawing from it, the nurse must set firm limits for the sexually aggressive individual so as to provide feedback regarding inappropriate behavior. This can be done by informing the cardiac patient that his sexual behavior makes others uncomfortable. He must be reassured that the members of the health care team accept him as he is but that sexually aggressive behavior is not acceptable or necessary for obtaining attention. As the individual feels more competent as a person he hopefully will find less of a need to prove his sexuality by being sexually aggressive.

The individual's sexually aggressive behavior provides the nurse with an overt clue to the patient's concerns and fears about sexual well-being. The nurse should explore with the cardiac patient what his behavior means to him. Does he perceive his M.I. as a threat to his sexuality? Is he attempting to counteract his fears of sexual inadequacy or impotence by being sexually aggressive? Many of the fears experienced by the cardiac patient and the sex partner about sexual activity after a myocardial infarction are created by misconceptions and the lack of knowledge about sexual capabilities.

The most common misconceptions include the beliefs that even mild exertion will kill the cardiac patient, sexual intercourse should never again be attempted, and repeated infarctions tend to occur at orgasm. Such misconceptions often lead to a decrease in sexual activity, with the sex partner of a cardiac patient becoming passive in response to sexual activity out of fear that it may be too strenuous for the postmyocardial infarction patient. This decrease in sexual activity tends to be more marked in older cardiac patients, but it is present in all age groups (Block, Maeder, and Haissly, 1975). Unless the cardiac patient and the sex partner are counselled on postmyocardial infarction sexual activity, unnecessary strains caused by suppressed sexual needs can be created (Papadopoulos, Larrimore, Cardin, and Shelley, 1980).

In an attempt to deal with suppressed sexual needs, most cardiac patients masturbate at some time prior to discharge from the hospital. The use of masturbation may prove helpful in providing visible proof that sexual function remains. Masturbation is a natural form of sexual self-expression and can be considered an acceptable activity when the cardiac patient is capable of walking two lengths of a hospital corridor without undue side effects.

Physicians often use the tolerance of exercise as a guideline for determining tolerance of sexual intercourse. According to Hellerstein and Friedman (1970), marital coitus for the postmyocardial infarction patient requires caloric expenditure of approximately 4½ calories, with peak effort at about 6 calories, for less than thirty seconds. The heart rate generally increases up to 117 beats per minute. This physical stress very closely equals the rapid ascent of two flights of stairs or a brisk walk down the street. The postmyocardial infarction patient's tolerance of such activity can be used as a guideline for determining tolerance of sexual activity which generally can be resumed from one to four months postmyocardial infarction (Hellerstein and Friedman, 1970; Puksta, 1977).

Before the patient is discharged from the hospital both the cardiac patient and the sex partner should receive verbal and written instructions on the important issues of sexual activity. The primary goals are to assist the individual and sex partner in reestablishing their pre-illness state of sexuality, to educate the couple about sexual adaptations imposed by the myocardial infarction, and to facilitate communications between the couple for optimal sexual satisfaction (McLane, Krop, and Mehta, 1980; Murillo-Rohde, 1980).

Some of the important points to include in the patient's sexual counselling and written going-home instructions are as follows:

1. Utilize positions and maneuvers that impose less strain upon the cardiac patient.

   (a) A back-lying position for the cardiac patient with the sex partner kneeling (so that full body weight is not upon the patient) is less demanding for the individual who has sustained a myocardial infarction. Some men, however, may find this position demeaning and unacceptable, especially if they identify their role as dominant and controlling. To enforce an abrupt change in sexual style or role could further disrupt the equilibrium of the sexual relationship. Therefore, other alternatives may be suggested during the recovery period, with encouragement to resume pre-illness sexual patterns as the patient's state of wellness progresses.

   (b) A side-lying position (rear and front entry) produces less strain on the cardiac patient.

   (c) Having the cardiac patient sit in an armless chair with the sex partner sitting on his lap and facing him tends to decrease strain on the cardiac patient. It is advisable, however, for the couple to use a chair that is low enough so that they can place their feet on the floor.

   (d) Encouraging the patient to concentrate on breathing regularly during coitus because breathholding prior to orgasm may trigger a Valsalva maneuver. This maneuver causes a transient decrease in venous return and precipitates hypotension and reflex tachycardia. These factors lead to inadequate coronary perfusion and hence may cause palpitations and anginal pain in the final stage of the sexual response.

   (e) Encourage the avoidance of acts, such as penial and digital insertion into the anus, that create vagal excitement and subsequent bradycardia.

2. Avoid intercourse in certain situations.

   (a) Coitus should be avoided when extremely fatigued, when emotionally upset, and for at least three hours after consuming a heavy meal or after drinking alcohol since each of these situations places an additional workload upon the cardiac system.

   (b) An environment in which there is excessive heat or excessive cold should not be used for sexual activity since the heart has to increase its activity to maintain the body's normal temperature.

   (c) Illicit sexual encounters are generally not advised during the recovery period from a myocardial infarction because they tend to increase the risk of reinfarction and death (Wagner and Sivarajan, 1979). "Death in the saddle syndrome" is thought to occur more frequently when the cardiac patient engages in sex with a much younger partner in an unfamiliar milieu. The danger to the cardiac patient is related to deviating from one's usual partner or usual sexual pattern, thereby increasing one's stress level.

3. Be aware of warning signals that may indicate a decreased tolerance of sexual activity.

   (a) Prolonged (more than fifteen minutes) rapid heart rate and rapid breathing after sexual intercourse (at rest) should be noted and reported.

   (b) An extreme feeling of fatigue on the day after intercourse should be noted and reported.

   (c) Chest pain during or after intercourse should be noted and reported. In some instances, individuals who experience anginal pain during and after intercourse are advised to take prophylactic nitroglycerine prior to the sex act.

Occupational Impact

The occurrence of an M.I. often creates a financial strain upon the family. The financial strain may occur because of a loss in family income, the expense of the hospitalization, the request for the cardiac patient to take an early retirement, and/or the reassignment of the cardiac patient to a less strenuous job with a reduced income. As a result of the financial strain, mortgage payments, home improvement costs, and school expenses for children may become difficult to meet. Savings may dwindle and the cardiac patient's spouse may feel the need to secure employment. The employment of the male cardiac patient's spouse may not defray expenses since her income often is well below that of her husband, especially if she has not worked before. The spouse may feel additional pressures going back to work and experience tension if assumption of all the domestic responsibilities continues.

Fortunately most cardiac patients are able to return to the same job after a myocardial infarction with little modification in responsibilities. A social worker, an occupational therapist, a rehabilitation counselor, or an occupational health nurse can increase the individual's chances of returning to work by dealing directly with the employer. The employer can be kept up to date on the medical status of the employee, the employee's physical capabilities, and the employee's projected date of return to work. With patient approval, the health care provider can discuss with the employer the cardiac patient's concerns about resuming occupational pursuits. The patient, the employer, and the health care provider together can identify stress provoking situations within the work environment which may require alteration. Should it be impossible to alter the stress provoking situations, the cardiac patient may need to consider changing jobs or job activities.

The greatest single physical factor related to a safe return to work is the ability to resume gradually those activities which were usual for the post-myocardial infarction patient prior to the illness. For example, the cardiac patient may want to start out by working several hours a day, advance to half days, progress to three quarter days, and finally resume full day employment. Most individuals can return progressively to the job responsibilities they had prior to illness without angina, dyspnea, palpitations, or excessive fatigue. If any of these symptoms appear, they should be reported to the physician so that appropriate medical intervention and/or work-related alterations can be instituted. The patients who encounter difficulties in returning to the same job do so because of physical limitations or anxiety related to resumption of work responsibilities. These anxieties can be the individual's concerns or they can be concerns expressed by the spouse (Cay, 1982). It is not uncommon for the spouse to believe that the work situation was the greatest contributing factor to the occurrence of the myocardial infarction. A common statement expressed by the spouse is, "He or she just worked himself or herself into a heart attack." However, the spouse's anxiety generally diminishes markedly once the postmyocardial infarction patient *successfully* resumes work responsibilities.

The longer an individual is out of work after physical recovery is complete, the more difficult the rehabilitation process becomes. Individuals who encounter difficulties resuming work responsibilities generally require selective placement, psychiatric assistance, vocational counselling and testing, or job retraining. Such activities may be initiated by either a social worker, an occupational therapist, a rehabilitation counselor, or an occupational health nurse. Kjøller (1976) found that the incidence of recurrences of myocardial infarction was higher among individuals who had abandoned work after an M.I. than among those who resumed work shortly after recovery. Thus, resumption of meaningful and productive activity is important in the rehabilitative process for both the postmyocardial infarction patient and the family.

Social Impact

The nurse must not overlook the response of the cardiac patient's significant others toward a myocardial infarction. The spouse, children, and even friends tend to respond to the occurrence of the myocardial infarction with guilt feelings and overprotective behavior. The wife of a male cardiac patient may express her guilt feelings by blaming herself for her husband's illness and make such statements as: "I never should have let him work that hard. Maybe I nagged him too much?" Because of her feelings of guilt, the spouse often searches for a cause of the illness and frequently identifies it as overwork. In response to this identification, the spouse feels a need to protect her husband so that there will not be a recurrence. The following comments express a sense of overprotection: "I will never let him work that hard again." "I'll make sure that he relaxes more." Such maneuvers as listening for her husband's heartbeat and breathing while he sleeps are common. Some wives even have gone to the extreme of awakening their husbands to make sure that they are still alive and well. The male cardiac patient's wife does not want her husband to overexert and she does not want anything in the environment to upset him. As a result, she may assume the role of both decision maker and major breadwinner. This overprotective manner may further intensify the cardiac patient's feelings of dependence and helplessness. He may respond to this overprotective behavior with either anger or a demonstration of excessive helplessness and dependency.

Often the overprotective behavior of the spouse and the excessively dependent or angry behavior of the cardiac patient are the result of a lack of understanding about the illness and the prescribed health care regimens. The cardiac patient often is afraid to share fears with family members and becomes resentful and angry with others when they attempt to shield him or her from unpleasant information. Therefore, detailed home care instructions are necessary for both the patient and the family. The instructions should include the amount of activity to engage in at a prescribed stage of recovery and include a means of assessing the tolerance of the increased activity (e.g., changes in pulse rate and respiratory rate).

Since family members may be expected to make role and interactional changes because of the M.I., they require assistance from members of the health care team. Family members must be encouraged to verbalize their fears, concerns, and feelings of anger. The spouse especially must be encouraged not to internalize any hostile feelings. Instead he or she must be encouraged to vent feelings to members of the health care team and to examine what it is about the myocardial infarction experience that makes him or her angry. Once the anger provoking aspects of the myocardial infarction have been identified the spouse needs to examine alternatives for dealing with these situations. Support groups comprised of spouses and/or family members have proven helpful in examination and discussion of ways to deal with the myocardial experience (Razin, 1982). These groups often are available through the hospital, a rehabilitation center, or a local chapter of the American Heart Association. A member of the health care team generally serves as the group leader, whose role involves encouraging and supporting group members as they express and share their experiences with each other.

In addition, the spouse should be encouraged to discuss feelings with the cardiac patient, especially since he or she has experienced loss—loss of the mate's wellness and loss of the sense of strength that the partner once represented. Reactions to these losses frequently are exemplified by sleep disturbances and alterations in appetite. Both the spouse and the cardiac patient are better able to cope with the cardiac patient's loss of wellness when each of them is aware of the other's feelings. Since both may be reluctant to express themselves openly, each may internalize feelings that further add to manifestations of anger and guilt. Thus both require assurance that open discussion between them is much better than silence that leads to internalization of feelings.

SUMMARY

Western society's increased standard of living has led to more comforts and luxuries. No longer do people have to fight the elements for survival, but Western society's luxurious living has brought an increased incidence of coronary heart disease. Today coronary disease constitutes the leading cause of incapacitation and death in Europe and the United States. Coronary disease has become the illness of the leisure person.

When coronary heart disease, such as a myocardial infarction, results, the impact of the illness is multidimensional. The individual afflicted is faced with alterations in his or her psychological well-being, somatic identity, sexuality, occupational identity, and social role. The role of the health care team is to help the cardiac patient and the family identify the alterations in life-style that will be necessary as a result of the illness and to assist them in incorporating these alterations into their activities of daily living.

Patient Situation   Mr. C. P. is a fifty-three-year-old, married, certified public accountant who has one daughter who is currently enrolled in medical school. He is employed by a large accounting firm and has been very busy the past few months completing clients' income tax forms. Five days ago while rushing home for a quick dinner before returning to the office to complete some urgent work he suffered severe chest pains. When he arrived home, he told his wife, who encouraged him to notify the family physician about the complaint. The family physician instructed him to go directly to the community hospital emergency room. Upon examination, Mr. C. P. was diagnosed as having sustained a myocardial infarction and subsequently was admitted to the coronary care unit.

Now that his condition is stable, Mr. C. P. is being transferred from the coronary care unit to the cardiac step-down unit. One of the staff nurses from the cardiac step-down unit has just interviewed Mr. C. P. and his wife. During the interview the nurse identified problems related to Mr. C. P.'s psychological well-being, somatic identity, sexuality, occupational identity, and social role.

Following are Mr. C. P.'s nursing care plan and patient care cardex which deal with the above mentioned areas of concern.

NURSING CARE PLAN

Nursing Diagnoses	Objectives	Nursing Interventions	Principles/Rationale	Evaluations
Psychological Impact Anxiety manifested by expressed concern about being transferred from the coronary care unit to the cardiac step-down unit.	To increase Mr. C. P.'s knowledge of the reason for transfer from the coronary care unit to the cardiac step-down unit.	Explain to Mr. and Mrs. C. P. that transfer from the coronary care unit to the cardiac step-down unit is a positive progression toward recovery.	Understanding that transfer from the coronary care unit is standard procedure and a sign of progression toward recovery can aid in decreasing an individual's anxiety about his transfer.	The nurse would observe for: Mr. C. P.'s expression that his anxiety about being transferred from the coronary care unit has decreased.
	To decrease Mr. C. P.'s anxiety about the transfer from the coronary care unit to the cardiac step-down unit.	Provide Mr. and Mrs. C. P. with information about the cardiac step-down unit. For example, explain the environment and routines and how they differ from the coronary care unit.	An individual provided with information about an impending, unfamiliar situation is less likely to become anxious due to fear of the unknown.	Mr. C. P.'s increased ease with the nursing staff of the cardiac step-down unit.
		Encourage Mrs. C. P. to be present, if possible, during Mr. C. P.'s transfer from the coronary care unit to the cardiac step-down unit.	Having a family member present during transfer from the coronary care unit provides additional support and comfort for the patient.	
		Transfer Mr. C. P. during the daylight hours.	Moving a patient during the night from familiar surroundings to unfamiliar surroundings tends to increase anxiety and disorientation.	Mr. C. P.'s increased ease in the environment of the cardiac step-down unit.

(cont.)

NURSING CARE PLAN (cont.)

Nursing Diagnoses	Objectives	Nursing Interventions	Principles/Rationale	Evaluations
		Remove Mr. C. P.'s cardiac monitor several hours prior to transfer from the coronary care unit.	Some patients develop a great attachment to the cardiac monitor and feel that their heart's function is dependent upon the machine, even after it is explained to them that it is not. Removing the monitor several hours before transfer allows the patient time to deal with the fact that one can survive without the monitor.	
		Encourage the nursing staff of the coronary care unit to visit Mr. C. P. after his transfer to the cardiac step-down unit.	Patients often become emotionally attached to the nursing staff in the coronary care unit. Therefore, a patient may find it easier to relate to the nursing staff of the cardiac step-down unit if there is no feeling of abandonment by the staff of the coronary care unit.	
Somatic Impact Unresolved body image perception manifested by the belief that he is a "cardiac invalid" (passive-dependent behavior).	To assist Mr. C. P. in integrating his changed body image into his life-style.	Provide Mr. C. P. with limits in which to function. For example, instruct him on what physical activities are expected of him and encourage him to carry them out.	Setting limits for an individual provides a structured environment and communicates what is expected.	The nurse would observe for: A decrease in Mr. C. P.'s passive-dependent behavior.
		Provide positive feedback for achievements in physical activity.	Receiving positive feedback enhances an individual's feelings of self-worth.	An increase in Mr. C. P.'s independence.

	To direct Mr. C. P.'s focus from somatic concerns to other objectives.	Encourage Mr. C. P. to verbalize how he feels about himself. For example, does he view himself as incapacitated and less than acceptable to himself and others or does he feel his illness has affected his relationship with others? Point out to Mr. C. P. the positive aspects of his life—for example, possible ways in which he can carry out some of his public accountant responsibilities at home.	Determining how an individual feels about himself or herself as a result of his illness assists the health care team in identifying ways of helping the individual deal with his or her feelings. Emphasizing to the cardiac patient the positive aspects of life demonstrates that, with alterations, many pre-M.I. activities can be carried out. In addition, when an individual develops the ability to focus attention from somatic concerns to other objectives that individual more readily demonstrates the ability to return to work.	An increase in Mr. C. P.'s interest in concerns other than those of somatic nature.
Sexual Impact Potential sexual dysfunction manifested by verbalized fear about being unable to resume sexual activity.	To clarify possible misconceptions that Mr. and Mrs. C. P. may have about post-M.I. sexual activity.	Inform Mr. and Mrs. C. P. that resumption of sexual activity will be determined by the physician, but it is usually dependent upon the patient's ability to tolerate the rapid ascent of two flights of stairs.	Providing the cardiac patient and his or her sex partner with information about the patient's sexual capabilities in the post-M.I. recovery period assists in preventing the couple from avoiding sexual encounters and aids in assisting the couple in achieving their pre-illness state of sexuality.	The nurse would observe for: Mr. and Mrs. C. P.'s verbalization about their decreased fear related to engaging in sexual activity.

(cont.)

NURSING CARE PLAN (cont.)

Nursing Diagnoses	Objectives	Nursing Interventions	Principles/Rationale	Evaluations
	To provide Mr. and Mrs. C. P. with information about sexual activity in the post-M.I. recovery period.	Provide Mr. and Mrs. C. P. with the following information both in written and verbal form: 1. Utilize positions and maneuvers that impose less strain upon the cardiac patient. (a) A back-lying position for the cardiac patient with the sex partner kneeling (so that full body weight is not upon the patient) is less demanding. (b) A side-lying position (rear and front entry) is less strenuous than many other positions. (c) Having the cardiac patient sit in an armless chair with the sex partner on his lap and facing him tends to decrease strain on the cardiac patient. The couple, however, must be encouraged to use a chair that is low enough so that they can place their feet on the floor. (d) Encourage the patient to concentrate on breathing regularly during coitus.	Knowing that certain alterations in sexual activity can reduce the strain upon the heart may increase the cardiac patient's likelihood of engaging in sexual activity.	

(cont.)

2. Avoid intercourse in certain situations.
(a) Coitus should be avoided when extremely fatigued, when upset, and after consuming a heavy meal or after drinking alcohol.
(b) Environments in which there is excessive heat or excessive cold should not be used for sexual activity.
(c) Illicit sexual encounters generally are ill-advised during the recovery period.
3. Be aware of warning signals that may indicate a decreased tolerance of sexual activity.
(a) Prolonged (more than fifteen minutes) rapid heart rate and rapid breathing after sexual intercourse should be noted and reported to the physician.
(b) An extreme feeling of fatigue on the day after intercourse should be noted and reported to the physician.
(c) Chest pain during and after intercourse should be noted and reported to the physician.

Knowing that certain situations place an additional workload upon the heart increases the cardiac patient's likelihood of avoiding such situations prior to coitus.

Knowing the warning signals that may indicate a decreased tolerance to sexual activity may aid in decreasing the incidence of subsequent cardiac complications.

NURSING CARE PLAN (cont.)

Nursing Diagnoses	Objectives	Nursing Interventions	Principles/Rationale	Evaluations
Occupational Impact Potential impairment of job management manifested by ex-pressed concern about being unable to re-turn to work.	To decrease Mr. C. P.'s concern about being incapacitated be-cause of his myocardial infarction.	Inform Mr. C. P. that most cardiac patients are able to re-turn to the same jobs with lit-tle modification in responsibilities.	By knowing that the odds of an individual's returning to work after an M.I. are very good, the cardiac patient is less likely to become extremely anxious about the work situa-tion.	The nurse would observe for: Mr. C. P.'s verbalization of possible ways to alter his work situation so that he can gradually return to work.
		Encourage Mr. C. P. to think of ways he can alter his work pattern so that he can make a gradual return to his work re-sponsibilities (e.g., doing book work and making business phone calls at home).	The greatest single physical factor related to a safe return to work is the ability to re-sume gradually activities that were usual for the post-M.I. patient prior to illness.	Mr. C. P.'s verbalization that with alterations he feels that he will eventu-ally be able to resume many of his pre-M.I. work responsibilities.
		Contact social service, occu-pational therapy, a cardiac re-habilitation counselor, or an occupational health nurse about setting up communica-tions with Mr. C. P.'s em-ployer about Mr. C. P.'s return to work.	By utilizing members of the health care team prepared in occupational rehabilitation, the individual's chances of re-turning to work are increased because there are direct deal-ings with the employer. The employer is kept up to date on the employee's medical status, physical capabilities, and pro-jected date of work resump-tion.	

Social Impact			The nurse would observe for:
Self-esteem disturbance of significant other manifested by Mrs. C. P.'s expressed feelings of guilt about the occurrence of Mr. C. P.'s myocardial infarction.			
To assist Mrs. C. P. in dealing with her feelings of guilt.	Encourage Mr. and Mrs. C. P. to discuss their feelings with each other.	The wife who does not discuss personal feelings with her husband about her reaction to his myocardial infarction is likely to suppress her feelings. Also marital partners are better able to cope with the loss of wellness when each of them is aware of the other's feelings.	Open discussion of feelings between Mr. and Mrs. C. P. Mrs. C. P.'s verbalization that her feelings of guilt are beginning to subside.
	Encourage Mrs. C. P. to discuss her feelings with other members of the cardiac club.	Sharing feelings with individuals who have sustained the same loss often helps in identifying ways of coping with one's own loss.	
To assist Mrs. C. P. from becoming overprotective of Mr. C. P. because of her feelings of guilt.	Encourage Mrs. C. P. to avoid demonstrating overprotective behavior (e.g., assuming role of decision making) toward Mr. C. P.	Overprotective behavior on the part of the spouse can cause the cardiac patient to respond with impatience and extreme irritability because the patient may find such behavior or demeaning.	Mrs. C. P.'s encouraging Mr. C. P. to increase his independence as he progresses toward recovery.
	Provide Mr. and Mrs. C. P. with well-defined home-going instructions related to Mr. C. P.'s prescribed therapies. They should include the amount of activity to engage in at each prescribed stage of recovery and how to assess exercise tolerance.	Overprotective behavior on the part of the spouse is caused by lack of understanding about the cardiac patient's prescribed therapies.	

PATIENT CARE CARDEX

PATIENT'S NAME: _____ Mr. C. P. _____

AGE: _____ 53 years _____

MARITAL STATUS: _____ Married _____

SIGNIFICANT OTHERS: _____ Wife and daughter _____

MEDICAL DIAGNOSIS: _____ Myocardial Infarction _____

SEX: _____ Male _____

OCCUPATION: _____ Certified public accountant _____

Nursing Diagnoses	Nursing Approaches
Psychological: Anxiety manifested by expressed concern about being transferred from the coronary care unit to the cardiac step-down unit.	1. Explain that transfer from the coronary care unit to the step-down unit is a positive progression toward recovery. 2. Provide information about the routines and environment of the step-down unit. 3. Encourage Mrs. C. P. to be present during transfer to the step-down unit. 4. Transfer during the daylight hours. 5. Remove the cardiac monitor several hours before the transfer from the coronary care unit. 6. Visit after transfer from the coronary care unit.
Somatic: Unresolved body image perception manifested by the belief that he is a "cardiac invalid" (passive-dependent behavior).	1. Define expected physical activities. 2. Provide positive feedback for achievements in physical activities. 3. Encourage verbalization of feelings about self. 4. Point out positive aspects of life (e.g., ways to do job-related activities in the home).
Sexual: Potential sexual dysfunction manifested by verbalized fear about being unable to resume sexual activity.	1. Inform that resumption of sexual activity will be determined by physician and may depend upon physical tolerance of rapid ascension of two flights of stairs. 2. Inform of sexual maneuvers that prevent extensive cardiac strain:

(a) Utilize a side-lying coital position (rear or front entry).
(b) Utilize a back-lying coital position with the sex partner kneeling.
(c) Utilize a sitting position in an armless chair with the sex partner on the lap of the patient. (Be sure that a low chair is used so that it allows for both individuals to place their feet on the floor.)
(d) Encourage to concentrate on breathing regularly during coitus.

3. Encourage to avoid intercourse in certain situations.
   (a) When extremely fatigued, when upset, and for at least three hours after consuming a heavy meal or after drinking alcohol.
   (b) In excessively warm or cold environments.
   (c) Illicit sexual encounters.

4. Inform of warning signals that may indicate intolerance of sexual activity:
   (a) Prolonged (more than fifteen minutes) rapid heart rate and rapid breathing after sexual intercourse.
   (b) Extreme fatigue on day after intercourse.
   (c) Chest pain during and after intercourse.

1. Inform that majority of cardiac victims are able to return to same job with little modification of responsibilities.
2. Encourage to think of ways to alter work pattern to allow for a gradual return to work responsibilities.
3. Contact social service, occupational therapy, cardiac rehabilitation counselor, or occupational health nurse about setting up communications with employer about patient's resumption of work responsibilities.

1. Encourage discussion of feelings between patient and wife.
2. Encourage wife to discuss her feelings with other members of a cardiac club.
3. Encourage wife to avoid overprotective behavior.
4. Provide with detailed home-going instructions on prescribed therapies.

Occupational: Potential impairment of job management manifested by expressed concern about being unable to return to work.

Social: Self-esteem disturbance of significant other manifested by Mrs. C. P.'s expressed feelings of guilt about the occurrence of Mr. C. P.'s myocardial infarction.

REFERENCES

ALONZO, A. *Illness behavior during acute episodes of coronary heart disease.* Unpublished Ph.D. thesis, University of California, Berkeley, 1973.

BIGOS, K. Behavioral adaptation during the acute phase of a myocardial infarction, *Western Journal of Nursing Research,* 1981, *3* (2), 150–171.

BLOCK, A., MAEDER, J., and HAISSLY, J. Sexual problems after myocardial infarction, *American Heart Journal,* 1975, *90* (4), 536–537.

CAY, E. Psychological problems in patients after a myocardial infarction, *Advances in Cardiology,* 1982, *29,* 108–112.

CROOG, S., SHAPIRO, C., and LEVINE, S. Denial among male heart patients, *Psychosomatic Medicine,* 1971, *33* (5), 385–397.

ERIKSON, E. *Childhood and society,* New York: W.W. Norton & Co., Inc., 1963.

FRIEDMAN, M. *Pathogenesis of coronary artery disease.* New York: McGraw-Hill, 1969.

GENTRY, W. Preadmission behavior. In W. Gentry and R. Williams, Jr. (Eds.), *Psychological aspects of myocardial infarction and coronary care.* St. Louis: C.V. Mosby, 1979.

GOLDSTEIN, S., MOSS, A., and GREEN, W. Sudden death in acute myocardial infarction, *Archives of Internal Medicine,* 1972, 129 (5), 720–724.

HAYNES, S., and FEINLEIB, M. Type A behavior and the incidence of coronary heart disease in the Framingham Heart Study. *Advances in Cardiology,* 1982, *29,* 85–94.

HELLERSTEIN, H., and FRIEDMAN, E. Sexual activity and the post-coronary patient, *Archives of Internal Medicine,* 1970, *125* (6), 987–999.

JENKINS, C. The coronary-prone personality. In W. Gentry and R. Williams, Jr. (Eds.), *Psychological aspects of myocardial infarction and coronary care.* St. Louis: C.V. Mosby, 1979.

KENIGSBERG, D., ZYZANSKI, S., JENKINS, C., WARDWELL, W., and LICCIARDELLO, A. The coronary-prone behavior pattern in hospitalized patients with and without coronary heart disease, *Psychosomatic Medicine,* 1974, *36* (4), 344–351.

KJØLLER, E. Resumption of work after acute myocardial infarction, *Acta Medica Scandinavica,* 1976, *199,* 379–385.

MCLANE, M., KROP, H., and MEHTA, J. Psychosexual adjustment and counseling after myocardial infarction, *Annals of Internal Medicine,* 1980, *92* (4), 514–519.

MURILLO-ROHDE, I. Sexual problems of the post coronary patient, *Imprint,* 1980, *27* (5), 32–33, 68–69.

MOSS, A., and GOLDSTEIN, S. The pre-hospital phase of acute myocardial infarction, *Circulation,* 1970, *41* (5), 737–742.

PAPADOPOULOS, C., LARRIMORE, P., CARDIN, S., and SHELLEY, S. Sexual concerns and needs of the postcoronary patient's wife, *Archives of Internal Medicine,* 1980, *140* (1), 39–41.

PROTOS, A., CARACTA, A., and GROSS, L. The seasonal susceptibility to myocardial infarction, *Journal of the American Geriatric Society,* 1971, *19* (6), 526–535.

PUKSTA, N. All about sex after a coronary, *American Journal of Nursing,* 1977, *77* (4), 602–605.

RAZIN, A. Psychosocial intervention in coronary artery disease: a review, *Psychosomatic Medicine,* 1982, *44* (4), 363–387.

ROSENMAN, R., and FRIEDMAN, M. Association of specific behavior patterns in women with blood and cardiovascular findings, *Circulation,* 1961, *24* (11), 1173-1184.

TJOE, S., and LURIA, M. Delays in reaching the cardiac care unit: an analysis, *Chest,* 1972, *61* (7), 617-621.

WAGNER, N., and SIVARAJAN, E. Sexual activity and the cardiac patient. In R. Green (Ed.), *Human sexuality—a health practitioner's text.* Baltimore: Williams & Wilkins, 1979.

11 ||||||||||||||||||||||||||||||||||||||||||||||||||||||

CHRONIC OBSTRUCTIVE PULMONARY DISEASE

INTRODUCTION

Although respiration is essential to life, the ability to breathe generally is taken for granted by most individuals. People tend not to be aware of respiratory function until they consciously change their breathing patterns to meet their needs, such as taking a deep breath before diving into a pool of water. The individual suffering from chronic obstructive pulmonary disease (COPD), however, has frequent thoughts about the ability to breathe. Since respiratory function is impaired, many, if not all, of the COPD patient's daily activities are affected by the inability to breathe effectively and efficiently.

Chronic obstructive pulmonary disease is a term applied to respiratory alterations that involve persistent obstruction of bronchial airflow. Various diseases are associated with chronic obstructive pulmonary disease, but the conditions that most frequently give rise to COPD are bronchial asthma, chronic bronchitis, and pulmonary emphysema. Each of these disorders can occur independently or in combination, with bronchitis and emphysema coexisting most frequently.

Nearly 14 million people have been identified as having some form of COPD with approximately 30 thousand dying annually (Silverberg, 1983). Following heart disease, pulmonary emphysema is the second leading cause of disability among American workers receiving Social Security disability payments. Respiratory conditions create an economic impact on the individual, on the family, and on society, with the total annual cost of pulmonary emphysema and other chronic respiratory disease being more than 2 billion dollars a year (Tashkin, 1982).

ETIOLOGIC FACTORS

Although the exact causes of COPD have not been identified, various etiologic factors are considered of importance in the development of chronic obstructive pulmonary disease. These factors include: smoking, air pollution, recurrent or chronic respiratory infections, occupational exposure to irritating fumes and dusts, genetic factors, aging, and allergic factors. Of these factors *smoking* has been identified as the greatest contributor in the development of chronic obstructive pulmonary disease (American Lung Association, 1981; Spain, Siegel, and Bradess, 1973).

An unfortunate factor in COPD is that early detection is difficult and afflicted individuals often are unable to recognize the development and progression of this respiratory disorder. By the time an individual is seen in the physician's office, the structural damage to the lungs is irreversible and the individual no longer has adequate cardiopulmonary reserve to meet his or her physiological needs. Only when adequate and consistent preventive measures for facilitating respiratory function are enforced will the incidence of COPD be reduced. Therefore, the public must be educated about factors that contribute to formation of COPD with particular emphasis upon the hazards of pulmonary irritants and the necessity of prompt treatment of respiratory disorders.

Individuals afflicted with COPD are required to make many alterations in their life-styles as the disease process progresses. The impact of this chronic illness is extensive and affects the individual's psychological well-being, somatic identity, sexuality, occupational identity, and social role. The remainder of this chapter will address each of these areas of concern and how members of the health care team can assist the individual and his or her family in dealing with the multiple ramifications of the disease process.

IMPACT OF CHRONIC OBSTRUCTIVE PULMONARY DISEASE

Psychological Impact

The individual with a chronic respiratory alteration commonly experiences a variety of emotional responses due to the presence of increased weakness, dyspnea, cough, and sputum production. These responses may include anger, fear, apathy, and/or depression: anger because of the inability to carry out daily activities as others do; fear of smothering to death because of impaired respiration; anxiety about what the future will hold as a result of the chronic illness; apathy toward therapies which may seem, at times, to do little good; and depression as the individual moves between exacerbations and remissions of the disease process. Unfortunately, these responses only create additional stress for the individual's already inefficient respiratory system.

Anxiety, anger, and fear are responses that tend to be associated with *increased* skeletal muscle activity and *increased* energy expenditure that can lead to an elevated ventilatory rate and an increase in oxygen consumption. Since the individual with COPD has an inefficient respiratory system, he or she is unable to supply the air exchange necessary to meet the metabolic demands of the increase in energy expenditure brought about by such responses. By contrast, apathy and depression are responses associated with *decreased* skeletal muscle activity and *decreased* energy expenditure which leads to a ventilatory volume below that which is necessary for the provision of sufficient oxygen intake and carbon dioxide removal. A decrease in ventilatory volume associated with depression is insufficient to maintain homeostasis and the individual with chronic obstructive pulmonary disease may experience additional insult to an already compromised respiratory system. Emotional responses, whether they increase or decrease energy expenditure, can rapidly upset the precarious cardiopulmonary system in the individual with chronic obstructive pulmonary disease. The end results are respiratory imbalance and decompensation (Dudley, 1981).

In an attempt to prevent the emotional stimulation that may lead to symptom production and physiological decompensation, the individual often develops obsessional traits and compulsive rituals or retreats into isolation. The individual may internalize emotional feelings in order not to evoke a physiological response within his or her body. As a result, the individual with COPD literally lives in an "emotional straitjacket." The individual's rigid avoidance of emotionally charged situations and the use of obsessional patterns tend to perpetuate those frustrations which the individual finds he or she cannot manage adequately. In turn, the inability to handle feelings of frustration creates an increased metabolic demand that requires additional oxygen consumption. Symptoms of respiratory distress are provoked and a vicious cycle ensues. Unless the individual with chronic obstructive pulmonary disease learns techniques for handling changes in his or her emotional state, he or she will be unable to maintain the therapeutic regimen and will decrease the chances for long-term survival.

It is the responsibility of the nurse to work with the individual having COPD and with the family on ways of coping with emotionally charged situations. It is vital that the individual with respiratory problems ventilate feelings to members of the health care team and to the family. By so doing, situations that provoke emotional responses can be identified and appropriately modified. For example, anger may occur if other members of the family use the family bathroom during the time the patient usually attends to morning hygiene. Members of the family should be encouraged to discuss with the COPD patient various ways of dealing with such a situation (McDonald and Hudson, 1982). One possible solution is to set up a realistic time schedule for each individual family member's use of the bathroom.

In addition to identifying and dealing with situations that provoke emotional responses, the individual with COPD needs encouragement to verbalize his or her feelings about the illness. It must not be forgotten that the individual with COPD has a chronic illness and, as a result, must repeatedly deal with the impact of loss of wellness. Since COPD frequently fluctuates between periods of remission and exacerbation, the individual affected may reexperience the stages of loss (repudiation, recognition, and reconciliation) each time an exacerbation of symptoms occurs (see Chapter 3). This needs to be explained to family members so they are better prepared to understand why their loved one may have variations in emotional responses. When symptoms of dyspnea, weakness, cough, and sputum production become acute, the respiratory patient may exhibit more intense responses of anger, fear, anxiety, apathy, or depression. Knowing that emotional responses become more acute during periods of exacerbation, family members and the respiratory patient may desire to be more active in identifying and in avoiding situations that provoke undue emotional stimulation for the afflicted individual.

Somatic Impact

The individual with COPD is well aware of the changes that have occurred in his or her appearance and may be self-conscious about these changes. Common bodily changes may include the presence of a barrel-shaped chest, excessive sputum production, pallor or an ashen tint to the skin, noisy respirations, and the assumption of a leaning-forward, arms supported, sitting position.

The presence of a barrel chest may embarrass the afflicted individual who finds his or her appearance grotesque and verbalizes anger with such comments as, "I feel like a walking beer keg!" or "I look like an upside down Coke bottle!" In addition, the individual with a barrel chest may encounter difficulties in obtaining clothing that accommodates the enlarged upper torso while remaining attractive and becoming in appearance.

Excessive sputum production may hinder the individual with COPD from engaging in social contacts if he or she feels that frequent coughing and expectorating are not conducive to social conversation. The COPD patient may feel that members of society find the frequent expectoration distasteful and hence avoid him or her. Skin color change, another body alteration, is a difficult manifestation to hide. Each time the individual looks in the mirror, the pallor or the bluish tint to the skin may be noted. As a result, the individual may not wish to look in the mirror or be seen by others.

Noisy respirations and a sitting position of leaning forward with the arms supported may create difficulties for the individual with COPD. He or she may avoid social contacts due to the feeling that noisy respirations might be distracting to others and that the unusual sitting position could be interpreted as disinterest in social conversation, since the individual looks ready to leap from the chair.

How well the adult experiencing any of these bodily changes can cope is affected by how effectively he or she handled earlier developmental stages of life. If the individual progressed through childhood and adolescence with a favorable view of self, he or she will be better able to cope with the difficulties imposed by chronic obstructive pulmonary disease. Therapies will be adhered to more readily and periods of exacerbations will be approached with a feeling of optimism. If difficulties were encountered during the developmental stages of childhood and adolescence, feelings of helplessness, weakness, and depression are more likely to occur. The demanding qualities of the child who feels miserable and guilty about the illness may be demonstrated. The individual may express feelings of anger toward others and verbalize having been mistreated by those upon whom he or she depends (health team members and family). As a result, tensions are created, relationships become strained, and emotional responses which can lead to respiratory difficulties may be triggered.

As discussed in Chapter 2, the stage of development being experienced by the adult with COPD has an effect upon his or her ability to cope with bodily changes brought about by the illness. During the stage of young adulthood (eighteen to forty-five years) intimacy with others is of importance (Erikson, 1963) both in friendship and in a mutually satisfying sexual relationship. If the individual feels his or her bodily appearance (barrel-chest, noisy respiration, or expectoration) is displeasing to others, he or she is likely to retreat into isolation. The female with COPD may be more concerned about her outward appearance as a result of her illness, while the male is more likely to be concerned about how his respiratory function affects his ability to achieve. The stage of adulthood (forty-five to sixty-five) brings the need to establish and guide future generations in the hope of bettering society (Erikson, 1963). The adult suffering from COPD, however, may view the future bleakly and consider himself or herself as an invalid undergoing economic ruin and premature death. The stage of maturity (sixty-five years and over) is a time when the individual sees contemporaries dying and begins to contemplate his or her own death. The individual with COPD may feel extreme loneliness, express feelings by being cantankerous, and estrange himself or herself from those to whom he or she looks for friendship and assistance. The COPD patient may find this developmental stage especially difficult since the individuals he or she tends to ostracize are the very ones relied upon for assistance in carrying out therapeutic regimens and meeting needs.

The role of the nurse and other members of the health team, when dealing with the somatic impact of COPD on an individual, involves encouraging the individual to verbalize feelings, to identify ways of dealing with expressed feelings, and to formulate ways of contending with the alterations in body image. To facilitate verbalization of feelings, the COPD patient may require encouragement to express specifically how he or she feels. Does the individual feel displeasing to look at, feel like an invalid, or feel lonely and isolated? As the individual expresses his or her feelings about bodily appearance, it is helpful to include the family in the validation of the reality of these feelings. For example, if the COPD patient feels displeasing to look at, family members should be encouraged to point out to the individual that such a fact is not based on reality. This can be done by demonstrating to the COPD patient that he or she is an acceptable and worthwhile individual. Including the COPD patient in family decision making, touching, and recognizing him or her are but a few ways of demonstrating acceptance.

The nurse can assist the COPD patient in the formulation of ways to contend with the alterations in body image by pointing out that the appearance of the barrel chest, the excessive sputum production, the presence of noisy respirations, and the skin color changes are expected occurrences in the disease process. Simply realizing that his or her bodily appearance is not unusual for an individual with COPD may lessen anxiety. Encouraging the individual to carry out pulmonary hygiene routinely can aid in reducing noisy respirations and excessive sputum accumulation. The individual needs encouragement to carry out pulmonary hygiene in the privacy of the bathroom or in the bedroom, thus avoiding the concern and embarrassment of wondering how others will react to his or her appearance at that time.

Clothing can play an important role in how the individual with COPD appears to others. Encouraging the individual with a barrel chest to avoid wearing tapered and form-fitting clothing that accentuates the shape of the chest can prove beneficial. Colors that accentuate ashen or pale skin color should be avoided. Since these colors depend upon natural skin tones, they may vary among individuals. Therefore, the person may have to experiment with clothing colors in order to determine which ones look best on him or her.

Since the individual with COPD often is concerned about how others interpret his or her body position while sitting, the nurse can point out that this assumed posture is necessary to facilitate respiratory function and to decrease the workload of breathing. The individual may find that maintaining eye contact with others while communicating can decrease some of the concerns of appearing inattentive during social conversation.

Sexual Impact

The sex act involves an increase in energy expenditure, an elevated ventilatory rate, and an increase in oxygen consumption. Since the individual with chronic obstructive pulmonary disease has an inefficient respiratory system, he or she may encounter difficulties in supplying the air exchange needed to meet the metabolic demands of the increased energy expenditure created by the sex act. This does not mean that an individual with COPD cannot take part in sexual expression, but alterations in the manner of expression may be necessary.

The individual with chronic obstructive pulmonary disease may demonstrate a progressive decrease in the frequency of sexual encounters since COPD is a *chronic* condition and physiologic changes tend to occur over a period of time. Such a decrease may not be readily evident to the individual with COPD since it has occurred over the years. However, if openly approached about the frequency of coitus, the individual with chronic obstructive pulmonary disease usually will identify that his or her sexual activity has diminished with the progression of the disease process. The diminution of sexual activity may cause the male to feel that he is "less than a man" and the female to believe that she has lost her "powers of femininity."

Unless sexual function of the respiratory patient is openly dealt with, it can create difficulties in a sexual relationship. The sex partner may become frustrated because of the respiratory patient's decreased ability to take part in the sex act. He or she inadvertently may sabotage the sexual relationship by carrying out acts, prior to coitus, which increase anxiety in the environment of the respiratory patient. Using an aerosol product which elicits respiratory difficulties because of its irritating effects or alluding to the respiratory patient's incapacity because of the illness are two such examples. The outcome is the creation of additional energy expenditure and oxygen consumption which further decreases the respiratory patient's already altered ability to tolerate the demands of the sex act. On the other hand, the sex partner may avoid sexual encounters with the respiratory patient if it is believed that such activity will create undue stress for the individual. Frustrations and feelings of rejection may result for the individual with COPD; the feelings in turn, can lead to an increased energy expenditure and oxygen consumption.

The members of the health care team can assist the respiratory patient in dealing with the altered abilities to tolerate sexual activity by encouraging the patient to discuss the sex act with the sex partner. The primary goal is to encourage the individual with COPD and the sex partner to identify methods that are comfortable, tolerable, and satisfying for both of them. Possible methods which can be suggested include:

1. Avoiding activities prior to coitus which tend to create an increase in respiratory rate and shortness of breath.

2. Utilizing rest periods just prior to coitus.

3. Avoiding coitus in the morning just prior to rising if pooling of respiratory secretions is a problem. If pooling of respiratory secretions is not a problem, morning coitus may prove most desirable since the individual with COPD may be well rested.

4. Avoiding coital positions that place excessive pressure on the thorax and abdomen since these positions tend to decrease the thorax's ability to expand to its optimum. Some couples may find the "doggy-fashion" position most desirable.

5. Breathing slowly and rhythmically during the sex act. Purse lips during expiration in order to prevent bronchiole constriction and subsequent respiratory distress.

6. Encouraging the sex partner to avoid using scents, body powders, or aerosol products that might elicit sneezing or coughing.

If the individual with chronic obstructive pulmonary disease finds that he or she is unable to tolerate the additional demands placed upon the respiratory system by the sex act, the individual may find manual stimulation (masturbation) satisfying as a means of sexual expression. Oral-genital sex also is a possibility; however, since individuals with COPD often become mouth breathers it may be an undesirable method of sexual expression. Again, manual stimulation may be a preferable alternate method.

Occupational Impact

One of the greatest impacts of chronic obstructive pulmonary disease is the change it imposes upon the individual's work role. Pulmonary emphysema, a condition associated with COPD, tends to affect individuals in the fourth to fifth decades of life—a time when a working individual frequently is at the peak of his or her career. Family economic responsibilities are high at this time since offspring often are attending college, getting married, or being assisted in their careers. Since the physiologic consequences of COPD produce a decrease in energy level, the individual affected often is required to make alterations in occupational pursuits. These alterations may be minor or major and may cause a change in the individual's standard of living.

Minor alterations can occur in any job setting and generally involve minimal changes in the work environment. A minor alteration may be removing the individual from an environment that contains irritating airborne pollutants or sudden temperature changes and placing the individual in a setting that does not contain substances or temperature settings which are irritating to the respiratory tract. For example, having the individual with COPD work in an office where smoking is not permitted may be one such minor occupational alteration. If the respiratory patient is working on a factory assembly line that has irritating fumes, he or she should be moved to an assembly line that does not have such fumes. The farmer with COPD needs to consider harvesting with an air-conditioned tractor cab and wearing a scarf or mask of some type over the mouth and nose when going out into cold weather. Each of these alterations is minor in that the individual still is able to carry out basically the same occupational tasks.

Another minor alteration may include reorganizing the approach to the individual's job by simplifying and pacing activites. For example, instead of carrying a heavy object (such as an electric typewriter) across the room, the individual should put it on a cart and roll it to its destination in an attempt to maximize economy of effort. By pacing activities for the conservation of energy, the individual with COPD can continue to perform many occupational responsibilities. To illustrate, the housewife can do a few household chores that require physical exertion and then sit down and rest while she mends clothes or writes letters.

Major alterations in occupational pursuits may include changing one's job or being forced into early retirement. If the severity of the disease process (as in the case of acute episodes of asthma or bronchitis) causes frequent lost working days, the individual with COPD may find his or her job in jeopardy unless the loss of work time can be resolved. The chance of obtaining another job may be minimal since letters of recommendation sent from one employer to another often allude to missed work days. As a result, the potential employer might consider the individual with chronic obstructive pulmonary disease an economic risk and refuse to hire him or her.

The nurse's primary role in dealing with the occupational impact of chronic obstructive pulmonary disease is to assist the individual in identifying necessary alterations in the work pattern and in developing means of maintaining adequate respiratory function. Assisting the individual and the family in recognizing *potential* situations and problems in one's work that may contribute to respiratory difficulties is essential. Since each individual is different and occupations are diverse, problems related to occupational respiratory hazards will vary. Encouraging both the patient and the family to describe the occupational environment and to identify situations that they feel potentiate respiratory difficulties is a helpful beginning. Once situations which incite respiratory difficulties are identified, appropriate interventions to deal with these situations can be carried out. In addition, approaching the employer, the industrial nurse, or company physician about alterations in the respiratory patient's work situation can prove beneficial since these individuals can be directly involved in initiating necessary changes.

Encouraging the respiratory patient and his or her family in an ongoing effort to identify ways of conserving energy is vital for preventing undue stress on the individual's compromised respiratory system. If the work environment cannot allow for energy conservation; major alterations in occupational pursuits are necessary. The nurse's role is to contact members of the health care team prepared in occupational rehabilitation. Such individuals may include the social worker, the occupational therapist, or the rehabilitation counselor. Above all, the individual with COPD must be kept as active as his or her physical ability allows to facilitate adequate functioning of the respiratory system. The nurse must encourage the respiratory patient and his or her family to avoid overprotecting the patient and placing him or her in a state of dependency by not allowing engagement in any form of physical activity or by continually assisting with every physical movement.

The use of breathing retraining is necessary in increasing the individual's exercise tolerance. The individual with chronic obstructive pulmonary disease should be instructed how to allow for maximum descent of the diaphragm and to use the diaphragm and abdominal muscles to aid in emptying the lungs. The respiratory therapist is a valuable member of the health care team prepared in teaching the respiratory patient diaphragmatic strengthening exercises. The basic principle involved is relaxation during controlled coordinated respiration. The individual with COPD is instructed to use a period of short inspiration and to allow for maximum descent of the diaphragm. This maneuver is then followed by contraction of the abdomen during expiration and exhalation against pursed lips. This simple technique improves the efficiency of ventilation and gas transport, resulting in increased effectiveness in respiratory function.

Once the individual with COPD has established effective bronchial hygiene to promote the reduction of airway resistance and has learned breathing retraining, a graded exercise program should begin. Improving the individual's exercise capacity is possible despite the irreversible lung damage that is present as a result of the disease process. If the respiratory patient is not kept active, he or she is likely to become immobilized both physically and emotionally. Both states of immobility can hasten the progression of the already chronic condition. Lack of physical activity leads to stasis of respiratory secretions and to subsequent respiratory infections and distress. Emotional immobility leads to boredom which, in turn leads to physical immobility and subsequent respiratory complications.

Social Impact

Reduction in social and recreational activities often are the first noticeable changes in the life-style of the individual afflicted with chronic obstructive pulmonary disease. The individual with COPD frequently finds that he or she does not have the energy to become involved with others emotionally or in activities requiring physical expenditures. Not only is it difficult to take part in physical activities, but even talking may prove exhausting. As a result, the individual withdraws from others and may become an isolate. Since the progression of COPD occurs over a period of years, the individual afflicted may not be aware of the progressive changes occurring in his or her social activities. As the withdrawal from social contacts and involvement progresses, the individual also may become increasingly depressed as a result of the ensuing loneliness and boredom (Dudley, Glaser, Jorgenson and Logan, 1980).

In order to prevent progressive withdrawal and subsequent depression, the individual with COPD must be encouraged to take part in social activities. Alterations in activities pursued may, however, be necessary so that the individual's energy is conserved. The individual with COPD can be advised to take part in activities in which energy expenditure is not excessive, such as attending the theater or watching a sports event. The kind of social event engaged in should be discussed by the respiratory patient and his or her family prior to attendance. Whether the activity is advisable for the individual should be determined ahead of time because some social activities may elicit emotional responses such as excessive laughter, excitement, or anger which can prove deleterious to respiratory function.

To facilitate enjoyment of the social event, the individual with COPD should be advised of ways to prepare himself or herself prior to the engagement. Carrying out good pulmonary hygiene to clear the respiratory tract before going out for an evening of entertainment can aid in preventing the occurrence of accumulated respiratory secretions and subsequent respiratory difficulty during social interactions. Lying down for a period of rest prior to a social function also aids in preventing physical exhaustion and subsequent respiratory distress.

The individual with COPD may need encouragement to avoid certain social functions, such as those involving large crowds during peak periods of upper respiratory infections (early fall, midwinter, and early spring) and those taking place where excessive air pollutants exist (smoke-filled rooms). To aid in dealing with these situations, individuals with COPD are encouraged to obtain flu shots for the prevention of upper respiratory infections, to sit in the non-smoking sections of vehicles, offices, and restaurants to decrease contact with air pollutants, and to travel by car in metropolitan areas before morning and evening rush hour traffic to increase avoidance of airborne irritants.

If the individual wishes to vacation, he or she should be alerted to the fact that visiting areas that have temperatures over ninety degrees Fahrenheit can be harmful since high temperatures increase metabolism which leads to an increase in oxygen consumption. If such circumstances are unavoidable, arrangements should be made for the provision of an air conditioner. By the same token, exposure to very cold weather can be harmful and elicit respiratory distress since cold weather can irritate the respiratory tract and lead to bronchospasms. If these temperatures are unavoidable, covering the mouth and nose with a scarf to warm the air that enters the respiratory tract is helpful. Since allergies can produce respiratory difficulties for the individual with COPD, the areas to be visited need to be identified. For example, ragweed, a common source of allergic reactions, is prevalent in the central and eastern parts of the United States, but it does not grow in the far west and south. Therefore, during the flowering season of ragweed, it would be preferable for the individual with COPD to take a trip to California or southern Florida. The individual with COPD also needs to be sensitive to areas of high altitude. Travel in places such as Pikes Peak and some passes through the Rocky Mountains may prove hazardous to the individual with COPD because of the decreased prevalence of oxygen. The individual should check with his or her physician to determine which altitude is advisable.

In addition to dealing with allergens, excessive temperature changes, and altitudes, the individual with COPD needs to be sensitive to the deleterious effect smoking has upon his or her respiratory tract. Since smoking is a habit often cultivated during social interaction, the individual with COPD may find it difficult not to smoke if everyone else is smoking. If the individual has been smoking for a number of years, it may prove difficult to alter his or her smoking habit. To aid in altering smoking habits, the following suggestions may prove helpful:

1. Place cigarettes in an inconvenient location.
2. Hide ashtrays.
3. Buy one pack of cigarettes at a time.
4. Do not carry matches or a cigarette lighter.
5. If the urge to smoke occurs, wait a few minutes and then immediately change the activities or thoughts being pursued.
6. Try to go longer each day without a cigarette.
7. Slowly stop smoke-linked habits such as a cup of coffee and a cigarette, a meal and a cigarette, or a party and a cigarette.
8. Stop smoking while in bed with an illness.
9. Stop smoking during vacation or on a relaxing day if the habit of smoking is associated with stressful situations.
10. Have a friend stop smoking at the same time.
11. Attend a smoking cessation course.
12. Utilize a replacement for the oral gratification obtained from smoking. For example: chewing gum, chewing toothpicks, or sucking hard candy.

The patient with COPD who is attempting to stop smoking may require a replacement—such as chewing gum, chewing toothpicks, or sucking hard candy—for the oral gratification obtained from smoking. Unfortunately, some individuals may increase their food consumption as a means of oral gratification replacement once they stop smoking, with resultant weight gain. If the individual with COPD is unable to stop smoking completely, he or she can decrease exposure to respiratory irritating smoke. Acts to decrease the hazards of smoke inhalation include:

1. Selecting a cigarette with less tar and nicotine.
2. Smoking half the cigarette and discarding the other half.
3. Taking fewer and smaller puffs on each cigarette.
4. Cutting down on inhaling.

Above all, encouragement from family, friends, and members of the health care team is necessary as the individual alters smoking habits. Encouragement to alter smoking habits and praise for progress made toward alterations in smoking habits are helpful. If possible family, friends, and members of the health care team should avoid smoking in the presence of the individual with COPD since the smoke is a respiratory irritant and having a smoker present may increase the individual's desire to smoke. If appropriate precautions are carried out to avoid respiratory irritants and infections and if the conservation of energy is kept in mind, the individual with COPD can engage in a fulfilling and enjoyable social life.

SUMMARY

Respiration is a vital activity; therefore, alterations in respiratory function can affect man's ability to carry out the activities of daily living. The individual with chronic obstructive pulmonary disease is continually aware of the effect that the disease process has upon his or her life-style.

Chronic obstructive pulmonary disease (COPD) is a term applied to respiratory alterations that involve persistent obstruction of bronchial airflow. Bronchial asthma, chronic bronchitis, and pulmonary emphysema are the three conditions that most frequently give rise to COPD.

The exact cause(s) of COPD is not known. However, various etiologic factors are considered important in the development of the condition. Of all the etiologic factors, research has identified smoking to be of greatest importance in the development of the chronic illness.

Since one's respiratory function can have an affect upon the ability to carry out activities of daily living, the impact of this chronic condition can affect psychological well-being, somatic identity, sexuality, occupational identity, and social role. Members of the health care team need to assist the individual with chronic obstructive pulmonary disease in identifying how the presence of this chronic respiratory illness affects the individual's everyday life and to aid him or her in dealing with each of these alterations.

Patient Situation   Mr. P. E. is a sixty-seven-year-old retired sawmill employee with a history of chronic obstructive pulmonary disease. He has been smoking 2½ packs of cigarettes a day for the past 30 years. He and his wife live with their divorced daughter and her three teenage children. Since neither Mr. P. E., Mrs. P. E., nor their daughter works, the family is supported by welfare assistance.

Mr. P. E. is currently being treated for an acute respiratory infection in the county welfare clinic on an outpatient basis. Mrs. P. E. and daughter bring Mr. P. E. to the clinic weekly for a checkup. During the assessment the clinical nurse was able to identify patient-centered problems related to Mr. P. E.'s psychological well-being, somatic identity, sexuality, occupational identity, and social role.

Below are Mr. P. E.'s nursing care plan and patient care cardex dealing with each of these areas of concern.

NURSING CARE PLAN

Nursing Diagnoses	Objectives	Nursing Interventions	Principles/Rationale	Evaluations
Psychological Impact Anger manifested by expressed disgust about teenage grandchildren occupying the bathroom for extended periods of time.	To decrease Mr. P. E.'s anger. To assist Mr. P. E. in appropriately expressing his anger.	Encourage Mr. P. E. to verbalize his anger to his family.	A family aware of situations that provoke emotional responses in the individual with chronic obstructive pulmonary disease is better prepared to identify ways of dealing with emotionally charged situations.	The nurse would observe for: Increased verbalization between Mr. P. E. and his family about situations that provoke an emotional response.
	To prevent respiratory distress caused by feelings of anger.	Encourage Mr. P. E.'s family to identify and discuss with Mr. P. E. ways in which they can alleviate the difficulties of shared bathroom usage (e.g., set up a time schedule for extended periods of bathroom use).	Actively involving the entire family in making a decision about a matter that affects each family member facilitates the likelihood that each member will adhere to the final decision. Appropriately expressing emotional feelings instead of internalizing them aids in decreasing the likelihood of respiratory symptoms and physiological decompensation in the individual with COPD caused by an emotional reaction.	A lack of or a decrease in Mr. P. E.'s respiratory symptoms during episodes of anger.

(cont.)

NURSING CARE PLAN (cont.)

Nursing Diagnoses	Objectives	Nursing Interventions	Principles/Rationale	Evaluations
Somatic Impact Body image alteration manifested by verbalization that sputum production is disgusting and displeasing.	To assist Mr. P. E. in dealing with his altered body image.	Point out to Mr. P. E. that the presence of his excessive sputum production is an expected change related to chronic obstructive pulmonary disease.	Realizing that certain bodily changes tend to occur with COPD helps decrease anxiety related to an altered body image.	The nurse would observe for: Decreased expression by Mr. P. E. that his bodily appearance is disgusting.
		Encourage Mr. P. E. to carry out his pulmonary hygiene routinely and whenever he expects or notes a buildup in respiratory secretions.	Pulmonary hygiene aids in decreasing the accumulation of respiratory secretions and subsequent embarrassment as a result of excessive expectoration.	Mr. P. E.'s routine adherence to good pulmonary hygiene.
		Encourage Mr. P. E. to carry out his pulmonary hygiene in the privacy of his room or in the bathroom.	Privacy during pulmonary hygiene helps decrease the concern and embarrassment of wondering how others will react to bodily appearance at this time.	
		Encourage Mr. P. E. to verbalize how he feels about himself.	Open ventilation of feelings about bodily appearance can aid in the individual's ability to identify ways of coping with these changes.	Open expression by Mr. P. E. about his self-image, and likely methods for dealing with his altered bodily appearance.
	To assist Mr. P. E. from isolating himself from others.	Point out to Mr. P. E.'s family that Mr. P. E. harbors concerns about his bodily appearance and requires expressions of acceptance.	Expressions of acceptance by family members toward the individual with COPD who is undergoing a change in body image assists in preventing the patient from isolating himself or herself from others as a result of feelings of rejection.	A decrease in Mr. P. E.'s attempts to isolate himself from others.

Sexual Impact				
Sexual dysfunction manifested by expressed concern about a decreased tolerance of sexual activity because of shortness of breath.	To enhance Mr. P. E.'s feelings of masculinity.	Encourage Mr. P. E. to discuss openly with Mrs. P. E. his concerns about his sexual capabilities.	Unless sexual functions of the individual with COPD are openly dealt with, difficulties in a sexual relationship can result. By openly discussing their sexual activity, the individual with COPD and his or her sex partner are more likely to identify and prevent the occurrence of sexual sabotaging acts that may unknowingly be carried out prior to coitus.	The nurse would observe for: Mr. P. E.'s verbalization of an increased satisfaction in his sexual relationship with his wife.
	To facilitate a satisfying sexual relationship for both Mr. and Mrs. P. E.	Encourage Mr. P. E. to: 1. Avoid activities prior to coitus that tend to create an increase in respiratory rate and shortness of breath. 2. Utilize rest periods prior to coitus. 3. Avoid coitus in the morning just prior to rising if pooling of respiratory secretions is a problem. If pooling of respiratory secretions is not a problem, morning coitus may prove most desirable since Mr. P. E. would be most rested at this time. 4. Avoid coital positions that place excessive pressure on the thorax and abdomen.	Preventing excessive demands upon the respiratory tract prior to coitus enhances the respiratory patient's ability to tolerate intercourse. Preventing pressure on the abdomen and rib cage enhances the thorax's ability to expand to its optimum, thereby decreasing the chances of respiratory distress.	

(cont.)

NURSING CARE PLAN (cont.)

Nursing Diagnoses	Objectives	Nursing Interventions	Principles/Rationale	Evaluations
		5. Breathe slowly and rhythmically during the sex act. Purse lips during expiration.	Breathing maneuvers that enhance respiration prevent respiratory distress and assist in increasing the respiratory patient's ability to tolerate sexual activity.	
		6. Advise Mrs. P. E. not to use perfumes, body powders, or aerosol products that elicit sneezing or coughing episodes.	Avoiding air pollutants prior to and during coitus aids in preventing the occurrence of respiratory difficulty caused by irritation of the respiratory tract.	
Occupational Impact Decreased activity tolerance manifested by expressed concern about the occurrence of fatigue and respiratory distress after carrying out odd jobs around the house.	To reduce the incidence of fatigue and respiratory distress after work.	Encourage Mr. P. E. to plan ahead in order to maximize economy of physical effort (e.g., instead of carrying a heavy object across the room placing it on a cart with wheels and rolling it to its destination). Encourage Mr. P. E. to pace his activities (e.g., work for thirty minutes and rest for ten minutes).	Planning and spacing activities for the conservation of energy can prevent undue respiratory distress. Planning and spacing activities for the conservation of energy can enhance the individual's ability to continue to carry out many occupational responsibilities.	The nurse would observe for: Mr. P. E.'s verbalization that by properly carrying out acts of energy conservation his respiratory distress and fatigue are decreased.

Nursing Diagnosis	Goal	Nursing Interventions	Rationale	Evaluation
	To maintain Mr. P. E.'s optimal level of physical performance.	Encourage Mr. P. E. to build up gradually his level of physical activity each day (e.g., increasing the distance walked by a few yards). Encourage Mr. P. E. to avoid completely stopping his physical activity.	Gradually increasing an individual's exercise capacity can decrease the chances of respiratory distress resulting from overexertion. Immobilization leads to stasis of respiratory secretions and subsequent respiratory infection and distress.	Mr. P. E.'s verbalization that he has gradually increased his physical activity with minimal resulting distress.
Social Impact Health management deficit manifested by verbalized anxiety about inability to stop smoking.	To assist Mr. P. E. in decreasing his cigarette consumption.	Encourage Mr. P. E. to: 1. Place cigarettes in an inconvenient location. 2. Hide ashtrays. 3. Buy one pack of cigarettes at a time. 4. Avoid carrying matches or a cigarette lighter. 5. Wait a few minutes and then immediately change the activities or thoughts being pursued if the urge to smoke occurs. 6. Try to go longer each day without a cigarette. 7. Slowly stop smoke-linked habits such as a cigarette and a meal or a cigarette and a cup of coffee. 8. Stop smoking while in bed with an illness. 9. Stop smoking during vacation or on a relaxing day if the habit of smoking is associated with stressful situations.	Increasing understanding about factors that contribute to smoking can enhance the desire to control smoking habits. Increasing the difficulty to smoke can decrease the desire to smoke. Decreasing the availability of smoking materials may decrease the frequency of smoking.	The nurse would observe for: Mr. P. E.'s verbalization about a decrease in the number of cigarettes that he is smoking.

(cont.)

NURSING CARE PLAN (cont.)

Nursing Diagnoses	Objectives	Nursing Interventions	Principles/Rationale	Evaluations
		10. Have a friend stop smoking at the same time. 11. Attend a smoking cessation course. 12. Utilize a replacement for the oral gratification obtained from smoking, for example, chewing gum, chewing toothpicks, or sucking hard candy.	Interacting with individuals attempting to alter a similar habit can provide emotional support and may facilitate the alteration of the habit. Developing adaptive responses to the oral need of smoking can facilitate in altering one's desire to smoke.	
		Encourage Mr. P. E.'s family to support him in his efforts to alter his smoking habits.	Support from significant others facilitates in the accomplishment of the alteration of a habit.	
		Encourage Mr. P. E.'s family to provide positive feedback for his attempts and accomplishments made in the alterations of his smoking habit.	Positive feedback for accomplishments facilitates feelings of self-worth.	

224

PATIENT CARE CARDEX

PATIENT'S NAME: _____ Mr. P. E. _____   MEDICAL DIAGNOSIS: _____ Chronic obstructive pulmonary disease _____

AGE: _____ 67 years _____   SEX: _____ Male _____

MARITAL STATUS: _____ Married _____   OCCUPATION: _____ Retired sawmill employee _____

SIGNIFICANT OTHERS: Wife, daughter, and three teenage grandchildren

Nursing Diagnoses	Nursing Approaches
Psychological: Anger manifested by expressed disgust about teenage grandchildren occupying the bathroom for extended periods of time.	1. Encourage verbalization of anger to family. 2. Encourage family and patient to identify and discuss ways of alleviating the bathroom difficulties.
Somatic: Body image alteration manifested by verbalization that sputum production is disgusting and displeasing.	1. Point out that excessive sputum production is an expected change related to COPD. 2. Encourage use of pulmonary hygiene on a routine basis and whenever sputum buildups are expected. 3. Encourage to carry out pulmonary hygiene in the privacy of the bathroom or bedroom. 4. Encourage verbalization of feelings about self. 5. Point out to family that patient harbors concerns about bodily appearance and requires expression of their acceptance.

(cont.)

PATIENT CARE CARDEX (cont.)

Nursing Diagnoses	Nursing Approaches

Sexual: Sexual dysfunction manifested by expressed concern about a decreased tolerance of sexual activity because of shortness of breath.	1. Encourage open discussion between patient and wife about patient's sexual capabilities.
	2. Encourage:
	  (a) Avoidance of activities prior to coitus that create an increase in respiratory rate and shortness of breath.
	  (b) Utilization of rest periods prior to coitus.
	  (c) Avoidance of coitus in morning if pooling of secretions is a problem.
	  (d) Avoidance of coital positions that place excessive pressure on the thorax and abdomen.
	  (e) Use of slow and rhythmical breathing using pursed-lip breathing during the sex act.
	  (f) Avoidance of the use of perfumes, body powders, or aerosol-applied products by wife prior to coitus that elicit sneezing or coughing.

Occupational: Decreased activity tolerance manifested by expressed concern about the occurrence of fatigue and respiratory distress after carrying out odd jobs around the house.	1. Encourage to plan ahead in order to maximize economy of physical effort. 2. Encourage to pace activities. 3. Encourage to gradually build up level of physical activity each day. 4. Encourage to avoid completely stopping physical activity.

Social: Health management deficit manifested by verbalized anxiety about inability to stop smoking.	1. Encourage to:
	  (a) Place cigarettes in inconvenient place.
	  (b) Hide ashtrays.
	  (c) Buy one pack of cigarettes at a time.
	  (d) Avoid carrying matches or a cigarette lighter.
	  (e) Wait a few minutes and then change activity or thoughts being pursued when urge to smoke occurs.
	  (f) Try to go longer each day without a cigarette.
	  (g) Slowly stop smoke-linked habits (e.g., a cigarette and a cup of coffee).
	  (h) Stop smoking while in bed with an illness.
	  (i) Stop smoking during vacation or on a relaxing day if smoking tends to be associated with stressful situations.
	  (j) Have a friend stop smoking at the same time.
	  (k) Attend a smoking cessation course.
	  (l) Utilize a replacement for the oral gratification obtained from smoking (e.g., gum chewing).
	2. Encourage family to be supportive during patient's efforts to alter smoking habits.
	3. Encourage family to provide positive feedback for attempts and accomplishments made by the patient in alterations in smoking habit.

REFERENCES

American Lung Association. *Chronic obstructive pulmonary disease.* New York: American Lung Association, 1981.

DUDLEY, D. Coping with chronic COPD: therapeutic options, *Geriatrics,* 1981, *36* (11), 69–74.

DUDLEY, D., GLASER, E., JORGENSON, B., and LOGAN, D. Psychosocial concomitants to rehabilitation in chronic obstructive pulmonary disease: Part I—Psychosocial and psychological consideration, *Chest,* 1980, *77* (3), 413–419.

ERIKSON, E. *Childhood and society.* New York: W.W. Norton and Co., Inc., 1963.

McDONALD, G., and HUDSON, L. Important aspects of pulmonary rehabilitation, *Geriatric,* 1982, *37* (3), 127–132, 134.

SILVERBERG, E. Cancer statistics, 1983, *Ca-A Cancer journal for clinicians,* 1983, *33* (1), 9–25.

SPAIN, D., Siegel, H., and BRADESS, V. Emphysema in apparently healthy adults, *Journal of the American Medical Association,* 1973, *224* (3), 322–325.

TASHKIN, D. Chronic obstructive pulmonary disease: management after diagnosis. In P. Selcky (Ed.), *Pulmonary disease.* New York: John Wiley, 1982.

12 ‖‖‖

DIABETES
MELLITUS

INTRODUCTION

Metabolic alterations, such as Addison's disease, hyperthyroidism, hypothy-
roidism, Cushing's syndrome, and diabetes mellitus, constitute some of the major health care problems in the United States today. Since diabetes mellitus is
one of the most commonly encountered metabolic disorders, this chapter will
deal exclusively with the impacts created by this disease.

Diabetes mellitus is defined as a chronic metabolic alteration involving a
disorder in carbohydrate metabolism which eventually leads to derangement of
protein and fat metabolism. The exact cause of diabetes mellitus is unknown;
however, the condition inevitably develops as a result of persistent insulin deficiency. Not only is this a chronic condition requiring lifelong therapy, but frequently it is associated with the major causes of death in the United States:
ischemic heart disease, hypertension, and renal failure (Silverberg, 1983). Certain individuals are identified as being especially susceptible to diabetes, including older people, obese people, women who have had many children, and
people who have diabetic relatives.

Between 4 million and 6 million individuals in the United States have
diagnosed diabetes mellitus with approximately 34 thousand dying each year
from complications of the disease (Silverberg, 1983). It is evident that an increasing number of people are diagnosed each year. No doubt this is related to
the facts that people live longer, a large proportion of more susceptible individuals are alive, diagnostic tests continually are being improved, and the
public is becoming increasingly aware of this alteration.

CLASSIFICATION OF DIABETES MELLITUS

Juvenile diabetes and adult-onset diabetes are the two identifiable types of diabetes. In juvenile diabetes the condition generally appears before the age of fifteen years, manifests an absolute deficiency in insulin, and can be controlled by insulin injections along with a therapeutic diet and exercise program. By comparison, adult-onset diabetes usually occurs in obese individuals over forty years of age, manifests a partial insulin deficiency, and often is controlled by diet and oral hypoglycemic agents.

Although juvenile and adult-onset diabetes may differ in age of onset, etiology, and means of treatment, both tend to demonstrate the same four cardinal symptoms: polyuria, polydypsia, weight loss, and polyphagia. Polyuria (frequent urination) occurs as a result of decreased water reabsorption by the renal tubules due to osmotic activity of the increased blood glucose levels. Polydypsia (excessive thirst) results from polyuria which can create a state of dehydration and subsequent thirst. Weight loss may result since glucose is not available to the cells and since fat and protein stores are broken down and utilized for energy. Polyphagia (excessive hunger) occurs as a result of tissue breakdown and wasting which, in turn, creates a state of starvation compelling the individual to eat in excess.

Regardless of whether the adult sustained the diabetes during childhood or during adulthood, many of the ramifications of the impact of the illness are the same. Diabetes mellitus has an effect upon the stricken individual's psychological well-being, somatic identity, sexuality, occupational identity, and social role.

IMPACT OF DIABETES MELLITUS

Psychological Impact

Studies to determine exactly which behavioral manifestations set the diabetic apart from other individuals have been pursued by researchers. Their findings have identified behaviors such as passivity, dependency, immaturity, insecurity, indecisiveness, and masochism, all of which are characteristics found in individuals with other chronic illnesses (Dunn and Turtle, 1981; Hann, 1979; Wilkinson, 1981). Clinicians therefore refute the association of any specific personality traits with diabetes mellitus and feel that behavioral manifestations exhibited by the diabetic are reactions to the condition itself.

How the newly diagnosed diabetic responds to the illness is of importance to all members of the health care team. The individual's response to the stress can be predicted somewhat by how he or she has dealt with stress in the past. Has the individual been able to deal with prior losses? What have been his or her responses to previous stressors? For some diabetics the presence of the illness serves as an outlet for feelings of frustration and inadequacy while for others it may provide a fast means of reestablishing a nurturing relationship. When assessing the diabetic's response to illness, the nurse should be cognizant of the role diabetes mellitus plays in the life of the individual affected.

Often the newly diagnosed diabetic views the illness as a lifelong disability that negatively affects every aspect of his or her life. Such a response can create difficulties for the nurse when attempts are made to teach necessary health care therapies. If the meaning of food goes beyond that of meeting one's nutritional needs, it may be extremely difficult for the diabetic to make alterations in eating habits. Before initiating instructions on necessary therapies, such as dietary alterations and insulin injections, it is advisable for the nurse to assess the meaning the therapy holds for the diabetic. Does he or she view dietary restrictions as punishment? Does he or she perceive taking insulin as an unwanted burden? During the assessment process the nurse can obtain data to address these issues. Once the meaning which the therapy holds for the diabetic has been identified, the nurse and the diabetic can proceed with the necessary health care instruction.

As the therapies are carried out, the meaning which they hold must be incorporated into the diabetic's therapeutic program. For example, if dietary habits have religious or cultural connotations, the patient, the nutritionist, and the nurse can plan the diet with these considerations in mind. Many clinicians have found that a more liberal approach to the diabetic diet is better because the diabetic is more likely to adhere to it than to a strictly regimented approach. If the diabetic demonstrates passivity and dependency about injecting himself or herself, the nurse must structure the teaching plan accordingly. On the first teaching encounter, the nurse can assume the entire task of insulin administration. With each subsequent insulin injection, the diabetic should be encouraged to assume more responsibility for the drug administration. As the diabetic progresses toward independence in self-administration of insulin, positive feedback needs to be provided. This teaching approach should continue until the diabetic can independently administer his or her own insulin. In order to provide appropriate teaching of insulin administration in the acute care setting the educational process cannot be left until the day prior to discharge. In addition, as the diabetic is instructed about diet and drug therapy, family members need to be included since they serve both as augmentors and backups for the diabetic as he or she carries out health care regimens.

The effect that stress has upon the diabetic is of extreme importance in planning and dealing with his or her care. Stress may include experiences such as a vacation, a job change, pregnancy, an infection, surgery, trauma, or loss of a loved one. Stress, either physiological or psychological, can evoke bodily reactions that are unfavorable to the control of diabetes. The sympathetic nervous system is activated in times of stress resulting in an increased production of epinephrine. This increased epinephrine production activates glycogenolysis and a subsequent increase in blood glucose. During stress an acceleration of biologic forces opposing the peripheral tissue utilization of insulin occurs along with an increased release of hepatic glucose. The result again is an increased blood glucose. These normal responses to stress can upset the diabetic's precarious metabolic state and have been known to be precipitating factors that have led to the diagnosis of diabetes mellitus in some individuals (Luckmann and Sorensen, 1980).

To assist the diabetic and the family in coping with stress, the nurse needs to encourage them to identify and discuss any situation which is stressful for the diabetic. To illustrate, if the diabetic finds certain food preparations repulsive, he or she and members of the family may wish to discuss how best to prepare the food to enhance its palatability for everyone. If frequent telephone calls from friends during mealtime produce stress for the diabetic, the nurse should encourage the family to investigate alternatives to prevent disruptions during family dining. Regardless of which situations are stressful to the diabetic, they must be identified and dealt with by the diabetic and the family. If they are ignored, the diabetic's metabolic state is likely to be in a constant state of instability.

While initiating diabetic care and teaching, the nurse must consider the occurrence of behavioral responses to an alteration in glucose level. Behavioral changes, which might occur prior to a metabolic upset could include nervousness, difficulty in concentrating, mood swings, irritability, shakiness, and drowsiness. If any of these behavioral responses is identifiable, the diabetic's physical state should be assessed. Issues to be addressed should include whether the diabetic has taken insulin or hypoglycemic agents, has eaten too much or too little, has recently engaged in excessive exercise or encountered a stressful situation. Once the answer to these issues is addressed and the diabetic's presenting signs and symptoms (e.g., hunger, excessive perspiration, thirst, headache) are evaluated, it can be determined whether a state of hyperglycemia or hypoglycemia is occurring. When the metabolic state is identified the appropriate medical regimens can be instituted.

While assessing the diabetic's behavioral responses, the nurse needs to be aware of whether the diabetic is attempting to gain control of others or of the environment. In other words, is the diabetic using the illness as an excuse to manifest irritability or overt anxiety? In an attempt to determine if the illness is being used for secondary gains, the nurse, the diabetic, and the family should discuss the diabetic's behavioral reactions. Should the diabetic be using the illness for secondary gains, this fact needs to be pointed out and the diabetic should be encouraged to examine why he or she finds it necessary to use the illness as an attention-seeking device. More appropriate means of obtaining attention from others should be identified and ways of obtaining this attention should be delineated. If the behavioral reactions related to secondary gains are not dealt with openly, the diabetic is likely to increase turmoil within the family structure, thus increasing the possibility of stressful situations. These situations, in turn, upset the diabetic's already precarious metabolic state.

Somatic Impact

Somatic alterations caused by diabetes mellitus may range from no outward changes in bodily structure to loss of an entire body part, such as an extremity. When assessing the somatic impact of diabetes, the nurse must assess bodily changes brought on by the disease process, as well as the meaning that each required health care therapy holds for the individual. Some of the most frequently encountered somatic alterations brought on by the disease process include loss of sensation in peripheral body parts, ulceration formation, and blindness. These alterations create unique impacts upon the diabetic's somatic integrity; therefore, each will be discussed separately.

When loss of sensation in peripheral body parts occurs due to neuropathy, the diabetic no longer perceives his or her body structure as it once existed since retraction in body boundaries is likely to prevail. One of the greatest problems that develops with loss of sensation to body parts is the potential for injury. When the body parts no longer have normal sensation, the diabetic is more likely to burn, cut, or injure himself or herself. Therefore, the diabetic and the family require assistance in identifying and carrying out ways of preventing injury. Measures to prevent injuries include not using heating pads to warm the feet, not going barefoot, and not reusing disposable needles for insulin injections. Burns and infections resulting from injuries can have devastating effects since the diabetic's healing process is impaired as a result of altered blood glucose levels.

Ulcerations, especially to the lower extremities, are another bodily alteration brought on by the diabetic disease process. The ulcerations are a result of vascular changes and can range from small to very large wound sites. The diabetic's response to the ulcerations tends to be anger due to the perception of having lost control of one's bodily functions. To deal with the loss experienced by the individual with diabetes mellitus, the content presented in Chapter 3 should be utilized. In addition, to facilitate the diabetic's resumption of control, the patient should be provided with self-care activities involving the ulcerations. Such activities can include the application of medication and dressings to the ulcerated site. Demonstrating care of the wound to the diabetic and the family and requiring a return demonstration proves most helpful. The nurse working in the community setting may find it necessary to make frequent home visits until the diabetic and the family feel comfortable in dealing with wound care.

Giving encouragement about the improvement in the healing of the ulceration also is beneficial. However, at no time should the diabetic receive false reassurance. When stating that improvement has occurred in the wound, it is best for the nurse to state the improvement in specific terms, such as: "The ulceration appears less inflamed", "The ulceration has more granulation tissue", or "The tissue surrounding the ulceration has a healthy color." Unfortunately, some diabetics require amputations because ulcerations and/or vascular

changes have become uncontrollable. Such a procedure creates a major alteration in body boundaries and subsequent alterations in body image. The reader
is advised to consult Chapter 4 for material related to the care of an individual
undergoing an amputation.

Blindness is another bodily change brought on by the vascular changes
resulting from the disease process of diabetes mellitus. Approximately 10 percent of blindness (in all age groups) is a result of diabetic retinopathy. For individuals between the ages of forty-five and seventy-four, 20 percent of all new
cases of blindness are a result of diabetic retinopathy. When blindness occurs,
one's body image is altered since sensory reception is affected. To aid the
diabetic in dealing with alterations in visual function, the reader is advised to
consult Chapter 9 for appropriate material.

The diabetic's response to loss of sensation in peripheral body parts, ulceration formation, amputation, or blindness is affected by the diabetic's developmental stage at the time of the body alteration. If the diabetic is in the
stage of young adulthood (eighteen to forty-five years), he or she may find such
complications hinder the formation of intimate relationships with others
(Erikson, 1963). He or she may believe that the ulcerated or missing extremity
or the visual impairment makes him or her less than perfect and, therefore, an
undesirable companion in both friendship and in a sexually satisfying relationship. The female diabetic may find ulcerations more difficult to deal with since
she tends to devote more attention to her body than does the male diabetic. On
the other hand, the male diabetic may encounter more difficulty in coping with
blindness since he is more likely to interpret such a change as an impediment to
achievement.

The diabetic experiencing the stage of adulthood (forty-five to sixty-five
years) may encounter difficulties in achieving the task of generativity (Erikson,
1963). Ulcerations, an amputation, or blindness may lead the diabetic to believe
that he or she is ill-equipped to guide future generations with the hope of improving society. An ulcerated or missing limb or blindness may be interpreted
as a prelude to premature old age, and as a result the diabetic may retreat into
isolation and self-pity.

The stage of maturity (sixty-five years and older) brings with it the task of
ego integrity (Erikson, 1963). If the mature adult has developed a strong sense
of self-worth and is able to place value in past life experiences, he or she most
likely will not develop a feeling of despair. But if the individual has not
developed a strong sense of self-worth, he or she may view bodily changes, such
as an amputation or blindness, as signs of premature death. Frequent thoughts
of death are not uncommon for adults in the stage of maturity. The diabetic encountering complications of the illness may experience even more frequent
thoughts of death. The mature adult diabetic may feel great despair, manifested
by demonstrations of disgust.

The individual who is capable of controlling diabetes mellitus merely by
diet will undoubtedly feel differently about his or her body image from the in-

dividual who is required to control diet, regulate exercise, and inject himself or herself every day with insulin. Therefore, the nurse must be cognizant of what each required health care therapy means to the individual afflicted with diabetes mellitus. If the diabetic requires daily injections of insulin, the nurse needs to assess how the diabetic perceives the act of sticking himself or herself with a needle and placing medication into body tissues. It must not be forgotten that injecting oneself with a needle is an invasion of body boundaries and the diabetic may view it as just that. Although the act of injecting oneself with a needle is relatively painless, the diabetic may view the insulin injections as an assault upon body structure and hence upon body image.

In order to deal with the somatic impact imposed by insulin therapy, the diabetic requires encouragement to verbalize what it means to him or her to be on insulin. Does the individual perceive insulin therapy as an assault to the body's integrity? Does the diabetic feel that "sticking" himself or herself is punishment for some wrongdoing? These are issues that need to be addressed as the diabetic verbalizes his or her feelings. With the assistance of the nurse, these concerns need to be examined so that the diabetic has a realistic view of their appropriateness.

When the diabetic has uneasy feelings about invading body boundaries and inflicting discomfort due to insulin therapy, the nurse may find it helpful to reinforce proper injection technique. Many clinicians have found it helpful to demonstrate insulin administration and to have the diabetic do a series of return demonstrations until he or she feels confident and comfortable with the new skill. Providing the diabetic with positive reinforcement on the use of proper injection technique aids in decreasing anxiety, enhancing self-esteem, and increasing adherence to proper insulin administration.

Teaching the diabetic to use proper wrist action when injecting helps to avoid unnecessary discomfort caused by gradual entry of the needle into the skin. It is of great importance to instruct the diabetic to inject the insulin deep into the subcutaneous tissue, not to use cold insulin, and to rotate injection sites in an attempt to avoid the development of lipodystrophies. Lipodystrophies can be an additional unwanted change in body image since they create a noticeable thickening or dimpling of body tissue.

Sexual Impact

Sexual dysfunction is a common complication of diabetes mellitus for both men and women. All too often this fact is overlooked by health care professionals as they plan and initiate diabetic health care therapies. Researchers have found that the most frequent sexual dysfunction in the male diabetic is impotence. (Abelson, 1975; Krosnick and Podolsky, 1981) with a reported incidence of 40 to 60 percent (Ellenberg, 1979; Kolodny, Kahn, Goldstein, and Barnett, 1974). Although the incidence of impotence tends to increase with age, there does not appear to be any relationship between the frequency of impotence and the duration of the diabetes (Kolodny, Masters, Johnson, and Biggs, 1979; Tattersall, 1982).

Extensive research has been conducted in an attempt to identify the mechanisms involved in the diabetic's impotence. Investigators have found that the major cause is diabetic neuropathy, a process of microscopic damage to nerve tissue that occurs throughout the body of the diabetic. The basic physiological change which results is a thickening and beading of the penile nerves. In addition many men experience calcification of scrotal vessels, a decrease in penile blood pressure and blood flow (Kolodny, Masters, Johnson, and Biggs, 1979; Krosnick and Podolsky, 1981), impaired sperm motility, normal to low ejaculate volume, and normal to high sperm counts (Bartak, Josifko, and Horackova, 1975). Impaired sperm motility appears to be the most consistent finding in the analysis of the ejaculate. It is believed that the head and tail of the sperm separate as a result of higher than normal fructose levels in the semen making normal motility impossible (Unsain and Goodwin, 1982).

Ejaculation malfunction is another possible sexual disorder that can occur in the diabetic male. Premature ejaculation and retrograde ejaculation (ejaculation into the bladder) are the two ejaculatory difficulties that occur. Premature ejaculation is felt to be brought on by emotional disturbances, whereas retrograde ejaculation is the result of pathologic damage to the sympathetic innervation of the internal urethral sphincter with failure of bladder neck closure (Wabrek, 1973).

The evidence of sexual dysfunction in male diabetics is well-known but few studies have been published documenting the incidence of such problems in diabetic females. Several researchers have noted that orgasmic dysfunction is significantly more prevalent among diabetic women than among nondiabetic women (Kolodny, 1971; Ustov, 1978). In addition, it has been found that the appearance of sexual dysfunction in diabetic women correlates with the duration of the illness. However, no association with age, insulin dose, or complications (e.g. nephropathy, neuropathy, or vaginitis) exists.

When identifying the presence of a sexual dysfunction, such as impotence, the possibility of psychogenic factors should be considered. Since there are no data that reflect the frequency of psychogenic versus organic impotence, psychogenic factors should be considered as a possible cause. If the sexual dysfunction is automatically ascribed as being organic without proper assessment and it is, in fact, psychogenic, a treatable symptom may go unmanaged.

Once the type of sexual dysfunction is identified (organic or psychogenic), appropriate therapy may be initiated. In the case of organic impotence, most therapies have proven to be limited in their success, but this does not mean that the diabetic's problem simply should be dismissed. The problem is very real to the individual and one of the major functions of the nurse is to assist the diabetic in coping with organic impotence. Encouraging the diabetic to verbalize feelings to health care members and to the sex partner is vital. It is extremely important for the diabetic and the sex partner to discuss openly the diabetic's feelings about the sexual dysfunction. Does the male see himself as less than a man? Does the male diabetic think that he is imperfect? When the sex partner is aware of the male diabetic's feelings about the sexual dysfunction, emotional support is more likely to be provided by the sex partner. In addition, the affected male diabetic requires reassurance that the occurrence of impotence is not unique to him but tends to be present in a large percentage of diabetics. Simply realizing that he is not the only individual affected can aid in relieving some anxiety.

Whether the impotence is organic or psychogenic, the diabetic needs to be reassured that sexual activity can continue. Although caressing body parts may prove sexually satisfying for some individuals, using the "stuffing technique" (simply stuffing the penis into the vagina) may be desirable for other couples. The important part is for the diabetic and the sex partner to find a mutually satisfying means of sexual expression (Unsain, Goodwin, and Schuster, 1982). Some couples may encounter difficulties in identifying ways of achieving sexual satisfaction and, as a result, require sex counseling. After sex consultation, the use of a collapsible Silastic penile implant that allows for erection by means of manual control may be suggested (Siemens and Brandzel, 1982)

A fear of being unable to produce children may be an expressed concern of the male diabetic with sexual dysfunction. If the diabetic's semen quality is adequate, fertilization is very possible. In cases of retrograde ejaculation, bladder washings to retrieve sperm for artificial insemination have proven successful. If, however, the diabetic male encounters fertility problems, he should be advised to seek fertility counseling. Above all, the diabetic male needs reassurance that the children conceived by diabetic fathers are not discernibly different from those of nondiabetic fathers.

Diabetic females may express concern about their ability to conceive children. Since stillbirths, abortions, and large birth-weight babies are more frequent among diabetic women than nondiabetic women, such facts must be shared with the diabetic female contemplating a family. If the diabetic female becomes pregnant, the necessity for close medical supervision should be stressed in order to maintain the health of both the expectant mother and child. Both diabetic men and diabetic women must be aware that diabetes can be genetically transmitted. Therefore, genetic counseling is necessary so that both partners recognize the problems of disease transmission.

Since the susceptibility toward infection is higher in the diabetic, the occurrence of vaginitis may be common in the female diabetic. The presence of such a condition not only can prove uncomfortable for the female, but because of this discomfort, it may also affect her desire to partake in coitus. Thus, the diabetic female should be taught the necessity of good feminine hygiene.

The presence of a neurogenic bladder also may affect the diabetic's sexual activity. If the individual is not adequately instructed on the Credé maneuver, which aids in emptying the bladder, the chances of overflow incontinence can occur. If overflow incontinence occurs during sexual activity, either partner may find the accident unappealing and hence refrain from sexual contact.

Occupational Impact

How the diabetic is dealt with when he or she is seeking employment is affected by three major factors: the physical demands of the job, the work environment, and the individual's status of diabetic control. Physical demands of the job which involve heavy physical labor, rotating shifts, prolonged walking, or prolonged standing generally are ill-advised. Heavy physical labor and rotating shifts may make balancing activity level, food intake, and insulin administration a difficult task and subsequently place the diabetic's metabolic state in a precarious position. Prolonged walking or standing may place undue pressure on the feet which in turn may result in ulceration formation brought on by vascular insufficiency, a frequently encountered problem in diabetics.

The second factor influencing the diabetic's ability to maintain employment is the work environment. If the work environment involves operating dangerous machinery or working around hazardous objects, the diabetic may be considered unfit since an injury could prove fatal due to impaired healing ability. Work environments that are not conducive to allowing for insulin administration or required food intake also may prove unsafe since they do not enhance adequate physiological control of the disease process.

The third and most important factor for determining a diabetic's work placement is the status of diabetic control. Undoubtedly, the status of control is affected by the severity of the illness, the adequacy of medical management, and the presence of complications. Research has shown that diabetics miss fewer work days than nondiabetics (Moore, and Buschbom, 1974), therefore some industries and companies are becoming more lenient and more understanding about placing diabetics in jobs. The diabetic who is poorly controlled and/or suffers from complications will encounter problems in securing and maintaining employment.

In addition to the problems of securing and maintaining employment, the diabetic may have to deal with the lifelong financial burden of diabetes. Insulin, syringes, oral hypoglycemic agents, and materials for testing urine and/or blood glucose levels are an additional and lifelong expense. For diabetics who are on a low or fixed income, this financial burden can be overwhelming. Besides the cost of medications and materials needed for maintaining the diabetic disease process, the individual afflicted with diabetes is faced with the ongoing expense of medical consultation and, not uncommonly, hospitalization. With the rising cost of health care, the diabetic's financial savings can be depleted easily. For the diabetic who is in a stable state of diabetic control, the financial aspects will not be as overwhelming as for the diabetic who is in a continual state of metabolic flux.

The nurse's responsibilities in assisting the diabetic undergoing the occupational impact of the illness is to aid the diabetic in incorporating the required health care regimens into the demands of the work setting and to help him or her prevent diabetic complications that may be provoked by the job situation. Examining with the diabetic and members of the family what the physical and psychological demands of the job involve is the first step in incorporating the required health care regimens into the work environment. Once physical and psychological demands are identified, then planning must occur regarding what is needed in the diet to meet nutritional needs, how much insulin or hypoglycemic agent is required to maintain metabolic control of the disease process, and what types of physical and psychological activities are needed to enhance an adequate balance between diet intake and medication need. When all of these factors are appropriately dealt with metabolic control within the context of the work setting becomes a reality.

Assisting the diabetic in identifying job situations that can contribute to diabetic complications is vital. The occupational nurse is in an excellent position for this intervention. If the diabetic's job responsibilities encompass prolonged standing or walking, proper foot care should be encouraged since plantar ulceration can be a major complication (Stokes, Faris, and Hutton, 1975). If the diabetic must stand for prolonged periods of time, he or she should be instructed to carry out isotonic exercises to aid in facilitating venous return and to decrease the possibility of ulcer formation. If the diabetic works around objects that can create injury, such as glass, the use of protective devices (e.g. gloves) should be encouraged. Frequent examination of extremities for injury should be stressed with particular attention being paid to breaks in skin integrity. If there is a break in skin integrity, immediate treatment should be instituted to prevent the occurrence of an infectious process. Above all, the diabetic should be truthful with his or her employer about the presence of the illness since being untruthful could be life-threatening if ketoacidosis or hypoglycemia occur.

Social Impact

Often newly diagnosed diabetics may feel that due to their disease process, they will have to discontinue engaging in social activities. The diabetic and his or her family members need to be assured that such a practice is not necessary. The diabetic, with the assistance of the dietician, can learn how to select appropriate foods from restaurant menus and from a hostess' dining table. If the diabetic attends a banquet where the meal is already served on the plate, he or she can be instructed to eat appropriate portions to meet nutritional requirements and insulin demands. Regarding cocktail parties where alcoholic beverages and fancy foods are readily available, concerns expressed by the diabetic often are related to being tempted by the presence of many tasty foods and appearing unusual because others are drinking when they are not. Regarding beverage intake, the nurse may suggest that the diabetic who is planning to attend a cocktail party include in the daily nutritional requirements a fruit juice drink or a low-caloric drink. The fruit juice drink or the low-caloric drink can be garnished with orange slices and cherries so that it provides the ambiance of being like others. In dealing with the presence of many tempting foods, the diabetic can utilize maneuvers that decrease contact with foods, such as not standing close to the table containing the tempting culinary delights. The diabetic may want to use maneuvers often suggested for the obese individual who is attending a party. For further details on these maneuvers the reader is advised to consult Chapter 7.

Travel may present questions concerning health maintenance for some diabetics. The most frequently expressed concerns deal with the fear of loss of diabetic control and with the transport of insulin. To aid in preventing loss of control, the diabetic should maintain regularity in medication, diet, and physical activity during travel. Simply carrying out the diabetic routine as usual will tend to prevent the occurrence of difficulties. The transportation of insulin need not create undue difficulties for the traveling diabetic. Manufacturers of insulin state that insulin kept at room temperature will not undergo significant lowering of activity during the period of time that a single vial is in use. Of course, this assumes that the vial will be exhausted within a few weeks since insulin preparations are stable at room temperature for one to three months. In fact, it is better for the diabetic to administer room-temperature insulin because it reduces the chances of lipodystrophies.

The traveling diabetic is advised to carry an extra vial of insulin in case something should happen to the vial being actively used (e.g., breakage of the vial or appearance change of the insulin due to possible heat exposure). The extra vial may be kept at room temperature and then stored in a cool place, such as a refrigerator, once the diabetic reaches his or her travel destination. If the diabetic is camping for extended periods of time, keeping the extra vial of insulin in an ice chest or in an insulated bag proves workable. As a safety precaution, the traveling diabetic should obtain an extra written prescription from his or her physician in case additional insulin is needed during the trip. The potential problem of being without necessary medications is thus alleviated.

The diabetic should carry and/or wear some kind of identification indicating that he or she is a diabetic and how he or she is maintained (e.g., insulin dosage and/or oral hypoglycemic agents). This is advisable for all diabetics, but especially for the traveling diabetic. Various forms of "medical alert" jewelry (e.g., necklaces or bracelets) are available which have the appropriate diabetic information inscribed. Some diabetics may express concern about wearing a bracelet with this information because the bracelet draws attention to their illness and, as a result, makes them feel uncomfortable. If the diabetic expresses such concerns, the nurse might encourage the wearing of a long-chained necklace with a medallion containing the necessary information. The necklace would not be very noticeable because it could be worn under clothing.

The diabetic may withdraw from social interactions if physical complications such as ulcerations and failing vision occur. He or she may feel that the ulcerations are unsightly and/or the poor vision is a hindrance to social interaction. The nurse should encourage family members to be aware of the possibility of withdrawal if such complications are present and to actively engage the diabetic in social contacts. For further information about dealing with individuals who are manifesting withdrawal due to alterations in skin integrity and impaired visual function, the reader is advised to consult the somatic impact section of Chapter 8 and the social impact section of Chapter 10.

SUMMARY

Diabetes mellitus, one of the most commonly encountered metabolic disorders, affects between 4 million and 6 million individuals in the United States with evidence that it is increasing in prevalence. No doubt this is related to the facts that people live longer, larger proportions of more susceptible individuals are alive, diagnostic tests continually are being improved, and the public is becoming increasingly aware of the alteration.

An individual afflicted with diabetes mellitus is either of the juvenile-onset type or the adult-onset type. Regardless of the type of diabetes experienced by the individual, the illness creates multiple impacts upon life-style. When an individual is faced with diabetes, his or her psychological well-being, somatic identity, sexuality, occupational identity, and social role are affected. To aid an individual in dealing with each of these areas of concern, the nurse must identify how the illness affects each component of the diabetic's life and then assist him or her in dealing with each impact to the best of his or her ability.

Patient Situation   Mr. D. M., a fifty-four-year-old, married, lathe operator for a furniture company, has been a diabetic for the past eight years. Over the past six months he has encountered difficulties with diabetic control while on a regulated diet and oral hypoglycemic agents. Therefore, one month ago Mr. D. M.'s family physician placed him on insulin and a regulated diet. Mrs. D. M. has been administering the insulin to her husband since it was prescribed.

Mr. D. M. is now in the furniture company's dispensary after having experienced a state of hypoglycemia during work. He is being treated for the hypoglycemia by the company's occupational health nurse. During the intervention the nurse notes that Mr. D. M. is encountering difficulties with his illness related to his psychological well-being, somatic identity, sexuality, occupational identity, and social role.

Following are Mr. D. M.'s nursing care plan and patient care cardex dealing with each of these areas of conern.

NURSING CARE PLAN

Nursing Diagnoses	Objectives	Nursing Interventions	Principles/Rationale	Evaluations
Psychological Impact Fear manifested by expressed feelings of dread about future bouts of hypoglycemia.	To decrease Mr. D. M.'s fear.	Encourage Mr. D. M. to verbalize how he feels about his illness and the related therapies.	Verbalization assists in decreasing one's fears. Identifying how a diabetic feels about the illness and its related therapies assists in planning future approaches to nursing care.	The nurse would observe for: Mr. D. M.'s verbalization about feeling secure with controlling his diabetes.
		Review with Mr. D. M. the aspects of proper diabetic control (e.g., relationship of dietary intake, insulin therapy, and exercise regime). Reassure Mr. D. M. that, with proper control, the chances of complications, such as hypoglycemia, are reduced.	Increasing and reinforcing one's knowledge about one's illness and its related therapies can aid in decreasing fear.	
Somatic Impact Potential body image alteration manifested by expressed feelings of uneasiness about injecting himself with insulin.	To decrease Mr. D. M.'s feelings of uneasiness about administering his own insulin.	Encourage Mr. D. M. to verbalize how he views his insulin injections.	Diabetics may view insulin injections as an assault upon their body structure and body image since the act of injecting insulin invades body boundaries. Verbalizing aids in decreasing one's anxieties and in examining the appropriateness of such concerns. Knowing how the diabetic perceives insulin injections aids in developing an appropriate approach to teaching the therapy.	The nurse would observe for: Mr. D. M.'s verbalization of increased feelings of competence about injecting himself with insulin.

(cont.)

NURSING CARE PLAN (cont.)

Nursing Diagnoses	Objectives	Nursing Interventions	Principles/Rationale	Evaluations
	To increase Mr. D. M.'s feelings of competence about administering his own insulin.	Review with Mr. D. M. proper injection therapy (e.g., use of wrist action and deep subcutaneous injection).	Reinforcing one's knowledge about one's therapies can aid in decreasing anxiety related to fear of the unknown.	Mr. and Mrs. D. M.'s verbalization about Mr. D. M.'s taking an active role in his insulin administration.
		Demonstrate the technique of insulin injection and have Mr. D. M. do a series of return demonstrations.	Having an individual demonstrate, under supervision, progressive abilities in carrying out insulin injections can aid in increasing a sense of security about medication self-administration.	
		Provide positive reinforcement on the use of proper injection technique.	Positive reinforcement for a job well done aids in enhancing one's feelings of self-worth.	
		Encourage Mrs. D. M. to urge her husband to carry out his own insulin injections.	Encouragement from significant others to do one's own insulin injections helps prevent the occurrence of secondary gains from the illness.	
		Encourage Mrs. D. M. to provide her husband with positive reinforcement on his administration of insulin and his use of proper injection technique.	Positive feedback from significant others aids in enhancing feelings of self-worth.	

Sexual Impact Sexual dysfunction manifested by expressed feelings of emasculation caused by impotence.	To enhance Mr. D. M.'s feelings of manliness.	Encourage Mr. D. M. to verbalize his feelings to his wife.	A sex partner who is aware of a diabetic's feelings about sexual dysfunction is more likely to provide emotional support.	The nurse would observe for: Mr. D. M.'s verbalization that he has fewer feelings about being less than a man.
		Reassure Mr. D. M. that this problem is not unique to him but that it is present in a large percentage of diabetics.	Realizing that one is not the only individual afflicted with a problem can aid in relieving anxiety.	
		Encourage Mr. D. M. to see his physician so that the basis of his impotence can be identified (organic versus psychogenic).	In most cases of organic impotence caused by diabetes mellitus, past therapies have proven limited in their success. However, psychogenic impotence has proven to be a treatable symptom.	
		Encourage Mr. and Mrs. D. M. to identify means of achieving a mutually satisfying sexual experience (e.g., caressing of body parts, use of the stuffing technique). (If Mr. and Mrs. D. M. are unable to achieve sexual satisfaction, sex counseling may be suggested).	Satisfying sexual experiences can continue to exist in spite of the presence of impotence.	Mr. D. M.'s verbalization that he and his wife are achieving mutually satisfying sexual experiences.

(cont.)

NURSING CARE PLAN (cont.)

Nursing Diagnoses	Objectives	Nursing Interventions	Principles/Rationale	Evaluations
Occupational Impact Potential job management deficit manifested by expressed concern about being unable to maintain his position in the furniture company.	To decrease Mr. D. M.'s concerns about job security.	Encourage Mr. D. M. to carry out proper diabetic control (e.g., appropriate dietary regulation, insulin, and exercise).	Proper diabetic control can aid in decreasing the rapidity with which complications can occur.	The nurse would observe for: Mr. D. M.'s verbalization about job security.
	To facilitate Mr. D. M.'s ability to maintain his job as a lathe operator.	Encourage Mr. D. M. to recognize situations in his work environment that could provoke the incidence of diabetic complications and to carry out appropriate preventive measures (e.g., wearing gloves when handling splintered pieces of wood and wearing steel-toed shoes to prevent foot injury in case he drops a piece of wood on his foot).	Carrying out maneuvers for identifying work situations that could provoke diabetic complications aids in decreasing the possible incidence of these complications. A diabetic who suffers from diabetic complications is more likely to encounter difficulties in maintaining employment.	Mr. D. M.'s identification of work situations that could provoke diabetic complications and the institution of appropriate protective maneuvers.

Nursing Diagnosis	Goal	Nursing Intervention	Rationale	Evaluation
		Encourage Mr. D. M. to check his hands frequently for cuts and puncture wounds and to seek attention in the dispensary immediately if he is injured.	Identifying and treating a potential source of diabetic complications aids in decreasing the incidence and severity of that complication.	The nurse would observe for:
Social Impact Potential social isolation manifested by verbalized feelings of discomfort about attending parties that serve alcoholic beverages and fancy foods.	To increase Mr. D. M.'s feelings of comfort while attending parties that have food and alcoholic drink.	Advise Mr. D. M. that when he plans to attend a party where alcoholic drinks will be served he should include in his daily nutritional planning the allowance for a fruit juice drink or a low-caloric drink for party consumption.	Feelings of awkwardness provoked by not engaging in social drinking are decreased when the diabetic makes dietary allowances for the consumption of an allowed beverage for the social engagement.	Mr. D. M.'s verbalization about increased comfort when attending social engagements where food and alcoholic drink are to be served.
		Encourage Mr. D. M. to utilize maneuvers that decrease his contact with the fancy foods (e.g., not standing close to the serving table).	Decreasing the availability of tempting foods aids in preventing their consumption.	
	To prevent Mr. D. M. from withdrawing from social interaction.	Encourage Mr. D. M. to take part in social interactions.	Withdrawing from social interactions can lead to isolation which can lead to depression.	Mr. D. M.'s continuing to take part in social interaction.

PATIENT CARE CARDEX

PATIENT'S NAME: _____ Mr. D. M. _____   MEDICAL DIAGNOSIS: _____ Diabetes mellitus (insulin dependent)

AGE: _____ 54 years _____   SEX: _____ Male _____

MARITAL STATUS: _____ Married _____   OCCUPATION: _____ Lathe operator _____

SIGNIFICANT OTHERS: _____ Wife _____

Nursing Diagnoses	Nursing Approaches
Psychological: Fear manifested by expressed feelings of dread about future bouts of hypoglycemia.	1. Encourage verbalization of feelings about illness and related therapies. 2. Review aspects of proper diabetic control (relationship of dietary intake, insulin therapy, and exercise regime). 3. Point out that with proper control chances of complications are reduced.
Somatic: Potential body image alteration manifested by expressed feelings of uneasiness about injecting himself with insulin.	1. Encourage verbalization about feelings concerning insulin injections. 2. Review proper injection therapy. 3. Demonstrate injection technique and have patient do a series of return demonstrations.

4. Provide positive reinforcement on the use of proper injection technique.
5. Encourage wife to urge husband to carry out own insulin administration and to provide positive reinforcement when he does.

Sexual: Sexual dysfunction manifested by expressed feelings of emasculation caused by impotence.

1. Encourage verbalization of feelings to wife.
2. Point out that impotence is not unique to him but that it is present in a large percentage of diabetics.
3. Encourage to see physician about the basis of impotence (organic versus psychogenic).
4. Encourage with the wife to identify means of achieving a mutually satisfying sexual experience (use of caressing and stuffing technique). (Sex counseling may be in order.)

Occupational: Potential job management deficit manifested by expressed concern about being unable to maintain his position in the furniture company.

1. Encourage to carry out proper diabetic control.
2. Encourage to recognize situations in work environment that could provoke incidence of diabetic complications and to carry out appropriate preventive measures.
3. Encourage frequent checks of hands for puncture wounds and cuts and to seek appropriate treatment if there are injuries.

Social: Potential social isolation manifested by verbalized feelings of discomfort about attending parties that serve alcoholic beverages and fancy foods.

1. Advise that when he plans to attend a party where alcoholic drinks will be served he should include in his daily nutritional planning the allowance for a fruit juice drink or a low-caloric drink for party consumption.
2. Encourage to utilize maneuvers that decrease contact with fancy foods (e.g., not standing close to serving table).
3. Encourage to take part in social interactions so that he will not become an isolate.

REFERENCES

ABELSON, D. Diagnostic value of the penile pulse and blood pressure: a Doppler study of impotence in diabetics, *Journal of Urology,* 1975, *113* (5), 636–639.

BARTAK, V., JOSIFKO, M., and HORACKOVA, M. Juvenile diabetes and human sperm quality, *International Journal of Fertility,* 1975, *20* (1), 30–32.

DUNN, S., and TURTLE, J. The myths of the diabetic personality, *Diabetes Care,* 1981, *4* (6), 640–666.

ELLENBERG, M. Sexual diabetes: a comparison between men and women. *Diabetes Care,* 1979, *2* (1), 4–8.

ERIKSON, E. *Childhood and society.* New York: W.W. Norton and Co., Inc., 1963.

HANN, N. Psychosocial meanings of unfavorable medical forecasts. In G. Stone, F. Cohen, and N. Adler (Eds.), *Health psychology: a handbook.* San Francisco: Jossey-Bass, 1979.

KOLODNY, R. Sexual dysfunction in diabetic females, *Diabetes,* 1971, *20* (8), 557–559.

KOLODNY, R., KAHN, C., GOLDSTEIN, H., and BARNETT, D. Sexual dysfunction in diabetic men, *Diabetes,* 1974, *23* (4), 306–309.

KOLODNY, R., MASTERS, W., JOHNSON, V., and BIGGS, M. *Textbook of human sexuality of nurses.* Boston: Little, Brown, 1979.

KROSNICK, A., and PODOLSKY, S. Diabetes and sexual dysfunction: restoring normal ability, *Geriatrics,* 1981, *36* (3), 92–100.

LUCKMANN, J., and SORENSON, K. *Medical-surgical nursing: a psychophysiologic approach.* Philadelphia: Saunders, 1980.

MOORE, R., and BUSCHBOM, R. Work absenteeism in diabetics, *Diabetes,* 1974, *23* (12), 957–961.

SIEMENS, S., and BRANDZEL, R. *Sexuality: nursing assessment and intervention.* Philadelphia: Lippincott, 1982.

SILVERBERG, E. Cancer statistics. *Ca-A cancer Journal for Clinicians,* 1983, *33* (1), 9–25.

STOKES, I., FARIS, I., and HUTTON, W. The neuropathic ulcer and loads on the foot in diabetic patients, *Acta Orthopaedica Scandinavica,* 1975, *46,* 839–847.

TATTERSALL, R. Sexual problems of diabetic men, *British Medical Journal,* 1982, *2* (285), 911–912.

UNSAIN, I., and GOODWIN, M. Effects on sexual functioning. In D. Guthrie and R. Guthrie (Eds.) *Nursing management of diabetes mellitus.* St. Louis: C.V. Mosby, 1982.

UNSAIN, I., GOODWIN, M., and SCHUSTER, E. Diabetes and sexual functioning, *Nursing Clinics of North America,* 1982, *17* (3), 387–393.

USTOV, Z. Sexualni porucky u zen s uplavici cukrovou, *Ceskoslovenska Gynekologie,* 1978, *43,* 277–280.

WABREK, A. *Diabetes mellitus.* Edition 7, Revision 2. Indiana, Billy Research Laboratories, 1973.

WILKINSON, D. Psychiatric aspects of diabetes mellitus, *British Journal of Psychiatry,* 1981, *138,* 1–9.

13 ||||||||||||||||||||||||||||||||||||||||||||||||||||||||||||||

PEPTIC ULCER OR
ULCERATIVE COLITIS

INTRODUCTION

The prevalance of alterations in gastrointestinal (G.I.) function is well recognized by members of the health care system. The occurrence of gastrointestinal malfunctions, either independently or secondarily to other disease processes, is voluminous. Even the presence of diarrhea, as a result of stress, is not an uncommon occurrence for many individuals. Regardless of what G.I. malfunction occurs, its presence can have an impact on daily living.

Two relatively common gastrointestinal malfunctions that have long-term significance are peptic ulcers and ulcerative colitis. They affect different anatomical structures within the G.I. tract, but the impact that each has upon one's psychological well-being, somatic identity, sexuality, occupational identity, and social role is very similar.

ALTERATIONS IN GASTROINTESTINAL FUNCTION

Peptic ulcers are sites of ulceration formed in the mucosa, submucosa, or muscle layers of the distal esophagus, stomach, upper duodenum, or jejunum (following a gastroenterostomy). Ulcers can occur at any age, but duodenal ulcers tend to appear most often in individuals between the ages of thirty and fifty years while gastric ulcers are most prevalent in the forty to sixty age category. Approximately 10 percent of the population in the United States suffers from peptic ulcers with men being afflicted more often than women (Given and Simmons, 1979). It has been noted that the ratio of men to women suffering from gastric ulcers is two to one, whereas the ratio of those suffering from duodenal ulcers is seven to one.

The exact cause of peptic ulcers is unknown, but various factors have been identified as contributing to the development of the disease process. These factors include a source of irritation in the gastrointestinal tract, such as an increase in acid secretion with a decrease in alkaline mucous production, a breakdown in local tissue resistance, and the effects of heredity, hormones, personality, and environment. Even aspirin, cola beverages, coffee, and cigarettes have been found to increase the risk of peptic ulcer formation (Grossman, Guth, Isenberg, Passaro, Roth, Sturdevant, and Walsh, 1976).

The classic symptom of an uncomplicated peptic ulcer is gnawing, burning pain in the upper abdominal or epigastric region. The pain characteristically occurs one to two hours after meals and frequently awakens the individual at night. This gnawing, burning pain is usually relieved by food or antacids.

Ulcerative colitis is an inflammatory disease involving mainly the mucosa and submucosa of the colon, with bloody diarrhea being the primary clinical manifestation. Estimates of the number of individuals afflicted by this disease process vary widely since it generally tends to be an unreported condition in children when the symptoms are mild. However, it is believed that approximately 300,000 individuals suffer from this disease in the United States.

The majority of individuals suffering from ulcerative colitis have the initial onset between fifteen and forty-nine years of age with a peak age range of onset being sixteen to twenty years. Males and females tend to be equally afflicted by this gastrointestinal malfunction. However, a two-to-four times greater incidence of ulcerative colitis occurs in those of Jewish ancestry, with a distinctly lower frequency of occurrence among blacks and members of the Spanish-American population (Hertz and Rosenbaum, 1977).

Numerous theories concerning the etiology of ulcerative colitis exist. These theories have emphasized allergic, psychosomatic, vascular, genetic, immunologic, and microbiologic factors. It is felt that altered immunogenicity is most likely the cause of this disease process (Dworken, 1982).

It can been seen that a large proportion of individuals in the United States suffer from one of two major gastrointestinal malfunctions: peptic ulcer or ulcerative colitis. Although numerous research studies have been conducted on both disease entities, many questions remain unanswered. Regardless of which G.I. alteration the individual demonstrates, the impact of the illness upon the person can be overwhelming.

IMPACT OF A PEPTIC ULCER OR ULCERATIVE COLITIS

Psychological Impact

Persons that suffer from peptic ulcers tend to demonstrate a high degree of anxiety (Taylor, Gatchel, and Korman, 1982) related to their difficulty in expressing feelings of hostility or aggression, tend to have a great deal of initiative and drive, and are compulsive go-getters who usually are successful in their occupation (Wolcott, Wellisch, Robertson and Arthur, 1981). Their occupational fields of endeavor often are demanding and require quick decision making and the constant need to resolve problems. Since the ulcer patient tends to be a compulsive go-getter who is successful in his or her occupation, the occupational situation often has been identified as the sole contributor to the formation of the disease process. This is not necessarily true since the sufferer often is undergoing a conflict related to his or her dependence-independence status. The majority of individuals suffering from ulcers have an intense need to be independent and have developed a superego that forbids the expression of the need for dependence (Lyketsos, Arapakis, Psaras, Photiou, and Blackburn, 1982). As a result, the adult tends to overcompensate by giving the impression of being self-sufficient, ambitious, competent, aggressive, and independent. The individual may refuse to accept assistance from others and may burden himself or herself with excessive responsibilities. These responsibilities and the continual struggle to deal with them only reinforce the desire for a dependent relationship. Beneath the facade of self-confidence lies an individual with strong dependency needs.

One of the most devastating consequences of peptic ulcers is the widely held misconception that the gastrointestinal alteration is brought about exclusively by psychic stress. Members of the health care team who adhere to this belief are prone to blame the individual for creating the illness which, in turn, forces the ulcer-prone person to disguise his or her dependency needs in an attempt to cope with the disease process. The outcome is likely to be administration of ineffective therapy on the part of the health team member, feelings of guilt on the part of the ulcer patient, and additional unneeded stress in the environment.

Regardless of whether the dependence-independence conflict brought about the ulcer or the ulcer created the dependence-independence conflict, the presence of the conflict exists. In either situation, a vicious cycle ensues since one state tends to feed into the other. Unless this cycle is broken by appropriate intervention, the peptic ulcer sufferer's acute illness can result in a state of chronic illness.

Individuals suffering from ulcerative colitis are similar to persons afflicted with peptic ulcers in that they tend to manifest conflicting behavioral responses, the primary one being the existence of conflict between rebellion and compliance. The individual desires to be loved and accepted, but identifies in himself or herself unacceptable feelings of anger and resentment toward the very ones from whom love and acceptance are required. Some researchers believe that these conflicting feelings are brought about by unresolved loss. Such a loss could be a disruptive relationship with a mother, father, family member, or any other key person (Castelnuovo-Tedesco, Schwertfeger, and Janowsky, 1970).

Because of the individual's inability to deal with the conflicts of rebellion versus compliance, anger and resentment are not adequately expressed. The mucous membranes of the colon respond to these suppressed emotions and become inflamed and ulcerated. The typical patient often demonstrates immaturity, dependency, rigidity, perfectionism, and wariness of others (MacLean, 1976). The symptoms of the disease process tend to appear when the individual is confronted with a situation that appears uncontrollable to him or her. Along with the conflict between rebellion and compliance, the person afflicted with ulcerative colitis often manifests feelings of hopelessness and despair, subsequently feeling that his or her life situation has no chance of resolving itself.

Whether these behavioral manifestations occur prior to the disease process or after the illness remains a debate among clinicians and investigators. Psychological problems do occur in individuals with severe ulcerative colitis, but are these changes the consequence of the impact of the illness or the cause of the illness? Who would not be worn down both physically and psychologically by passing ten to fifteen blood-stained bowel movements each day?

The nurse's role in assisting the individual with gastrointestinal disorders such as peptic ulcer and ulcerative colitis is to encourage and allow verbalization of feelings to assist the individual in examining his or her behavior as it relates to the illness, and to provide guidance in modifying illness - provoked behavior. The person with a peptic ulcer requires encouragement to express his or her feelings in an attempt to identify dependency needs and to recognize what these needs mean to the individual. While the individual is verbalizing how he or she feels, the nurse should at no time make judgmental responses about the individual's need to be dependent. Rather, the nurse should have the individual examine what about being dependent bothers him or her and what alternatives might be used in place of the dependent behavior.

The ulcer patient also may require encouragement to express the reasons for having to push so vigorously. For example, what does it mean to the individual if he or she does not obtain a job promotion within the next six months? What will happen to the individual if he or she does not obtain a desired position in the work setting? As the patient explains the rationale for the need to create the impression of self-sufficiency, assertion, and independence, it will prove helpful to have him or her examine personal goals. Encouraging the individual to evaluate whether these goals are realistic, forces him or her to contend with the vicious cycle of dependence versus independence. As the individual reestablishes personal goals in a more realistic light, positive feedback is valuable since it provides the person with a sense of achievement.

When dealing with the individual afflicted with ulcerative colitis, the need to verbalize also is extremely important. This verbalization may have to be channelled in the direction of expressing feelings of rebellion. Since the person afflicted with ulcerative colitis often encounters difficulty in opposing others in thoughts and actions, he or she may require encouragement to express an opposing view. The individual should be told that it is alright to disagree with others and should not be reprimanded when disagreement occurs. As the person with ulcerative colitis expresses rebellion, he or she should receive positive feedback about the increased ability to appropriately verbalize opposing viewpoints.

Family members of individuals suffering from gastrointestinal alterations play a vital role in the health care of their loved one. Family members often require information about the importance of encouraging the ulcer patient's need to express feelings of dependence and the ulcerative colitis patient's need to verbalize feelings of rebellion. As the individual with gastrointestinal alterations verbalizes these feelings, family members may encounter difficulties in dealing with them and require assistance on how to deal with their own feelings about the illness. For example, do family members see the individual as weak, do they feel that the illness places a stigma upon them, or do they feel responsible for the illness? If difficulty in dealing with the illness is expressed by family members, these feelings need to be examined and alternatives for dealing with these feelings need to be explored. Above all, the family requires information on the disease process and its long-term consequences.

In times of stress, the individual with gastrointestinal alterations often undergoes an acute crisis in the disease process. Symptoms such as gnawing, burning, abdominal pain, or an increased frequency of bloody diarrhea may appear. Therefore, both the patient and the family should be encouraged to identify those situations which they believe, or know, to be stressful for the patient. If taking part in a golf tournament or hosting a dinner party exacerbates the symptoms, it may be advisable to avoid such activities. If the patient and the family are cognizant of how stress can increase the chances of symptom exacerbation, they are more likely to avoid such circumstances. However, it must be realized that not *all* stressful situations can be avoided.

The person with alterations in G.I. function, such as peptic ulcers and ulcerative colitis, often requires guidance in carrying out maneuvers to enhance relaxation. Both the afflicted individual and the family need to identify the maneuvers that the patient finds relaxing. What one person finds relaxing another individual may find stress producing; therefore, personalized identification of such maneuvers is necessary. Some people find fishing, golfing, and hiking relaxing while others enjoy sauna baths, movies, and reading. Once relaxing maneuvers have been identified, the individual must be encouraged to carry them out. Family members play an important role at this point because they are most aware of the patient's reactions to tension and stress and of the need to take part in relaxing activities.

Since the need to rest is an important component of the health care of the patient with G.I. alterations, it is no wonder that bed rest may be ordered when the individual is admitted to an acute care facility during an acute attack of the disease process. Placing a patient who is in an acute crisis in the hospital setting encourages physical rest and often is an attempt to enforce mental relaxation. The nurse, however, needs to be aware of the patient's activities during hospitalization since mental relaxation may not be occurring. For example, how restful is the business person who has his or her secretary visit all day in order to continue to carry out business affairs from a hospital bed? In such a case, limit-setting may be necessary. The limits should not be rigid since rigidity may add to the person's already stressful state. Instead of refusing the secretary admission into the patient's room, it is better to discuss with the patient the advisability of the secretary's visiting for only a few hours each day.

When an individual with gastrointestinal alterations is admitted to an acute care setting, dependency needs may be increased. The desire to be waited on and cared for may be manifested both by the person with a peptic ulcer and the individual with ulcerative colitis. During the stage of repudiation and/or when the illness is in an acute state, dependency needs will have to be met. During these periods the individual expends energy in denying and/or coping with the impact of the physical state. It is advisable to reassure the person that during this time it is acceptable to express dependency.

As the patient moves out of the stage of repudiation and/or progresses toward a more stable state of physical health, limits may have to be provided to decrease the patient's dependence. What is expected of him or her should be carefully described and health team members must be consistent in carrying out the requirements of these expectations. If a patient with a peptic ulcer avoids going for scheduled laboratory tests so that hospitalization and hence dependence are prolonged, limits must be provided. It may be advisable to encourage the individual to discuss with the nurse why he or she is avoiding the laboratory tests and how he or she might cope with the feelings of dependence. Limits, however, should not be extremely rigid. Rigidity often increases stress which can, in turn, lead to exacerbation of the symptoms. One of the difficulties in working with patients who have gastrointestinal alterations is identifying the fine lines between adequately set limits and rigidity, dependence and overdependence, and rebellion and compliance.

Somatic Impact

The impact that gastrointestinal alterations have upon an individual's somatic identity may not always be readily obvious to others. From all outward appearances no problem exists and only when complaints of burning abdominal pain are made or frequent trips to the bathroom are observed does the bystander recognize the existence of a problem.

The individual afflicted with a peptic ulcer projects his or her somatic focal point toward the gastrointestinal tract. The presence of a gnawing, burning, abdominal pain becomes uppermost in the individual's mind as he or she attempts to carry out his or her usual activities. Since the pain often is rhythmic in character, occurring one to two hours after eating, daily activities may become controlled by the usual time of the presence of pain. Life literally becomes controlled by "gut reactions" as the digestive tract works away at digesting itself. Once the individual with a peptic ulcer encounters bleeding of the G.I. tract, he or she may tend to focus attention on the appearance of his or her stools. Ritualistic observations for black, tarry-appearing bowel movements may be carried out by the individual. Again, the somatic focus is on the function of the gastrointestinal tract.

The somatic focal point of the individual with ulcerative colitis also tends to be directed toward the gastrointestinal tract. His or her existence during acute attacks of the disease process revolves around the frequent excretion of waste. There is constant fear that soiling of clothing will occur and that the accident will become obvious to others. The individual continually is concerned about emitting a stool odor as a result of improper cleansing after a bowel movement or as a result of a diarrhea accident. Diarrhea accidents often lead to feelings of regression since the individual believes that he or she has reverted back to the toddler stage when toilet training has not yet been accomplished. This may be common when the individual has encountered frequent soiling episodes.

How the person with a gastrointestinal alteration responds to the somatic impact of the illness can be affected by the developmental stage being experienced at the time of the illness. During the stage of young adulthood (eighteen to forty-five years) the incidence of both peptic ulcer and ulcerative colitis is common. Peptic ulcers tend to occur more often in the last half of young adulthood, while the peak age of onset of ulcerative colitis tends to occur in the early years of young adulthood. It is during this developmental stage that the task of establishing a meaningful relationship with others, both in friendship and in a mutually satisfying sexual relationship, become important (Erikson, 1963). The individual sustaining alteration in gastrointestinal function may encounter difficulties in accomplishing a state of intimacy and may retreat into isolation. This is especially true when the person afflicted with a gastrointestinal malfunction finds his or her body image displeasing.

The individual in the age category of forty-five to sixty-five years is experiencing the developmental stage of adulthood in which the primary task is generativity. During this time interests outside the home become important and the adult strives to establish and guide future generations (Erikson, 1963). If the individual in adulthood is afflicted with a gastrointestinal alteration, a sense of stagnation may result. The physiologic changes occurring as the result of the altered G.I. function (pain or diarrhea) may be interpreted as premature old age. As a result, the afflicted person may retire to a rocking chair before his or her time and become self-absorbed.

The person sixty-five years and over is in the stage of maturity. It is during this time that the adult withdraws body boundaries to more internal sites (Fisher and Cleveland, 1968) and may become fixated upon his or her gastrointestinal function. The presence of G.I. alterations, such as peptic ulcers or ulcerative colitis, may intensify the withdrawal of these body boundaries. Since frequent thoughts of death are common during this developmental stage, the existence of a gastrointestinal malfunction may intensify the frequency of these thoughts and, as a result, the person may enter a state of despair.

The nurse's role in dealing with the somatic impact of a gastrointestinal alteration is to assist the afflicted individual in coping with the altered body image. In order to deal with an altered body image, the person with a G.I. alteration should be educated about the basis of the disease process. He or she needs to know what the illness entails and what factors contribute to its existence. If the individual has a peptic ulcer, the importance of taking antacids or food on time in order to prevent the occurrence of abdominal pain should be stressed. It has been demonstrated that the kind of food consumed is of little importance as long as the individual can tolerate the food eaten. This should be pointed out to the person with a peptic ulcer, as well as to his or her family. To aid in relieving anxiety associated with abnormal stools, he or she should be reassured that it is alright to monitor stool appearance since it aids in identifying the presence of gastrointestinal bleeding. However, the person should be informed about drugs and foods that may darken the color of stools (i.e., iron, bismuth, and beets).

Assisting the individual with ulcerative colitis to deal with the altered body image is mainly focused on coping with diarrhea stools. Using a sitz bath and/or washing the perineal and rectal area after each stool can help to decrease the occurrence of odors. In addition, using soft, high-quality toilet tissue for cleansing and applying a lubricant, such as A & D ointment or Vaseline, to the rectal area can facilitate in decreasing skin irritation. Encouraging the individual to identify stressful situations and foods that tend to bring on bouts of diarrhea can be helpful. If possible, such situations and foods should be avoided.

If the person with ulcerative colitis expresses concern about soiling himself or herself, plastic-covered underwear or a perineal pad may be beneficial. Before suggesting such a maneuver, it is well-advised for the nurse to encourage the afflicted person to express his or her feelings about wearing such devices. Plastic underwear can intensify feelings of regression and a perineal pad can be emasculating to the male patient. If such feelings exist, it would be ill-advised to encourage the wearing of such apparel.

Sexual Impact

The individual with a peptic ulcer may encounter difficulty achieving a satisfying sexual experience if he or she is suffering from a gnawing, burning pain during sexual activity. Not only is the pain distracting and uncomfortable, but it may decrease libido and postpone or completely eliminate the sexual experience. If the ulcer patient encounters a stressful situation prior to the sexual experience or considers the sexual experience stressful, the likelihood of pain becomes greater. For example, if the person is engaging in an illicit sexual experience or feels the pressure of having to perform adequately during the sex act, chances of abdominal pain may increase.

In addition to a gnawing, burning, abdominal pain, the presence of burping may create additional problems during the sexual experience. The ulcer victim may not feel sexually desirable if he or she has to burp during the sexual encounter. The sex partner also may find eructation annoying and distracting if it occurs during the sex act and, therefore, may not achieve a satisfying sexual experience.

Research conducted on individuals with ulcers has dealt primarily with fertility. Kubicková and Veselý (1974) noted that ulcer patients had a 25 percent reduction in fertility compared to nonulcer controls. The investigators believed that this lower fertility rate was a result of a higher incidence of childless marriages and a smaller number of children per family. Since ulcer patients often have been identified as having a high drive to achieve, the presence of children may very possibly be seen as a deterrent to reaching their goals.

The nurse's responsibility in dealing with the sexual impact on the individual with a peptic ulcer is to assist him or her in decreasing the circumstances that hinder a satisfying sexual experience. Since abdominal pain and burping tend to occur when the stomach is empty, encouraging the consumption of antacids or food prior to engaging in a sexual experience can aid in preventing pain and eructation during the sexual encounter. Encouraging the sex partner not to stress the importance of performance during coitus can aid in decreasing the ulcer patient's anxiety about the need to perform during the sex act. Also, it may be advisable to point out to the ulcer patient that stressful situations prior to the sexual experience can contribute to the occurrence of pain during the encounter. With this information he or she is more likely to avoid stressful circumstances prior to a sexual encounter. If the ulcer patient finds the sexual experience stressful, the individual should be advised to discuss this openly with the sex partner. In some situations, however, the stress produced by a sexual experience may not be easily solved and sex counseling may be in order.

The sexual impact of ulcerative colitis is similar to that of peptic ulcers in that the difficulties encountered generally are related to symptoms of the disease process. Undoubtedly, one of the greatest concerns of the individual with ulcerative colitis is the fear of emitting a fecal odor or encountering a bout of diarrhea during the sexual experience. If either of these situations occurs, embarrassment and humiliation may result. Future sexual encounters may be avoided by both the ulcerative colitis patient and the sex partner for fear of a similar accident occurring; thus, stress is placed upon the sexual relationship.

If anal sex is practiced by the afflicted individual and the sex partner, this practice may have to cease or at least decrease during acute attacks of the illness. Since anal stimulation may lead to a bout of diarrhea, this practice would be ill-advised for the ulcerative colitis patient. During acute states of diarrhea the ulcerative colitis patient probably will not engage in sexual activity because he or she fears soiling himself or herself and the sex partner. Also the patient usually is physically exhausted from the acute state of illness.

Research on the sexual ramifications of ulcerative colitis has been limited.

Since the ulcerative colitis patient has been found to suffer from a conflict between rebellion and compliance, it should be of value to note whether the ulcerative colitis patient or the sex partner is the aggressor during the sexual encounter. One might predict that most of the time, the ulcerative colitis patient is not the aggressor in the sexual encounter. Knowing the role of the individual with ulcerative colitis in a sexual relationship is of value when sex counseling is being planned and implemented.

One of the nurse's roles is to assist the individual with ulcerative colitis to cope with the sexual impact of the illness. Encouraging verbalization between the patient and the sex partner about the fear of diarrhea and/or fecal odor during the sexual encounter is beneficial for identifying and planning alternatives for dealing with the situation. During verbalization both the individuals may require guidance on how best to handle the presence of diarrhea or a fecal odor during a sexual experience. For example, if the sex partner can remain very matter-of-fact about a diarrhea accident, a great deal of the ulcerative colitis patient's embarrassment and humiliation may be decreased. Placing an absorbent towel or pad on the bed in the buttocks region of the sexual partners can be helpful in decreasing a "messy situation" if diarrhea does occur. Readily available tissues or washcloths can help eliminate chaotic commotion of a diarrhea accident, while burning incense or using an air deodorizer in the bedroom can aid in decreasing the awareness of fecal odor.

The ulcerative colitis patient should be encouraged to identify stressful situations that could elicit bouts of diarrhea and, if possible, he or she should avoid these circumstances prior to a sexual experience. In some relationships spontaneity of a sexual encounter may be advisable since spontaneity tends to decrease anxiety brought on by preparing for the sexual activity. Sex counseling, in some cases, may be the only answer for dealing with the sexual impact of ulcerative colitis.

Occupational Impact

The existence of gastrointestinal disorders creates an economic impact, not only upon the individual afflicted, but also upon society in general. The presence of peptic ulcers or ulcerative colitis leads to manpower waste in all occupational activities that rely upon man's ability to perform. Ways in which gastrointestinal alterations affect manpower include:

1. Rejection from employment due to a code of physical standards for job applicant.
2. Time lost from work due to hospitalization, doctor's appointments, illness time spent at home, diagnostic tests, and convalescent periods.
3. Substandard performance due to decreased productivity.
4. Termination of occupation due to gastrointestinal disability.
5. Draining of company funds due to compensation claims.

In addition to the aforementioned factors that contribute to manpower waste, it must not be forgotten that certain occupations contribute to the incidence of gastrointestinal alterations. The individual in an occupation in which important and/or costly decisions are required may suffer from a higher incidence of gastrointestinal disorders. Research has demonstrated that air traffic controllers manifest a higher incidence of peptic ulcers than other individuals because of the stresses of the job (Cobb and Rose, 1973). The hierarchial position held by the individual also may have an effect upon the incidence of the gastrointestinal disorder. When a person holds a high status position, positive feedback from others on a job well done generally is not forthcoming. He or she is so far up the "occupational ladder" that there is no one above to provide positive feedback on high quality performance. Thus, frustration and stress can occur as a result of the lack of praise.

In dealing with the occupational impact of gastrointestinal alterations, the nurse's role centers around encouraging the afflicted person to identify what situations in the occupational setting are stress-provoking and what actions can be taken to deal with these situations. Through open communication among the nurse, the individual, and the family, these situations can be made apparent. In some instances, the nurse may have to encourage the individual to alter or to change his or her job in an attempt to decrease excessive stress. For some individuals, job retraining may be in order. In addition, encouraging a regular work schedule is advisable. A continual change in work hours makes it difficult for the individual with a peptic ulcer to eat regularly and to take antacids regularly in an attempt to decrease the incidence of abdominal pain. By comparison, the ulcerative colitis victim will have difficulty regulating his or her work schedule around diarrhea stools if work hours are constantly fluctuating. The continual changes in working hours is in and of itself a stressor to which some individuals may encounter difficulty adapting.

Social Impact

For the individual afflicted with a peptic ulcer, the presence of the illness creates a social impact related to the activities confronted in a social situation. For example, since alcohol consumption is not advisable for the individual with an ulcer because of the potentiation of the secretion of gastric acid, social functions that serve alcoholic beverages may prove uncomfortable for the afflicted person. The ulcer patient may wish to be a part of the social activity and, therefore, feel awkward if he or she is not drinking something along with everyone else at the social affair. In addition to drinking alcoholic beverages, many people smoke at social encounters. Smoking is ill-advised for the ulcer patient since it tends to increase gastric motility. Thus, the ulcer victim's difficulties in a social situation often revolve around contending with activities that are not advisable for him or her.

The social impact of ulcerative colitis tends to be related to the consequences of the symptoms of the disease process. The afflicted individual's major social concerns are the fear of odor and excrement associated with the illness and the ways in which the illness restricts the use of his or her time for social purposes. For example, managing the frequent diarrhea stools and the presence of odor can be difficult, especially if bathroom facilities are not readily available. The ulcerative colitis patient's time for activities is limited and he or she must be flexible since plans may be subject to last minute change due to bouts of diarrhea.

The nurse's role in dealing with the social impact of gastrointestinal alterations is to assist the individual and the family in identifying and carrying out ways of dealing with social interactions. If alcoholic beverages are present at social engagements, the nurse should encourage the peptic ulcer victim to drink juice or soft drinks. Both generally are available when alcoholic beverages are served and can be disguised with garnishes of cherries or fruit slices. If other people's smoking tempts the individual with a peptic ulcer to smoke a cigarette, the individual can be instructed on how to decrease smoking. The reader is advised to consult Chapter 11 for a discussion of preventive tactics regarding smoking.

To assist the individual with ulcerative colitis to cope with the social impact of the illness, the nurse should aid the individual in identifying preventive strategies. For example, the afflicted person can carefully map a route for social engagements according to the accessibility of bathrooms. If the individual encounters a strange or new environment, he or she should identify the location of the toilets immediately upon arrival. Engaging in activities, such as long car rides, which prolong the inaccessibility to bathroom facilities, may need to be avoided.

Unless the individual with ulcerative colitis is in an acute state of illness, he or she should be encouraged to maintain social interactions. Having family and friends act as interactional allies is helpful. In other words, family and friends can aid by explaining or justifying the ulcerative colitis victim's unconventional behavior as he or she attempts to maintain activities despite frequent and abrupt exits. The afflicted person can learn to excuse himself or herself graciously from the company of others, quickly change clothing if needed, and rapidly repair a soiled environment. If the afflicted individual can remain calm about the situation, others are more likely to retain their composure following the accident. When family members and friends remain matter-of-fact about a diarrhea accident, less tension is created.

It must not be forgotten that family members may experience anxiety about attending a social function with a loved one with a gastrointestinal alteration. The frequent need to consume food or antacids or the frequent exits to the bathroom may elicit feelings of discomfort or disgust on the part of the family members. Should the social circumstances provoke anxiety, the afflicted person and the family may wish to identify alternate means of social interaction.

Encouraging the identification of an involvement in social affairs that are equally enjoyable for both the family member and the afflicted person can prove helpful. A family member may find attending a lecture series on art with the individual with G.I. alterations unpleasant since the individual's movements can be very obvious to others. Visiting an art museum may be more comfortable for both the family member and the afflicted person since the individual with G.I. alterations can consume antacids in the privacy of the bathroom or unobtrusively use the toilet. Thus, it is best when the social affair selected is a joint decision between the afflicted person and the family.

SUMMARY

Gastrointestinal alterations are well-recognized health care problems. Two of the more common G.I. alterations affecting the adult are peptic ulcers and ulcerative colitis. Peptic ulcers are sites of ulceration occurring in the mucosa, submucosa, or muscle layers of the distal esophagus, stomach, upper duodenum, or jejunum. The classic symptom of a peptic ulcer is gnawing, burning, epigastric pain often occurring one to two hours after eating. Ulcerative colitis is an inflammatory disease involving, mainly, the mucosa and submucosa of the colon. The classic symptom of this condition is bloody diarrhea.

Regardless of which gastrointestinal alteration affects an individual, impacts are created upon the individual's psychological well-being, somatic identity, sexuality, occupational identity, and social role. To aid the afflicted person in dealing with either one of these gastrointestinal malfunctions, the nurse needs to identify how the illness is affecting each component of the individual's life and then assist him or her in dealing with each impact to the best of his or her ability.

Patient Situation   Mr. D. U. is a forty-five-year-old single, investigative newspaper reporter who is very active in his work and often attends job-related cocktail parties. When at these parties he drinks alcoholic beverages and smokes from one to two packs of cigarettes. Mr. D. U. has experienced persistent gnawing, burning pain in the epigastric region over the past three months. His pain tends to occur one to two hours after eating. Because of persistent discomfort, Mr. D. U.'s male sex partner encouraged him to see his physician about the problem. As a result, Mr. D. U. was admitted to the hospital for a gastrointestinal work-up.

It is now three days postadmission and Mr. D. U.'s diagnostic tests indicate the presence of a duodenal ulcer. During the nursing assessment the nurse in charge of Mr. D.U.'s care identified patient-centered problems related to his psychological well-being, somatic identity, sexuality, occupational identity, and social role.

Following are Mr. D. U.'s nursing care plan and patient care cardex dealing with each of these areas of concern.

NURSING CARE PLAN

Nursing Diagnoses	Objectives	Nursing Interventions	Principles/Rationale	Evaluations
Psychological Impact Unresolved dependence/independence conflict manifested by refusal to carry out health care therapies without frequent encouragement and approval from the nursing staff.	To decrease Mr. D. U.'s need to be dependent.	Encourage and allow Mr. D. U. to express his feelings of dependence.	Verbalization of feelings of dependence can aid in the development of insight into one's behavior.	The nurse would observe for: Open communication between Mr. D. U. and the nursing staff about his feelings of dependence.
	To increase Mr. D. U.'s self-esteem.	Avoid judgmental responses when Mr. D. U. expresses his need to be dependent.	Judgmental responses are barriers to communications.	
		Encourage Mr. D. U.'s male sex partner to verbalize his feelings about Mr. D. U.'s expressions of dependence.	Being aware of significant other's feelings aids members of the health care team in assisting the significant other to deal and cope with his feelings.	Mr. D. U.'s sex partner's open communication to the nursing staff about his feelings about Mr. D. U.'s feelings of dependence.
		Provide Mr. D. U. with realistic limits (e.g., explain to Mr. D. U. what health care therapies he is expected to carry out).	Setting limits aids in decreasing an individual's dependence.	A decrease in Mr. D. U.'s dependent behavior.

Somatic Impact Body image alteration manifested by expressed feelings that his body is completely controlled by the presence of the duodenal ulcer.	To assist Mr. D. U. in coping with his altered body image.	Avoid rigidity in limit setting (e.g., do not enforce the consumption of antacids/milk exactly on the hour or half-hour).	Rigidity often increases stress which can lead to an exacerbation of symptoms.	Mr. D. U.'s identification and avoidance of stressful situations.
		Aid Mr. D. U. in identifying and avoiding, if possible, situations that produce stress for him.	Avoidance of stressful situations can aid in decreasing the incidence of ulcer symptoms (e.g., epigastric pain).	
		Encourage Mr. D. U. to verbalize how he feels his disease entity affects his body image.	Open ventilation of feelings about body image can aid in the individual's ability to identify ways of coping with bodily changes.	The nurse would observe for: Open expression by Mr. D. U. regarding how he feels his disease entity affects his body image with possible solutions of how to deal with his altered body image.
		Provide Mr. D. U. with sound education about the basis of his disease process (e.g., what the illness entails and what factors contribute to its existence).	Realizing that certain bodily changes tend to occur with peptic ulcer can help in decreasing one's anxiety about an altered body image.	
		Instruct Mr. D. U. on the importance of food/antacid consumption on a regular basis to prevent occurrence of epigastric pain.	Realizing that regular consumption of food/antacids aids in decreasing the incidence of epigastric pain can aid in the ulcer victim's likelihood of adhering to this health care therapy.	Mr. D. U.'s regular consumption of food/antacids.

(cont.)

NURSING CARE PLAN (cont.)

Nursing Diagnoses	Objectives	Nursing Interventions	Principles/Rationale	Evaluations
Sexual Impact Sexual dysfunction manifested by expressed concern that libido is decreased during and after gnawing, burning, epigastric pain.	To decrease the incidence of circumstances that hinder a satisfying sexual experience.	Encourage Mr. D. U. to remember to consume antacids or food prior to engaging in a sexual experience.	Having food or antacids prior to a sexual experience can aid in decreasing the incidence of pain during the sexual encounter.	The nurse would observe for: Mr. D. U.'s verbalization that he is experiencing satisfying sexual encounters.
		Encourage Mr. D. U. to identify and avoid stressful situations prior to a sexual encounter.	Stress prior to a sexual experience can contribute to the occurrence of epigastric pain during the sexual encounter.	
Occupational Impact Potential job management deficit manifested by the fact that epigastric distress often occurs while at work.	To assist Mr. D. U. in identifying situations in the work environment that may potentiate his epigastric discomfort.	Encourage Mr. D. U. to verbalize to members of the health care team and to his male sex partner how he feels about his job.	Verbalization about a job aids in assisting the individual to identify the possible stresses of the job.	The nurse would observe for: Mr. D. U.'s verbalization of job situations that may contribute to his epigastric discomfort.

Social Impact* Potential social isolation manifested by the fact that epigastric distress tends to occur while attending cocktail parties.	To inform Mr. D. U. of social activities that can increase the incidence of epigastric distress.	Encourage Mr. D. U. to avoid shift work, if possible.	Changing shifts makes it difficult for an ulcer victim to consume foods and antacid regularly in an attempt to decrease the incidence of abdominal pain.	The nurse would observe for: Mr. D. U.'s verbalization of how alcohol, smoking, and stress can affect his peptic ulcer.
		Encourage Mr. D. U. to avoid alcohol consumption and smoking.	Alcohol consumption and smoking are both ill-advised activities for the ulcer victim since they can potentiate epigastric discomfort.	
		Encourage Mr. D. U. to drink fruit juices or soft drinks garnished with cherries and fruit slices at cocktail parties.	Drinking soft drinks while others are drinking alcoholic beverages can aid in decreasing the ulcer victim's feelings of awkwardness at a cocktail party.	
		Suggest the use of tactics that attempt to decrease the incidence of smoking. (Refer to Chapter 11 for details.)	Smokers are more likely to smoke when in the presence of other smokers.	

*Social activities generally are considered a form of relaxation, but they can be stressful.

PATIENT CARE CARDEX

PATIENT'S NAME: _____Mr. D. U._____

AGE: _____45 years_____

MARITAL STATUS: _____Single_____

SIGNIFICANT OTHERS: _____Male sex partner_____

MEDICAL DIAGNOSIS: _____Peptic ulcer—duodenal_____

SEX: _____Male_____

OCCUPATION: _____Investigative newspaper reporter_____

Nursing Diagnoses

Psychological: Unresolved dependence/independence conflict manifested by refusal to carry out health care therapies without frequent encouragement and approval from the nursing staff.

Nursing Approaches

1. Encourage verbalization of feelings about dependence.
2. Avoid judgmental responses to expressions of dependence.
3. Encourage male sex partner to express feelings about partner's expression of dependence.
4. Provide with limits (e.g., describe expected behavior in regards to health care therapies).
5. Avoid rigidity in limit setting (e.g., do not force consumption of antacids/milk exactly on the hour).

6. Aid in identifying and avoiding stressful situations.

Somatic: Body image alteration manifested by expressed feelings that his body is completely controlled by the presence of the duodenal ulcer.

1. Encourage verbalization about how disease entity affects body image.
2. Provide with sound education about basis of disease process (e.g., what illness entails and what factors contribute to its existence).
3. Instruct on importance of regular food/antacid consumption.

Sexual: Sexual dysfunction manifested by expressed concern that libido is decreased during and after gnawing, burning, epigastric pain.

1. Encourage regular consumption of antacids or food prior to engaging in sexual experience.
2. Encourage the identification and avoidance of stressful situations prior to a sexual encounter.

Occupational: Potential job management deficit manifested by the fact that epigastric distress often occurs while at work.

1. Encourage to verbalize how he feels about his job.
2. Encourage to avoid shift work, if possible.

Social: Potential social isolation manifested by the fact that epigastric distress tends to occur while attending cocktail parties.

1. Encourage the avoidance of alcohol consumption and smoking.
2. Encourage to drink fruit juices or soft drinks garnished with cherries and fruit slices when at cocktail parties.
3. Suggest the use of tactics that attempt to decrease the incidence of smoking.

REFERENCES

CASTELNUOVO-TEDESCO, P., SCHWERTFEGER, H., and JANOWSKY, D. Psychological characteristics of patients with ulcerative colitis and patients with peptic ulcer: A comparison, *Psychiatry in Medicine,* 1970, *1* (1), 59–75.

COBB, S., and ROSE, R. Hypertension, peptic ulcer, and diabetes in air traffic controllers, *Journal of the American Medical Association,* 1973, *244* (4), 489–492.

DWORKEN, H. *Gastroenterology: Pathophysiology and clinical applications.* Boston: Butterworths, 1982.

ERIKSON, E. *Childhood and society,* New York: W.W. Norton and Co., Inc., 1963.

FISHER, S., and CLEVELAND, S. *Body image and personality.* New York: Dover, 1968.

GIVEN, B., and SIMMONS, S. *Gastroenterology in clinical nursing.* St. Louis: C.V. Mosby, 1979.

GROSSMAN, M., GUTH, P., ISENBERG, J., PASSARO, E., ROTH, B. STURDEVANT, R., and WALSH, J. A new look at peptic ulcer, *Annals of International Medicine,* 1976, *84,* 57–67.

HERTZ, D., and ROSENBAUM, M. Gastrointestinal disorders. In E. Wittkower and H. Warnes (Eds.), *Psychosomatic medicine: Its clinical applications.* New York: Harper & Row Pub., 1977.

KUBICKOVÁ, Z., and VESELÝ, K. Fertility and reproduction in patients with duodenal ulcers, *Journal of Reproduction and Fertility,* 1974, *36* (2), 311–317.

LYKETSOS, G., ARAPAKIS, G., PSARAS, M., PHOTIOU, I., and BLACKBURN, I. Psychological characteristics of hypertensive and ulcer patients. *Journal of Psychosomatic Research,* 1982, *26* (2), 255–262.

MACLEAN, G. An approach to the treatment of an adolescent with ulcerative colitis, *Canadian Psychiatric Association Journal,* 1976, *21* (5), 287–293.

TAYLOR, J., GATCHEL, R., and KORMAN, M. Psychophysiological and cognitive characteristics of ulcer and rheumatoid arthritis patients, *Journal of Behavioral Medicine,* 1982, *5* (2), 173–188.

WOLCOTT, D., WELLISCH, D., ROBERTSON, C., and ARTHUR, R. Serum gastrin and the family environment in duodenal ulcer disease, *Psychosomatic Medicine,* 1981, *43* (6), 501–507.

14 |||||||||||||||||||||||||||||||||||||||||||||||||

STROKE OR
SPINAL CORD
INJURY

INTRODUCTION

Among the most devastating health care problems affecting humans are those involving neurological function. When a neurological malfunction is present, an individual's ability to move about freely and safely often is affected. The afflicted individual may become dependent upon others for assistance in carrying out his or her daily activities. There are numerous conditions affecting the neurological system, but only two of the more common alterations, strokes or cerebrovascular accidents (CVAs) and spinal cord injuries, will be dealt with in this chapter. Members of the health care team, however, will find that the health care concepts in this chapter also may be applied to persons afflicted with other neurological alterations.

PATIENT PROFILE

Approximately one half million persons suffer from strokes or cerebrovascular accidents each year with almost 200,000 dying annually. Stroke is the third cause of death in women and the fourth cause of death in men in the United States (Silverberg, 1983). It is the second cause of chronic illness and disability with approximately 1,820,000 people being disabled to some extent by the residual effects (American Heart Association, 1980). Modern and effective rehabilitation, however, has made it possible for over three quarters of the individuals who have suffered from a stroke to care effectively for themselves.

By definition, a stroke is a condition brought about by an acute vascular lesion in the brain. The three most common causes of a stroke are thrombosis, embolism, and hemorrhage with thrombosis being the most common (Kinney and Schenk, 1983). Although men and women can be afflicted with a stroke at any age, the greatest incidence occurs after thirty-five years of age. The onset of the disease process may be mild, with the afflicted person experiencing transient symptoms such as slight disturbances in speech or mild mental confusion. On the other hand the onset of the illness may be violent, with the afflicted individual falling to the floor in a comatose state, breathing stertorously, and demonstrating paralysis on one side of the body (Swift-Bandini, 1982).

By comparison, approximately 10,000 individuals sustain a spinal cord injury each year in the United States. Sixty percent of all spinal cord injuries are a result of motor vehicle accidents, with diving accidents, gunshot wounds, and pedestrian traffic collisions being the next three leading causes. Four out of five spinal cord injuries are experienced by men, with the male age group of eighteen to thirty-five years of age accounting for the single largest category of afflicted persons (Conway-Rutowski, 1982). Age-adjusted incidence rates are highest for black males and lowest for males of Asian origin. In addition, single, divorced, or separated individuals have been reported to encounter a higher risk of spinal cord injuries than married persons. The incidence of spinal cord injuries among nonmarried persons may be due to greater probability of risk-taking.

The symptoms manifested by a spinal cord injury vary greatly since they depend upon the level, severity, and extent of the injury. The spinal cord may be completely severed or only partially destroyed. Damage of the cord may cause paralysis of the body part innervated by nerves leaving the cord below the level of injury. However, there is no significant difference in the incidence of paraplegia as opposed to quadraplegia (Conway-Rutkowski, 1982).

A stroke or a spinal cord injury can inflict alterations upon an individual's motor and sensory status. The degree of alteration depends upon the severity and extent of the illness. Impacts have been imposed upon the psychological well-being, somatic identity, sexuality, occupational identity, and social role of the person afflicted with a stroke or the individual who has sustained a spinal cord injury. The remainder of this chapter will discuss how both illnesses affect these areas of concern and how the family, the nurse and other members of the health care team can assist the afflicted individual in coping with the resulting impacts.

IMPACT OF A STROKE OR A SPINAL CORD INJURY

Psychological Impact

When an individual is afflicted with a stroke, the psychological response to the illness encompasses the individual's basic personality characteristics, the personality disturbances accompanying cerebrovascular disease prior to the stroke, and the mental symptoms resulting from the cerebral damage and physical disability of the stroke. It is not uncommon for the afflicted individual, prior to a stroke, to display affective and intellectual disturbances due to cerebrovascular disease, with impairment of abstract thought being the most characteristic feature. With a loss of the abstract thought process, the afflicted individual becomes more stimulus-bound, encounters difficulty with attention and judgment, and tends to react to stress in a patterned way. Irritability, inability to withstand stress at home or at work, emotional liability demonstrated by sudden tears or jocularity, and increased anxiety or depression are early expressions of cerebrovascular disease.

Once the person sustains a stroke, additional psychological responses occur. The sense of powerlessness tends to be one of the cardinal psychological reactions immediately following the illness. The feeling of powerlessness is intensified when the individual finds that he or she is unable to move, is incontinent of urine and feces, and is incapable of verbal communication in an understandable form. This sense of powerlessness often is compounded by the victim's fear of total loss of body function and by fear that death may be near. His or her self-image has sustained a major blow and the individual questions self-worth. Two questions often asked by the stroke patient are: "What will become of me?" and "What will others think of me now?"

The individual afflicted with a stroke undergoes two additional psychological reactions: anxiety and depression. The anxiety tends to be associated with an awareness of the presence of diminished cerebral function in addition to physical incapacitation. The victim may encounter difficulties in thinking clearly and becomes disoriented to time, place, and person. Attempts to communicate may be futile since others are unable to comprehend what he or she is attempting to say. As a result, the stroke patient's anxiety heightens and his or her attempts to communicate become increasingly incomprehensible. The family also may undergo anxiety which often is characterized by apprehension and uncertainty about the future integrity of the family unit. The family members may demonstrate anger at the stroke patient because of their own feelings of powerlessness about the illness.

To aid the stroke patient and the family in dealing with the sense of powerlessness and the feelings of anxiety, the nurse needs to assess and identify the coping mechanisms used by both the individual afflicted with the stroke and the family. Since every person goes through life developing various means of coping and adapting to stressful situations, the nurse and other members of the health care team must be cognizant of these mechanisms. In other words, "How did this individual deal with previous stresses, such as an illness?" "What are the individual's physical and mental strengths?" "What are the family's strengths?" Once the coping mechanism and strengths of the stroke patient and the family have been identified, the nurse can assist them in utilizing these behaviors to deal with the illness. For example, if the stroke patient or the family members have found crying a means of relieving anxiety, then such a maneuver should be encouraged as a means of coping with stress. Possibly the counsel of a clergyman has been effective for the afflicted person or the family when crisis situations have occurred. If so, the patient should be encouraged to seek counsel from such a person as he or she attempts to cope with the impact of a stroke.

Depression, a second psychological reaction to stroke, is generally a behavior manifested in those persons who have encountered little intellectual impairment. Once the acute stage of the stroke has passed and the afflicted person's behavior patterns have stabilized, the nurse and other health team members must determine which behaviors are a result of brain damage and which are not. For example, when the stroke patient bursts into tears, is the behavior the result of "organic crying," the result of motor discharge, or the result of thinking sad thoughts?

The afflicted person's feelings of depression may be brought about by numerous situations. The stroke patient may feel depressed at the thought of being unable to carry out his or her daily activities. No longer can the stroke patient take for granted walking, feeding, bathing, or dressing himself or herself. The stroke patient now is dependent upon others for assistance and has concerns about the family's welfare, finances, and job security which may precipitate feelings of depression.

To assist the stroke patient and family members in dealing with depression, reassurance about the availability of both physical and psychological assistance is in order, as well as positive feedback on all progress made. The nurse should point out to the stroke patient that he or she has assumed more responsibility in self-feeding or personal hygiene when it occurs and praise the individual when increased independence in getting from the bed into the chair is demonstrated. Above all, the afflicted person *never* should be reprimanded for expressing feelings of depression. Often family members become embarrassed if their afflicted loved one suddenly bursts into tears or into gales of laughter when neither sad nor happy environmental events are present. It should be explained to the family that the stroke patient frequently encounters difficulties in controlling emotions and that he or she always should be allowed to express feelings openly. If family members continue to encounter difficulty in dealing with their loved one's expression of feelings, they may require guidance in identifying what specifically about the emotional outbursts upset them, in examining what the outbursts mean to them, and in delineating available alternatives for contending with these outbursts. As family members begin to delineate possible alternatives for dealing with the stroke patient's expression of feelings, they need to be encouraged to verbalize how they plan to deal with the feelings the next time they are expressed.

In contrast, the psychological impact of a spinal cord injury tends to be of an intense nature since the afflicted individual generally is a young adult who has sustained a traumatic accident. Immediately following the injury the afflicted person experiences repudiation. As discussed in Chapter 3, the initial reaction to loss is shock with thought processes being slowed and the person appearing confused and numb. The spinal cord injury patient often is unresponsive and remote when questioned about the accident. Feelings typically are flat and vague since the afflicted person fails to comprehend the total impact of what has happened to him or her, with the primary concern being survival.

Following a reaction of shock, a denial of the total impact of the illness or injury may be exhibited by the patient. He or she finds it difficult to believe or accept that sensory and/or motor alterations are present. The inability to move around freely seems totally incomprehensible. The individual does not want to talk or think about the injury since false hopes often arise as the patient fantasizes about moving around without restriction. A statement such as, "I'm going to walk out of this hospital come hell or high water!" is a demonstration of the afflicted person's denial.

To aid the spinal cord injury patient during the stage of repudiation, it is best to allow him or her to deny, but by no means should the nurse join the individual in denial. To remove denial suddenly would be disasterous since it is his or her only means of coping at this time. Instead, the spinal cord injury patient should be provided with truthful information about the illness. The information, however, should not be so extensive as to intensify the use of further denial. For example, if the individual asks if he or she will walk again, a simple statement such as, "It is very unlikely" can suffice. Giving the individual a five minute explanation about the neurological reasons why he or she will not walk again will only overwhelm the individual's already taxed psychological state. Eventually the spinal cord injury patient's denial breaks down due to the discovery that wishful thinking is not coming true.

Following demonstrations of denial, the spinal cord injury patient enters the second stage of loss, recognition. It is during this stage of loss that the individual begins to face the reality of the permanent disability. This stage of loss is marked by anxiety, hostility, guilt, and depression. It is not uncommon for the spinal cord injury patient to believe that he or she is being punished by God for real or imagined sins. The afflicted person may feel that the fate that has occurred is self-imposed. He or she may withdraw, be uncommunicative, and lie quietly in bed with the sheets drawn over the head to hide weeping.

Suicide in nonspecific terms may be contemplated with remarks such as, "I would be better off dead" or "I would like to die" being expressed. If the suicidal ideation takes on a specific plan, such as how, when, and where the act will be carried out, immediate psychiatric intervention is mandatory. It is a grave mistake to believe that disability mechanically precludes an individual's ability to commit suicide. Suicide is a significant cause of death in this population.

Since the spinal cord injury patient may blame others for the loss, hostility may be manifested during the stage of recognition with members of the health team and family often being the targets of the individual's wrath. The afflicted person's language may become abusive as his or her behavior becomes demanding, intolerant, and impatient. He or she is likely to be physically and verbally assaultive. Although the spinal cord injury patient may demonstrate thoroughly disagreeable behavior during the stage of recognition, it is a most opportune time to make rapid gains in the rehabilitative process.

To utilize the spinal cord injury patient's negative behavior during the stage of recognition, the nurse needs to channel such behavior into constructive endeavors. During periods of hostile and aggressive behavior, the spinal cord injury patient needs to be provided with activities that appropriately and constructively refocus his or her energies. If the individual is physically capable, a punching bag to hit, materials for leather tooling, or materials for rug hooking should be provided. All of these activities require physical expenditure of energy and at the same time aid in building muscles in the upper extremities. The afflicted person also should be encouraged to express hostility verbally while being guided in recognizing that he or she is responsible and accountable for behavior exhibited. It also is helpful to point out to the afflicted individual his or her positive attributes during the stage of recognition. Making a point of referring to what the patient can do both physically and mentally and what plans exist for rehabilitation is most beneficial. These maneuvers are direct attempts to help rebuild the spinal cord patient's self-concept while providing goal-directed behavior.

Family members may encounter difficulties in dealing with their loved one's expressed feelings during the stage of recognition. Therefore family members should be encouraged to ventilate their feelings of helplessness and frustration to members of the health care team. Ways in which they can help to channel the afflicted person's energies into constructive endeavors should be suggested. For example, bringing in the person's T.V. so that he or she can expend energy while watching a boxing match or a competitive skiing event is one possible suggestion. If the family continues to encounter difficulty in coping with the spinal cord victim's feelings during the stage of recognition, counselling may be in order and the nurse must refer the family accordingly.

The spinal cord injury patient enters the third stage of loss, resolution, when he or she comes to accept himself or herself as a disabled person. During resolution the individual begins to obtain satisfaction from new positive experiences such as learning to drive a car with hand controls or carrying out self-transfer techniques from a wheelchair to a car. These positive experiences enable the afflicted individual to feel good about ''self'' while achieving a sense of mastery over the environment. As a result, the individual begins to view himself or herself as someone who has the ability to be independent, to make decisions, and to realistically become a responsible individual. It is during resolution that the person with a spinal cord injury demonstrates the capability for organizing and planning his or her life in such a manner as to enable movement toward a more functional level.

The nurse's responsibility does not end when the individual with a spinal cord injury reaches the stage of resolution. It is during this period that the nurse must be ever aware of the individual's need for honesty, support, and reassurance. Although the spinal cord injury patient may have reached the stage of resolution, he or she may demonstrate anxiety, hostility, and depression during times of stress. Professional intervention may be necessary to aid the individual in dealing with these feelings. The nurse is advised to use interventions previously presented in relationship to these behavioral manifestations.

Somatic Impact

The extensiveness of the stroke or the spinal cord injury will determine the types of bodily dysfunctions occurring. However, certain bodily alterations tend to occur commonly in both of these illnesses. These alterations and the impact they create upon one's body image will be presented in this section.

An individual afflicted with a stroke undergoes numerous assaults to his or her body image. Some of the more common assaults include an alteration in bladder and bowel function, a loss of motor and sensory function on one side of the body, and an alteration in verbal communication. Each alteration creates difficulties for the afflicted person atttempting to redefine and deal with the post-stroke body image.

Urinary incontinence, a common problem for the person afflicted with a stroke, is brought about by the fact that micturition consists of both voluntary and involuntary control. The voluntary control is regulated by the cerebrum, while involuntary control is regulated by the reflex arc of the spinal nerves. Because the person afflicted with a stroke has undergone an alteration in cerebral function, the bladder may empty when intrabladder pressure stimulates the spinal nerve reflex. For the stroke patient, the awareness of the need to void tends to occur almost simultaneously with the automatic reflex act. If voluntary emptying of the bladder does not take place when the urge to void occurs, involuntary emptying of the bladder results. By comparison, constipation, another excretory dysfunction facing the stroke patient, is brought about by the fact that colon motility decreases while water absorption from the fecal mass continues as long as the fecal contents are in the colon. If improperly dealt with, constipation can lead to fecal impaction.

The role of the nurse in aiding the stroke patient in dealing with excretory dysfunction involves regulating bladder and bowel control. Since bladder and bowel control are bodily habits dealt with early in childhood, their dysfunction during adult life can lead to feelings of humiliation and thoughts of regression. In the early course of recovery the use of external catheters for male patients and indwelling catheters for female patients may be necessary to prevent urinary incontinence and subsequent skin breakdown. However, once the acute crisis of illness is over, it is advisable to establish a routine schedule for bladder retraining. In other words, regularly and consistently involving the patient in an adequate intake of fluid, in a perineal muscle-strengthening exercise program, and in a carefully planned voiding schedule is necessary. The stroke patient should be encouraged (unless contraindicated) to drink between 2000 and 2500 ml. of fluid each day, to engage in perineal exercises* four to six times a day, and to be placed on the commode or toilet every thirty minutes to two hours. As the program progresses, the patient should be encouraged to hold his or her urine longer so that the time intervals can be lengthened. In the case of bowel dysfunction, giving the stroke patient a suppository (i.e. bisacodyl) approximately one-half to one hour before breakfast, having the individual eat breakfast, and sitting the person on the toilet or commode immediately after breakfast has proven very effective for alleviating constipation. This routine should be carried out every other or every third day. If the stroke patient finds the morning too rushed, he or she may find carrying out the bowel cleansing procedure in the evening more convenient. Routinely checking the afflicted person for an impaction decreases the likelihood of accumulation of hardened stool in the rectum. In some circumstances a cleansing enema may be necessary; however, administering large enemas that decrease bowel tone should be a practice of the past.

In the event the stroke patient soils himself or herself at anytime with either urine or feces, reassurance needs to be provided regarding the fact that pre-stroke control over elimination has been altered. The individual should be cleansed immediately, in a matter-of-fact fashion, and should never be reprimanded for the soiling. Provision for the release of feelings of humiliation and embarrassment about the loss of elimination function needs to be provided. During the expression of feelings, information needs to be shared concerning the fact that bladder and bowel retraining may be slow, but with time most afflicted persons can be kept free of elimination soiling.

Alteration in motor and sensory function on one side of the body is another impact imposed upon the stroke patient's body image. On the affected side, the afflicted individual may manifest homonymous hemianopia, impairment in depth and visual perception in the horizontal and vertical planes, a decrease or loss of sensory input, and/or a decrease or loss of motor control. Homonymous hemianopia, blindness in one-half of the same field of vision for both eyes, tends to occur when the individual has sustained a stroke involving the right middle cerebral artery. With a right-sided stroke the visual field cuts that result are left-sided. Thus the individual may neglect food on the left side of the tray, bump into environmental objects that are to the left of the body, and start reading in the center of the printed page. The individual needs to be taught compensatory mechanisms to deal with this alteration in visual function so that unnecessary injury and frustration can be prevented. Such mechanisms include instructing the individual to intentionally look to the left to scan the en-

---

*The reader is advised to consult a medical-surgical nursing textbook for techniques in carrying out perineal exercises.

vironment and increase the visual field, placing the individual's food tray or other objects within the right visual field, and encouraging others to approach the stroke patient on the right side to avoid startling him or her. It also is advisable to position the stroke patient so that the visual field is toward the center of activity in the room. By so doing the stroke patient receives maximum visual stimulation from the environment and subsequently does not feel isolated.

Depth and visual perception in the horizontal and vertical planes also may be impaired in the stroke patient who has sustained an alteration in motor function on one side of the body (hemiplegia). These perceptual alterations cause problems in the patient's gait and posture which, in turn, may increase vulnerability to accidents. The stroke patient with perceptual alterations benefits from simplicity. Clothing that is simply designed and easy to put on, directions that are brief and concise, and food trays that are set with a minimum number of dishes and utensils are easiest for the individual to deal with, since decision making and complexity are reduced.

A decrease or a loss of sensation on one side of the body creates an image of one-half a body for the stroke patient. The individual may describe the affected side as useless, no good, and nonexistent. The stroke patient actually may verbalize a desire to rid himself or herself of part or all of the affected side. Since the afflicted individual fails to perceive normal sensations from the affected side, the chances of accidental injury to that side are increased. Accidental burning or cutting of the skin on the affected side may go unnoticed since painful stimuli are not perceived. The nurse and other members of the health care team need to emphasize this fact to the afflicted person and to family members. Use of heating pads, hot bath water, and constricting shoes and clothing, staying in one position for a long period of time, and going barefoot should be avoided since each of these activities can be a source of injury to the affected side. Both the stroke patient and the family should be encouraged to examine daily the affected side for possible cuts, burns, or pressure areas. If any of these injuries is noted, appropriate care must be initiated.*

A decrease or loss of motor control on the affected side results in alterations in mobility, in facial appearance, and in ability to feed oneself. As a result, the stroke patient may find that he or she will have to undergo rehabilitative processes to learn to walk and to feed himself or herself again. The individual may require the assistance of a custom-built fork, a cane, a walker, or a sling. Since ambulatory aids and feeding devices are necessary for mobility and independence, they eventually become an integral part of the person's body image. The stroke patient sees these aids and devices as an extension of self, since without them he or she cannot function independently.

As a result of sensory and motor loss, facial drooping on the affected side is common. When viewing oneself in the mirror the stroke patient may feel

---

*The reader is advised to consult a textbook of medical-surgical nursing for physical care of the individual with a stroke.

uneasy about facial appearance since one-half of the face responds to voluntary control. The affected side demonstrates an unhappy or drooping appearance as a result of the loss of muscle function. The afflicted individual needs to be encouraged to verbalize both to the members of the health care team and to the family how he or she feels about facial appearance. In addition, expressions of acceptance by health team members and family members are vital. Including the afflicted person in decision making, directly looking at him or her during communication, and making body contact are but a few maneuvers to use to express acceptance. Above all, health team members and family members must avoid making derogatory comments or remarks about the stroke patient's facial appearance.

The stroke patient may drool and be unable to remove food from the cheek on the affected side due to loss of control of facial muscles. To aid in decreasing the obviousness of these two problems, the afflicted person should be encouraged to carry tissues (these can be tucked inside the arm sling), to wipe secretions, and to check the cheek for residual food after eating. The stroke patient can be instructed to turn away from others while carrying out these maneuvers so as to avoid attracting unnecessary attention.

A decreased ability to use body language also exists for the stroke patient since altered motor control is present. No longer can the individual freely move the affected arm and leg in nonverbal expression. As a result, the stroke patient's use of body language initially may diminish, but as the recovery and rehabilitative processes progress, there will be a more conscious use of the unaffected side for nonverbal expression. Hence, the afflicted individual needs reassurance that as independence and mobility increase, spontaneous body language also will increase.

Another impact upon the stroke patient's body image is aphasia, a defect in the utilization and interpretation of the symbols of language brought about by a dysfunction in the cerebral cortex. Aphasia may be *sensory* in nature (receptive aphasia) in that the afflicted individual encounters difficulties comprehending speech, or *motor* in nature (expressive aphasia) in that the ability to produce speech is impaired (Conway-Rutkowski, 1982). Some stroke patients afflicted with receptive aphasia may be able to follow simple verbal commands with relative ease, others may be able to follow verbal commands accompanied by gestures, while some may be unable to follow even one-word and one-gesture commands. Stroke patients with expressive aphasia vary from being able to say one word over and over to being unable to utter a sound. Such an individual often points, nods, shakes his or her head, and uses pantomime in an attempt to communicate. Since a major human need is to communicate effectively with others, the presence of either receptive or expressive aphasia can be stress provoking.

To facilitate communication, the family, the nurse, and other health team members need to keep the following basic techniques in mind when communicating with the aphasic patient:

1. Provide a variety of auditory and visual stimuli.
2. Speak directly to the person.
3. Encourage the individual to look directly at the speaker.
4. Use simple one-word commands and gestures.
5. Speak in a normal tone of voice and at a slower than usual pace.
6. Keep sentence structure brief and simple.
7. Allow the person time to respond if a response is expected.
8. Provide paper and pencil if the individual is able to write, so that a picture of the object wanted can be drawn if necessary.
9. Provide the person with a book containing pictures of all the items he or she may request. The individual can point to the picture of the item needed.
10. Be patient as the person atttempts to comprehend communication and/or express himself or herself.

For some stroke patients speech therapy may be necessary. In such a case, the nurse should contact the health team member who is qualified to carry out the necessary therapy.

The somatic impact of a spinal cord injury is similar, in some respects, to the somatic impact of a stroke. The individual who has sustained a spinal cord injury also views his or her body as being half of its original size. With the spinal cord injury patient, however, the missing body parts extend either from the waist down (paraplegia) or extend from the neck down (quadriplegia). The individual who has become a quadriplegic, as a result of the injury, may describe his or her body image as nothing more than a head and a chest.

To aid the afflicted person in coping with his or her body image, one must encourage the individual to verbalize to the nurse and family members how he or she feels about not being able to move one half or three quarters of the body. Does the individual consider himself or herself dependent upon others? As the individual discloses personal feelings, the strengths he or she possesses need to be emphasized, such as the ability to problem-solve or the ability to be innovative. In addition, the spinal cord injury patient requires reassurance that through rehabilitation he or she will be able to become more independent and mobile with the use of ambulatory aids. As the individual develops skills of mobility and self-care, some of the feelings about being only one half or three quarters of a person may subside.

The spinal cord injury patient spends a large amount of time sitting in a wheelchair. As a result, the plane of communication is altered. Instead of communicating face to face with others, the individual communicates face to chest or face to waist. The spinal cord injury patient literally is looked down upon during the communication process just as the young child often is looked down upon by the adult. This alteration in body image may seem demeaning and, for the male spinal cord injury patient, even emasculating. To aid the patient in coping with the feeling of being talked down to, one should encourage the individual to request others to pull up a chair and sit if a conversation is to extend for any length of time. Members of the health care team and family members also need to remember to carry out this maneuver.

Changes in the size of the muscle mass of the upper extremities can be an additional body image alteration for the spinal cord injury patient who is a paraplegic. Paraplegics learn to use the upper extremities for moving the paralyzed body from one location to another. As a result, muscles become strengthened and enlarged. Generally, this alteration does not create problems unless the afflicted individual considers this increased muscle mass grotesque. The male paraplegic often believes that an increased muscle mass is a mark of masculinity while the female paraplegic views that change as an unfeminine attribute. Explaining to the afflicted female the value and reason for the increased muscle mass and encouraging her to wear clothing that loosely covers the arms and chest to aid in concealing the enlarged muscle mass can prove beneficial.

Bladder and bowel alterations are additional assaults to the integrity of the body image of the spinal cord injury patient. The person becomes dependent upon an intermittent catheterization program during the early weeks after injury due to reflexive emptying brought on by bladder atony. However, the spinal cord injury patient eventually must learn other methods of emptying the bladder, with the objective being a catheter-free state. Such methods include rectal stretching, the crede maneuver, and the Valsalva maneuver, all of which increase intra-abdominal pressure on the bladder to promote emptying*. To facilitate the individual's incorporation of any one of these methods into his or her body image, proper teaching of the method used is essential, as well as appropriate timing of the administration of the method so as to avoid unnecessary soiling. Bowel alteration for the spinal cord injury patient is related to a decrease in gastrointestinal motility. If constipation is not adequately treated an impaction can occur. The approaches for dealing with this problem are the same as the approaches used for dealing with altered bowel function.

The developmental stage being experienced by the stroke patient and the spinal cord injury patient at the time of illness has an effect upon the afflicted person's body image. If a stroke or spinal cord injury occurs during the developmental stage of young adulthood (eighteen to forty-five years) when energies are centered around sharing oneself with others in both friendship and a mutually satisfying sexual relationship (Erikson, 1963) and if the afflicted adult encounters problems in dealing with the illness, a sense of isolation is likely to develop. The sense of isolation may be brought about by the afflicted person's inability to see his or her body as useful and /or attractive. The accep-

---

*For further information on these methods, the reader is advised to consult a textbook of medical-surgical nursing.

tance of one's body image plays a vital role in being able to relate successfully to others. For the female afflicted with a stroke or a spinal cord injury, her body image centers around the appearance that she believes her body presents. If she sees herself as unattractive, she is likely to retreat from others. The male, on the other hand, is more likely to define his body image in terms of achievement rather than bodily attributes. If the afflicted male believes that he cannot achieve because of his altered body image, he too may retreat from others and fail to establish either a meaningful friendship or a mutually satisfying sexual relationship.

The presence of a stroke or a spinal cord injury during the stage of adulthood (forty-five to sixty-five years), when energies are directed toward establishing and guiding future generations with the hope of bettering society (Erikson, 1963), may lead to feelings of defeatism and depression. Instead of attempting to guide others, the afflicted person may withdraw and isolate himself or herself in self-pity.

The presence of an altered body image as the result of a stroke or spinal cord injury during the stage of maturity (sixty-five years and over), when frequent thoughts of death occur, may intensify the frequency of such thoughts. The afflicted person may view the illness as the final prelude to terminating his or her existence and, as a result, enter into a state of despair. The individual may question self-worth and value to others.

To aid the afflicted individual regardless of developmental stage, the person must be made to feel that he or she has something positive to offer. Pointing out the person's assets and what can be done for self and for others through rehabilitation can help to prevent isolation, stagnation, and despair. If the afflicted person was an avid and critical reader, proofreading rough draft manuscripts may be a realistic endeavor. If the individual was an outstanding cook, putting recipes into written form for others to use is another example of utilizing one's positive assets. Thus, the family, the nurse, and other members of the health care team must be creative in aiding the afflicted person in recognizing his or her attributes and utilizing them to their fullest.

Sexual Impact

Sexuality neither begins nor ends in the bedroom; it involves more than just coitus and is therefore an ever-present part of life. Just because an individual has sustained a neurological alteration, by no means is he or she void of sexuality and/or sexual expression. The impact of a neurological alteration upon one's sexuality will vary depending upon the location, the extent, and the nature of the alteration. Therefore, the first task in dealing with the sexual impact of a neurological condition, such as a stroke or a spinal cord injury, is to assess and identify, with the aid of the afflicted individual and his or her sex partner, the changes in sexual behavior that have occurred or will occur as a result of the illness.

The sexual impact of a stroke often demonstrates itself by a lack of interest in sexual activity or the development of new sexual inhibitions. It is not uncommon for the sex partner of the afflicted person to make the following comments: "My lover just is not interested in sex anymore. We used to have such a fulfilling sex life." The lack of interest or development of new inhibitions often is related to the afflicted person's fear of being unable to perform sexually and the fear of being sexually undesirable. The fear of being unable to perform sexually tends to be more prevalent in the male afflicted with a stroke than in the female since men often perceive their bodies as means of achieving. The fear of lacking sexual desirability tends to be more prevalent in the female stroke patient than in the male since women place more value on their appearance.

The stroke patient suffers from a loss in the ability to feel physical contact and in the ability to support body weight on the affected side since alteration in sensory/motor function has occurred due to the disease process. As a result, it is difficult, if not impossible to derive pleasure from sexual tactile experiences on the affected side or to support the body weight on the affected side. Nevertheless, members of the health care team must not write off the afflicted individual's ability to take part in and derive satisfaction from a sexual experience. The nurse's role in dealing with the sexual impact of a stroke is to identify and to discuss with the afflicted person and his or her sex partner, potential difficulties and possible alternatives related to the sexual experience. This must be done prior to the afflicted person's discharge from the acute care setting.

One of the most frustrating factors for the sex partner is being unaware of the possible difficulties related to the afflicted person's sexuality. Therefore, it is important to encourage the stroke patient and his or her sex partner to identify and to discuss with each other sexual experiences which each finds pleasurable. For example, the stroke patient will find it helpful to point out to the sex partner that it is advisable to direct physical caresses toward the unaffected side for maximizing the sexual experience. Using the side-lying position for the sex act may prove more comfortable for both partners since the stroke patient may encounter difficulties supporting personal body weight if he or she assumes the superior position. Both partners need to be encouraged to experiment with various positions and maneuvers so that they can identify what acts are most pleasurable for them. The sex partner should be encouraged to reassure the stroke patient of his or her sexual desirability. Complimenting the stroke patient on appearance or simply saying how nice it is to be with the individual are but two such examples. In addition, the sex partner should be encouraged to avoid referring to the afflicted person's ability to perform sexually since comments to this effect only intensify existing fears of sexual inadequacy. If the sexual impact of the stroke becomes overwhelming and seems unresolvable for the couple, the nurse needs to encourage sex counselling by a qualified therapist.

The sexual impact of a spinal cord injury depends upon the location and extent of the lesion. It has been clinically noted, however, that three specific problems tend to occur for the male spinal cord injury patient: the absence of an erection; the absence of ejaculation; and the absence of orgasm. According to the frequently cited study of Bors and Comarr (1960), when a complete upper motor neuron lesion is present, erection (reflexogenic* only) is possible in approximately 93 percent of the victims, ejaculation is rare, and orgasm is absent. In males afflicted with an incomplete upper motor neuron lesion, erection is possible in 99 percent of the victims (reflexogenic in 80 percent and reflexogenic and psychogenic** in 19 percent), ejaculation is infrequent, and orgasm is present if ejaculation occurs. When a complete lower motor neuron lesion is present, erection and ejaculation are infrequent and orgasm is present if ejaculation occurs. With an incomplete lower motor neuron lesion, erection (psychogenic and reflexogenic) is possible in 90 percent of the victims, ejaculation is frequent, and orgasm is present if ejaculation occurs. Generally the afflicted person will know within six months of the injury how much sexual function will return (Comarr, 1971). To assess sexual potential, the spinal cord injury patient requires a complete neurological examination since lack of information on the person's sexual potential could lead to the dissemination of erroneous explanations and inappropriate counselling.

The nurse's role, in assisting the spinal cord injury patient in dealing with the sexual impact of the illness, is to aid the patient and the sex partner in maximizing the sexual experience based upon sexual potentials. Manual stimulation of the penis generally is an effective method for promoting erection when psychogenic stimulation is ineffective. The use of a condom stretched around the base of the penis and held in place with stretchable tape may be used to maintain engorgement and prevent detumescence before intromission. However, the spinal cord injury patient should be encouraged not to position the condom too tightly or to leave it in place for more than thirty minutes (Woods, 1979) since an alteration in blood supply to the penis could occur. Caressing the inner surfaces of the thighs and the lower abdomen also can lead to an erection (reflex) and can prove beneficial for some couples during their sexual experiences. In addition, the male patient should be cautioned against the use of drugs or alcohol prior to intercourse since they act as central nervous system depressants and, as a result, may act to eradicate an erection.

Alternate means to sexual stimulation may need to be suggested to the spinal cord injury patient and his or her sex partner. For example, oral-genital contact may be desirable for some couples while manual stimulation of the clitoris and the "stuffing-technique" may serve as substitutes for intromission for the male incapable of an erection (Woods, 1979). The use of prosthetic devices, vibrators, or fantasy materials as aids to sexual arousal may be prefer-

*Reflexogenic: in response to local stimulation.
**Psychogenic: in response to psychic stimulation.

red by some individuals. Regardless of what means of sexual expression are selected, the forms and frequency of sexual activity are individual and depend upon sexual appetite.

Positioning during coitus may be a concern of the spinal cord injury patient. If the patient is a quadriplegic, a supine position with the sex partner on top, providing all activity, may prove most successful. With the paraplegic male, the use of top, bottom, or side-lying positions are realistic possibilities. The position(s) of choice will depend upon what the spinal cord injury patient and his or her sex partner find most conducive to heightened sexual experience.

The presence of a urethral catheter is a matter with which some male spinal cord injury victims may have to contend. Some males find it desirable to leave the catheter in place by bending it over the end of the penis and stripping a condom over the penis and the catheter. Others may find this experience difficult since traction is placed on the catheter and subsequent aggravation of a urinary tract infection can occur. If the male uses an external catheter, it should be removed prior to coitus and replaced afterwards. To aid in avoiding urination during intercourse, individuals who remove their internal and external catheters or who utilize intermittent catheterization should be advised to empty their bladders prior to coitus (Comarr and Gunderson, 1975). The spinal cord injury victim usually is able to withdraw in time to avoid urination since the urge to micturate in most cases is indicated by bladder spasms. To deal with the possible presence of urination during coitus, it is advisable for the couple to place a heavy absorbent towel under the buttocks.

In addition, it is essential to instruct the male spinal cord injury patient in good perineal care since chronic bladder infections are not uncommon and are a potential source of infection for the sex partner. Careful cleansing and inspecting of the skin integrity of the penis is a must. If the male is not circumcised, retracting the foreskin for cleansing is necessary in maintaining good hygiene.

Although a spinal cord injury does not necessarily preclude reproduction, the afflicted male's chances may be decreased. If the male spinal cord injury patient is unable to ejaculate successfully, there is little chance of impregnating the sex partner. In such cases, it may be advisable to recommend semen analysis for the purpose of artificial insemination. If artificial insemination is inadvisable, adoption or donor insemination may be recommended as alternative approaches.

Limited research has been conducted on the sexual function and sexual activity of the female who has sustained a spinal cord injury. It is known, however, that in complete lesions of the spinal cord, the female does not experience vaginal sensations. Although she may experience emotional satisfaction from intercourse, little in the way of physical satisfaction is encountered. According to Jackson (1972), few such women experience orgasm and it remains doubtful whether a true physiological orgasm can occur in the female with a complete spinal cord lesion. Faking an orgasm is not an uncommon practice and this, no doubt, is due to the female's wishes to please her sex partner.

One should not assume that the female who has undergone a spinal cord injury will have fewer fears and concerns about her feminine sexual identity than her male counterpart. It has been noted that women appear to be less disturbed than men about maintaining their sexuality with the opposite sex. This probably can be attributed to the fact that women, in general, tend to assume a more passive role during coitus. However, at no time should members of the health team negate the existence of fear and concerns about sexuality in the female spinal cord injury patient.

Positioning for the female who has sustained a spinal cord injury generally is supine during intercourse. However, other positions are not unrealistic and the afflicted individual and her sex partner may desire to experiment with various positions in order to find the one(s) most desirable for their particular sexual experience.

The existence of an internal catheter may raise questions about what to do with it during coitus. Since the catheter is positioned in an orifice separate from the orifice used for intercourse, it need not be removed. If the female wishes to remove the catheter or if she is on intermittent catheterizations, she should be encouraged to empty her bladder prior to coitus in order to prevent urination during intercourse.

As part of the sexual experience, the ability to bear children may be a question raised by the female spinal cord injury patient. The female who is still menstruating can, of course, conceive and give birth to children. She must be informed, however, that her normal menstrual cycle may be disrupted for approximately six months following the injury. If she is in or near menopause, she probably will not menstruate after the injury. Most women should be able to deliver children vaginally and a Caesarean section generally is not necessary unless anatomical or physiological problems intervene.

For both the male and female spinal cord injury patient, communication between the patient and the sex partner is vital. It is essential for both to discuss with each other their fears, feelings, and desires. For example, if the spinal cord injury victim desires an oral-genital experience and the sex partner finds this unpleasant, they should discuss this matter. During this discussion they may identify an alternate means of sexual expression which is desirable for both of them. It is through communication that the sharing of activities which are most pleasurable takes place. To illustrate, the female spinal cord injury patient may find that placing pillows under her thighs to support her legs is not only comfortable, but that it also increases the enjoyment of her sex partner's sexual experience. What the spinal cord injury patient and his or her sex partner need to realize is what they together find enjoyable is what is important.

The impact that the spinal cord injury has upon the stability of the relationship between the patient and spouse may be a concern of the afflicted person. If the relationship was unstable at the time of the injury, the chances of separation or a divorce may be greater. The divorce and separation rate has been found to be significantly higher in those afflicted individuals who had been married more than once at the time of the injury and who were once employed but are not currently. Most divorces tend to occur within a five-year period following the injury (Ghatit, 1975). Research has suggested that the divorce rate for the spinal cord injury patient does not differ from the divorce rate throughout the United States. The separation rate, however, appears to be lower among spinal cord injury patients than among the general population (Deyoe, 1972; Ghatit and Hanson, 1976).

Occupational Impact

As with all other impacts created by a neurological condition, the extent of the deficit greatly affects what impact the illness will have upon the afflicted person's ability to function in an occupational role. If the afflicted individual is employed at the time of the stroke, the chance of being forced out of the job market due to being unable to move about freely and independently is increased. Should the individual be retired and have saved money for a reasonably comfortable and independent life-style, medical expenses are likely to deplete his or her savings. Generally the afflicted individual's job-related health insurance ends with retirement and, as a result, limited resources for adequate payment of health care or rehabilitation may be available. Thus the retired person may be forced to become a recipient of public financial assistance following a stroke.

In assessing the impact that the illness has upon the occupation, the nurse needs to know whether the afflicted person must have full use of all extremities to carry out occupational endeavors. For example, an individual with a "desk job" most likely will have less difficulty in maintaining an occupational position than the individual who is involved in manual labor. The nurse's role in dealing with the occupational impact of the stroke involves assisting the afflicted person and the family in identifying what alterations can be made so that the stroke patient can continue to pursue occupational endeavors.

The presence of the illness may make the afflicted person totally incapable of continuing his or her pre-illness occupation. When the afflicted person and the family begin to identify the impact that the stroke will have upon occupational activities, the nurse's actions should be directed toward contacting members of the health care team qualified in assisting the stroke patient to deal with the occupational impact of the illness. Such health team members include the occupational health nurse, the social worker, the rehabilitation counselor, and/or the occupational therapist. These health team members can contact the stroke patient's employer and, with the employer, identify what alterations, if any, can be made in the work environment to accommodate the stroke patient. If accommodations cannot be made, job retraining may be necessary.

The impact of a spinal cord injury may demand alterations in occupational goals since the individual afflicted generally is a young adult at the beginning of his or her career. Since the paraplegic has functional use of the upper extremities, he or she retains the ability to carry out many different jobs. Therefore, the nurse should encourage the afflicted person and the family to identify what alterations, if any, may have to be made so that the spinal cord injury patient can continue occupational endeavors. Occupations requiring four workable limbs obviously would be out of the question; however, a limitless number of jobs require the use of only the upper extremities. For example, if the afflicted person was a professional ball player, he may find it feasible to change his career to coaching. If alterations in the work situation are not feasible, then job retraining is in order.

For both the stroke patient and the spinal cord injury patient, encouragement to reenter the work force as soon as possible is necessary. The nurse and other health team members must inform the afflicted person and the family of the importance of resuming gainful employment. Not only does gainful employment provide much needed economic support, but it also aids in decreasing the incidence of depression (Feibel and Springer, 1982; Richards, 1982).

Alterations in family roles may occur as a result of a stroke or a spinal cord injury. Prior to the illness the afflicted person may have assumed total control of the family's financial matters. Following the illness, other family members may have to assume part or all of this responsibility. If this occurs, the afflicted person may feel that his or her self-worth is being threatened. Thus, the nurse should encourage the afflicted person and family members to discuss what means can be used to maintain realistic family roles. It is not advisable to exclude totally the afflicted individual from the role he or she led within the family before the illness, since it may create feelings of low self-worth. Examination by family members of each individual's contribution to the family's integrity and the allowance for each contribution is vital for family stability.

Social Impact

The effect a neurological alteration, such as a stroke or a spinal cord injury, has on an individual's social identity depends on the degree of neurological deficit and the amount of social encounter engaged in by the specific individual. If little neurological deficit exists, the afflicted person probably will not have to alter social activities in any way. When sensory and motor deficits cause the afflicted individual to be immobile, he or she may find it necessary to make alterations in social activities (Sjogren and Fugl-Meyer, 1982).

One of the most common reactions to the social impact of a stroke is the fear of not being a desirable participant in social interactions. The afflicted person may feel he or she is a burden to others due to difficulty with or alterations in mobility. The ultimate outcome of such feelings may be withdrawal from social interactions. In order to engage in the social activities once enjoyed, the stroke patient may find it necessary to modify social involvement. For example, if he or she was an avid square dancer or an active cross-country skier, these activities may have to be altered or dispensed with entirely. Instead of square dancing, the afflicted person may find ballroom dancing more desirable or may even enjoy sitting along the sidelines conversing while watching others dance. If cross-country skiing was a sport enjoyed by the person, he or she may find bird watching an enjoyable substitute since this activity places the individual in the out-of-doors, just as skiing did. If the afflicted individual took part in more sedentary activities prior to the illness, then card playing, stamp collecting, or coin collecting may be feasible social activities.

When the nurse is assessing the social impact created by the stroke, it is advisable to be aware of the person's social life before the illness. The major goal is to assist the afflicted person in attaining and maintaining his or her pre-illness social state. The nurse and other members of the health care team should assist the stroke patient and the family in identifying social activities in which the patient can partake. As the type of activities are identified, certain environmental factors must be assessed. For example, does the environment housing the social activity have numerous steps for the stroke patient to climb and, if so, is a ramp available? Do the bathroom facilities provide a commode with handrails and an elevated commode seat to facilitate getting on and off the commode? Once the environment of the social function is examined, the stroke patient and the family can decide on the feasibility of taking part in the social event.

The presence of ambulatory aids may create difficulties for some individuals in the social setting. Some stroke patients may find their walkers a hindrance in setting up a comfortable social distance. In such cases, the nurse should encourage the stroke patient to sit and place the walker to one side, thus preventing the blockage of potential personal body contact. Should the stroke patient feel the arm sling is a distraction, he or she can be encouraged to wear colorful or decorative slings. How colorful and decorative the afflicted person desires to be is strictly up to the individual.

In addition to wearing colorful and attractive arm slings, the stroke patient should be encouraged to buy clothing that is both becoming and easy to put on and take off (e.g., clothes that button and zip in the front). Often one of the greatest deterrents to taking part in social functions is the concern about how one looks to others. Clothing that is both becoming and comfortable for the individual and easy to get in and out of is more likely to be worn. If the person feels attractive to others, engaging in social events is more likely to occur.

The stroke patient and the family need to express to each other how they feel about taking part in social activities in which a handicapped individual is included. If the stroke patient feels like a burden in some social events, he or she should be encouraged to say so. If young grandchildren feel that their grandparent afflicted with a stroke is an unpleasant addition at certain social functions, they need to express these feelings. Once these feelings are expressed, the afflicted person and the family are more capable of appropriately selecting, together, social activities that can be enjoyed by all. In some situations, the stroke patient and the family may find it advisable to attend certain social functions separately, but it is better if this is a joint decision made within the family structure.

Often social events involving large crowds can create difficulties for the stroke patient. Crowding may cause the afflicted person to feel unstable on his or her feet and, as a result, he or she may fear falling. In such circumstances it is advisable to plan to arrive at the social function early and to leave after others have left in an attempt to avoid the pushing and shoving encountered by crowding.

The nurse may find it beneficial to encourage the stroke patient to take part in a stroke club. Such an organization can provide educational assistance and aid in offering a supportive milieu that helps the afflicted person resocialize. In addition to stroke clubs, senior citizen clubs, church groups, and retirement centers are other possible resources for socialization.

One of the most common social impacts of a spinal cord injury is how one contends with the presence of the much needed ambulatory aid, the wheelchair. Since the individual is dependent upon the wheelchair for mobility, the spinal cord injury patient will find it necessary to assess social activities engaged in prior to the illness in order to identify whether the wheelchair will in any way hinder specific social interactions. For example, can the wheelchair be maneuvered into the building that houses the social activity, e.g., are ramps available? Can bathroom facilities in the building accommodate a wheelchair? If the doors to the bathroom and the commode are large enough to allow the entry of the wheelchair, does the commode area allow for maneuverability of the wheelchair? Although many public facilities have made great strides in the construction of ramps and bathroom facilities for the handicapped, many public and private facilities remain inconvenient for the presence of the individual with a wheelchair.

The spinal cord injury patient may be required to alter a social activity because of the wheelchair. It should be pointed out to the patient and the family, however, that many social and sports events need not be eliminated because of the wheelchair. For example, the spinal cord injury patient (i.e., paraplegic) confined to a wheelchair can continue to bowl, take part in archery, play cards, and even play baseball and basketball. In fact, there are a number of sports tournaments ranging from track and field events to water sports for those confined to wheelchairs. With a little imagination and ingenuity, the wheelchair bound spinal cord injury patient can carry out an almost limitless number of social and sports activities. The nurse and other members of the health care team should encourage the afflicted person and the family to be imaginative so that the spinal cord injury patient can continue to enjoy social and sports activities.

The presence of a wheelchair during social events may create concern since the patient may fear that its presence is a deterrent to social interactions and that it draws attention to the disability. To aid in dealing with these feelings, the nurse can suggest that the spinal cord injury patient transfer from the wheelchair to a couch or chair at social gatherings. If the individual attends a concert or the theater, transferring from the wheelchair to an aisle seat and putting the collapsed wheelchair out of the way aid in decreasing the noticeability of the ambulatory aid during the social encounter.

What to wear when confined to the wheelchair may be an additional concern for the spinal cord injury patient. Females can be advised to wear slacks or pantsuits because they prevent unnecessary exposure during transfer to and from the wheelchair. If the woman does not like slacks or pantsuits, then long dresses or dresses with full skirts are an alternative means of avoiding unnecessary exposure during transfer. Coats can create difficulties in a wheelchair since their length can be a nuisance when assuming a sitting position; therefore, short jackets and ponchos are manageable possibilities. Clothing usually does not create problems for the male spinal cord injury patient who uses a wheelchair. Men, however, also are advised to wear jackets instead of long overcoats since they are easier to arrange and hence more comfortable. Both men and women spinal cord injury patients using wheelchairs are advised to wear attractive clothing that accentuates the torso (Bregman and Hadley, 1976). If the afflicted person feels attractive to others, he or she is less likely to avoid social contacts. To add to one's attractiveness, the nurse can suggest to the spinal cord patient the selection of an attractive wheelchair (e.g., a patterned design or a favorite color).

The spinal cord injury patient and the family should be encouraged to express to each other their feelings about taking part in social events. As with the stroke patient, situations identified as uncomfortable for either the afflicted person or the family should be discussed. Together they must decide on the most appropriate way to handle a specific social activity. Above all, the afflicted person and the family require encouragement from the nurse not to allow themselves to withdraw from social involvement and retreat into isolation.

SUMMARY

Alterations in neurological function can produce devastating impacts upon an individual's life-style. Two of the more common neurological disorders are stroke and spinal cord injury. Approximately one half million persons are afflicted yearly with a stroke and approximately 10,000 persons yearly sustain an injury to the spinal cord. A stroke is a condition brought about by an acute lesion in the brain. Both men and women can be afflicted by this illness, with the greatest incidence of occurrence being after thirty-five years of age. A spinal cord injury generally is brought about by trauma with men being afflicted four times more often than women. Individuals sustaining a spinal cord injury tend to be in the age group of eighteen to thirty-five years. Both conditions can produce a variety of neurological symptoms depending upon the location and extent of the cerebral or spinal cord involvement.

Regardless of whether an individual sustains a stroke or a spinal cord injury, the neurological deficits created by the illness place an impact upon the afflicted person's psychological well-being, somatic identity, sexuality, occupational identity, and social role. The nurse's role involves assisting the afflicted person and the family in identifying what impact the illness has upon each component of the individual's life and to aid him or her in dealing with each resulting impact.

Patient Situation Mr. C. A. is a fifty-seven-year-old art museum curator. He is married and the father of five children. Two of his children still reside at home with him and his wife. In conjunction with his job, Mr. C. A. is involved in many social activities including fund raising events for the art museum.

Eight days ago Mr. C. A. suffered a stroke while at work. He is now in an acute care center and plans are being made for his rehabilitation and discharge to home. The nurse in charge of Mr. C. A.'s discharge planning has identified problems related to Mr. C. A.'s psychological well-being, somatic identity, sexuality, occupational identity, and social role.

Following are Mr. C. A.'s nursing care plan and patient care cardex dealing with each of these areas of concern.

NURSING CARE PLAN

Nursing Diagnoses	Objectives	Nursing Interventions	Principles/Rationale	Evaluations
Psychological Impact Self-esteem disturbances manifested by expressed feelings about a sense of powerlessness.	To enhance Mr. C. A.'s feelings of self-worth.	Encourage Mr. C. A. and his family to identify coping mechanisms used by Mr. C. A. in the past (e.g., how did he deal with previous stressors, such as an illness?).	Every person goes through life developing various means of coping with stressful situations.	The nurse would observe for: Mr. C. A.'s increased verbalization about his self-worth (e.g., his positive attributes).
		Encourage Mr. C. A. to utilize coping mechanisms used in the past for dealing with stressful situations (e.g., crying or counsel of a religious leader).	Using coping mechanisms utilized in past stressful situations can aid the afflicted individual in coping with the present stress, a stroke.	
Somatic Impact Impaired verbal communication manifested by difficulty in expressing self in the verbal form.	To facilitate Mr. C. A.'s ability to communicate. To decrease Mr. C. A.'s anxiety as he attempts to express himself.	Encourage members of the health care team and family to carry out the following techniques: 1. Provide Mr. C. A. with a variety of auditory and visual stimuli.	A variety of auditory and visual stimuli prevent monotony which, in turn, enhances the likelihood of an increased comprehension of the stimuli.	The nurse would observe for: Mr. C. A.'s increased ability to communicate effectively. Mr. C. A.'s decreased anxiety during his attempts to communicate.
		2. Speak directly to Mr. C. A. 3. Encourage Mr. C. A. to look directly at the speaker.	Speaking directly to the stroke patient decreases the chances of misinterpretation of the spoken word.	

Intervention	Rationale
4. Use simple one-word commands and gestures.	Uncomplicated communication is easier to comprehend.
5. Speak in a normal tone of voice and at a slower than usual pace.	Normal voice tones and a slow speaking pace increase the likelihood of the stroke patient's comprehension of the spoken message.
6. Keep sentence structure brief and simple.	Simple sentence structure is easier to comprehend.
7. Allow time for Mr. C. A. to respond if a response is expected.	Providing adequate time for the stroke patient to respond aids in decreasing anxiety during attempts to communicate.
8. Provide Mr. C. A. with paper and pencil so that he can draw a picture of the object he wants.	Providing the stroke patient with a variety of ways to communicate aids in enhancing the ability to communicate effectively.
9. Provide Mr. C. A. with a book containing pictures of all the items he could possibly request so that he can point to the pictures of the items he needs.	Providing alternate means of communication aids in decreasing the stroke patient's anxiety when one means of communication proves ineffective.
10. Be patient with Mr. C. A. as he attempts to express himself.	Impatience demonstrated on the part of the health team members and family members when the stroke patient is attempting to communicate tends to increase the afflicted individual's anxiety.

(cont.)

293

NURSING CARE PLAN (cont.)

Nursing Diagnoses	Objectives	Nursing Interventions	Principles/Rationale	Evaluations
Sexual Impact Sexual dysfunction manifested by expressed lack of interest in sexual activity.	To decrease Mr. C. A.'s fear about being unable to perform sexually.	Encourage Mr. and Mrs. C. A. to ventilate openly their feelings with each other about the sex act.	Open ventilation between the stroke patient and sex partner aids in decreasing the afflicted person's anxiety about the sex act.	The nurse would observe for: Mr. C. A.'s verbalization about a more active interest in sexual activity with his wife.
		Encourage Mr. and Mrs. C. A. to identify and discuss with each other sexual experiences which each finds pleasurable (e.g., caressing Mr. C. A.'s unaffected side since sensory deficits exist on the affected side or using the side-lying position since Mr. C. A. may find it awkward to support his body weight in a superior position).	Identifying sexual experiences which both partners find enjoyable enhances the likelihood of a mutually satisfying sexual experience.	
		Encourage Mr. and Mrs. C. A. to experiment with various coital positions and sexual maneuvers.	Experimenting with various coital positions and sexual maneuvers can aid in identifying situations that enhance a mutually satisfying sexual experience.	

	To enhance Mr. C. A.'s feelings of sexual desirability.	Encourage Mrs. C. A. to reassure Mr. C. A. that he is sexually desirable (e.g., tell him how nice it is to be alone with him once again). Encourage Mrs. C. A. to avoid referring to Mr. C. A.'s ability to perform sexually.	Reassuring a stroke patient of sexual desirability helps enhance feelings of self-worth. Comments about a stroke patient's abilities to perform sexually can add to existing fears of sexual inadequacy.	The nurse would observe for: Mr. C. A.'s verbalization of how his illness may alter his occupational role.
Occupational Impact Job management deficit manifested by verbalized concern about being unable to maintain job responsibilities.	To facilitate Mr. C. A.'s ability to look realistically at the possibility of having to make alterations in his job situation.	Encourage Mr. C. A. and his family to identify what alterations in the work situation will be necessary in order for Mr. C. A. to continue his job as museum curator. Contact members of the health care team qualified in assisting Mr. C. A. to deal with the occupational impact of his illness (e.g., occupational health nurse, social worker, occupational therapist and/or rehabilitation counselor).	Stroke patients often are able to continue in their pre-illness occupational pursuits with only minor changes having to be made in the job environment. Health team members such as the occupational social worker, occupational therapist, and/or health nurse, rehabilitation counselor are in an excellent position to contact the stroke patient's employer and with his or her help, identify what alterations, if any, can be made in the work situation to accommodate the afflicted employee.	

(cont.)

NURSING CARE PLAN (cont.)

Nursing Diagnoses	Objectives	Nursing Interventions	Principles/Rationale	Evaluations
Social Impact Potential social isolation manifested by expressed concern about how he will appear to others during social engagements.	To prevent Mr. C. A.'s withdrawal from social interactions.	Encourage Mr. C. A. and his family to discuss how each feels about attending social engagements with a disabled person.	Verbalization between the stroke patient and the family about attending social engagements facilitates the selection of appropriate social activities which can be enjoyed by all.	The nurse would observe for: Mr. C. A.'s verbalization about enjoying social activities.
		Inform Mr. C. A.'s family about the importance of encouraging Mr. C. A. to take part in social activities.	Difficulty or alterations in mobility may cause the stroke patient to feel like a burden during social engagements and, as a result, cause the patient to withdraw from social encounters.	
	To increase Mr. C. A.'s comfort when attending social events.	Encourage Mr. C. A. and his family to assess the social environment for features that facilitate the stroke patient's independence (e.g., ramps instead of stairs and elevated commode seats).	Social events housed in environments that facilitate the stroke patient's independence are more likely to be attended by the afflicted person.	

Encourage Mr. C. A. to purchase clothes that are becoming and easy to put on and take off.	Clothing that is becoming and easy to put on and take off is more likely to be worn. In turn, if the stroke patient feels attractive to others, he or she is more likely to engage in social encounters.
When Mr. C. A. attends events where there are large crowds, encourage him to arrive early and to wait until the majority of the crowd has left before leaving.	Maneuvers that aid the stroke patient in avoiding pushing and shoving of large crowds helps the afflicted person to deal with the feeling of physical instability.
Suggest to Mr. C. A. the possibility of attending a stroke club.	Organizations, such as a stroke club, can provide a supportive milieu that aids in the stroke patient's resocialization.

PATIENT CARE CARDEX

PATIENT'S NAME: ___Mr. C. A.___   MEDICAL DIAGNOSIS: ___Stroke___

AGE: ___57 years___   SEX: ___Male___

MARITAL STATUS: ___Married___   OCCUPATION: ___Museum curator___

SIGNIFICANT OTHERS: ___Wife and five children (two living___

___at home)___

Nursing Diagnoses	Nursing Approaches
Psychological: Self-esteem disturbances manifested by expressed feelings about a sense of powerlessness.	1. Encourage identification of coping mechanisms used in past stressful situations. 2. Encourage utilization of coping mechanisms used in past stressful situations.
Somatic: Impaired verbal communication manifested by difficulty in expressing self in the verbal form.	1. Utilize the following techniques when communicating: (a) Provide with a variety of visual and auditory stimuli. (b) Speak to directly. (c) Encourage to look directly at the speaker. (d) Use simple one-word commands and gestures.

(e) Speak in a normal tone of voice and at a slower than usual pace.
(f) Keep sentence structure brief and simple.
(g) Allow time for a response if a response is expected.
(h) Provide paper and pencil for drawing a picture of items requested.
(i) Provide a book containing pictures of all items possibly needed. Have patient point at items needed.
(j) Be patient during attempts to express self.

Sexual: Sexual dysfunction manifested by expressed lack of interest in sexual activity.

1. Encourage to identify with wife sexual experiences each find pleasurable (e.g., caressing unaffected side of body or using side-lying position).
2. Encourage husband and wife to experiment with various coital positions and sexual maneuvers.
3. Encourage wife to reassure husband that he is sexually desirable.
4. Encourage wife to avoid referring to husband's ability to perform sexually.

Occupational: Job management deficit manifested by verbalized concern about being unable to maintain job responsibilities.

1. Encourage, along with family, to identify alterations in work setting that will be necessary in order to facilitate job as museum curator.
2. Contact members of the health care team qualified in dealing with the occupational impact of a stroke (e.g., occupational health nurse, social worker, occupational therapist, and/or rehabilitation counselor).

Social: Potential social isolation manifested by expressed concern about how he will appear to others during social engagements.

1. Encourage to discuss with family how each member feels about attending social engagements with a disabled person.
2. Inform family of importance of encouraging afflicted individual to take part in social activities.
3. Encourage, along with family, to assess social environments for features that facilitate a stroke patient's independence (e.g., ramps and elevated commode seats).
4. Encourage to buy clothes that are both becoming and easy to put on and take off.
5. Encourage when attending events where there are large crowds to arrive early and leave after most of the crowd has left.
6. Suggest involvement in a stroke club.

REFERENCES

AMERICAN HEART ASSOCIATION, *Heart Facts*. Dallas: American Heart Association, 1980.

BORS, E., and COMARR, A. Neurological disturbances of sexual function with special reference to 529 patients with spinal cord injury, *Urological Survey*, 1960,*10*, 191–221.

BREGMAN, S., and HADLEY, R. Sexual adjustment and feminine attractiveness among spinal cord injured women, *Archives of Physical Medicine and Rehabilitation*, 1976, *57* (9), 448–450.

COMARR, A. Sexual concepts in traumatic cord and equina lesions, *Journal of Urology* 1971, *106*, 375–378.

COMARR, S., and GUNDERSON, B. Sexual function in traumatic paraplegia and quadriplegia, *American Journal of Nursing*, 1975, *75* (2), 250–255.

CONWAY-RUTOWSKI, L. *Carini and Owens' neurological and neurosurgical nursing*. St. Louis: C.V. Mosby, 1982.

DEYOE, F. Marriage and family patterns with long-term spinal cord injury, *Paraplegia*, 1972, *10* (3), 219–224.

ERIKSON, E. *Childhood and society*. New York: W.W. Norton and Co., Inc., 1963.

FEIBEL, J., and SPRINGER, C. Depression and failure to resume social activities after stroke, *Archives of Physical Medicine and Rehabilitation*, 1982, *63* (6), 276–277.

GHATIT, A. Outcome of marriages existing at the time of a male's spinal cord injury, *Journal of Chronic Disease*, 1975, *28*, 383–388.

GHATIT, A., and HANSON, R. Marriages and divorce after spinal cord injury, *Archives of Physical Medicine and Rehabilitation*, 1976, *57* (10), 470–472.

JACKSON, R. Sexual rehabilitation after cord injury, *Paraplegia*, 1972, *10* (1), 50–55.

KINNEY, M., and SCHENK, E. Problems of the nervous system. In W. Phipps, B. Long, and N. Woods (Eds.) *Medical-surgical nursing: concepts and clinical practice*. St. Louis: C.V. Mosby, 1983.

RICHARDS, B. A social and psychological study of 166 spinal cord injured patients from Queensland, *Paraplegia*, 1982, *20* (2), 90–96.

SILVERBERG, E. Cancer statistics, *Ca-A Cancer Journal for Clinicians*, 1983, *33* (1), 9–25.

SJOGREN, K., and FUGL-MEYER, A. Adjustment to life after stroke with special reference to sexual intercourse and leisure, *Journal of Psychosomatic Research*, 1982, *26* (4), 409–417.

SWIFT-BANDINI, N. *Manual of neurological nursing*. Boston: Little, Brown, 1982.

WOODS, N. *Human sexuality in health and illness*. St. Louis: C.V. Mosby, 1979.

15 ⅠⅠⅠⅠⅠⅠⅠⅠⅠⅠⅠⅠⅠⅠⅠⅠⅠⅠⅠⅠⅠⅠⅠⅠⅠⅠⅠⅠⅠⅠⅠⅠⅠⅠⅠⅠⅠⅠ

RENAL FAILURE

INTRODUCTION

Historically, the concept of dialysis is not new to the world of health care. In the early 1900s attempts were made to devise the first prototype of the hemodialyzer (Abel, Rawntree, and Turner, 1913), but it has been within the past four decades that hemodialysis has become a well-established form of therapy for individuals afflicted with renal failure or irreversible kidney damage. There are approximately 35 thousand Americans maintained on hemodialysis, 15 percent of whom utilize home hemodialysis (Wineman, 1978). Thus, the professional nurse is responsible for working with individuals who are dependent upon a machine for sustaining life.

The basic goals of hemodialysis are: (1) to remove end-products of protein metabolism (urea and creatinine) from the blood; (2) to maintain a safe concentration of serum electrolytes; (3) to correct acidosis and replenish the blood's bicarbonate system; and (4) to remove excess fluid from the blood (Miller, 1983). These goals are accomplished by having the individual's blood flow from his or her body into a membrane package (the dialysis machine) and back again into the body. While the afflicted person's blood is in the dialysis machine diffusion takes place between the individual's blood and the dialysate solution across a semi-permeable membrane of the dialysis machine. In order to make an access to the patient's blood supply for the dialysis procedure, either an external arteriovenous shunt is inserted or an internal arteriovenous fistula is made.

Perhaps the greatest limitation imposed upon the person undergoing hemodialysis is the time involved in the therapy since the individual must spend approximately four to ten hours, two to three times a week, on the dialysis machine. Depending on hemodialysis for sustaining life has an impact on the afflicted person's psychological well-being, somatic identity, sexuality, occupational identity, and social role. The remainder of this chapter will discuss how hemodialysis can affect each of these areas of concern.

IMPACT OF HEMODIALYSIS

Psychological Impact

An individual afflicted with renal failure or irreversible kidney damage is faced with a life-threatening situation. Something must be done about the condition or the individual will die. Hemodialysis has saved many lives and continues to save lives, but the psychological impact of kidney malfunction does not end when the afflicted individual begins dialysis. The individual undergoing hemodialysis becomes a marginal person since he or she is neither ill nor well and is forced to become committed to the dialysis machine for survival (Rajapaksa, 1979).

Because of this commitment, three stages of adaptation tend to be experienced—the "honeymoon" period, the period of disenchantment and discouragement, and the period of long-term adaptation (Reichsman and Levy, 1972). The "honeymoon" period occurs one to three weeks after the individual's first dialysis treatment and lasts from six weeks to six months. It is during this stage of adaptation that the individual demonstrates a marked improvement both physically and psychologically. Confidence, hope, and a relative lack of perception of personal limitations and the hardships that accompany the therapy are manifested. Most afflicted persons readily accept their intense dependence upon the dialysis machine, the dialysis procedure, and the professional staff. However, individuals who dislike being dependent initially encounter more difficulties in coping with the "honeymoon" period than the individual who enjoys a state of dependence.

Few individuals experience basic displeasure during the "honeymoon" period; however, this period of adaptation is not free of problems. Many afflicted persons experience repetitive, intense periods of anxiety and fear. When questioned about their feelings, they tend to refer fears related to mechanical failure at the shunt site, to running out of shunt sites, to machine failure, to life expectancy, and to the ability to return to work (Jennrich, 1975). Despite some expressed anxieties and fears during this period of adaptation, the "honeymoon" period is dominated by feelings of contentment, confidence, and hope. The afflicted person basically repudiates his or her loss of wellness.

The nurse's role in assisting the individual to cope with the "honeymoon" period involves encouraging the individual to express his or her anxieties and fears about the dialysis process. As the patient discloses personal feelings, information needs to be provided concerning how the machine functions and what mechanisms exist to assure the safety and well-being of the patient. The patient's confidence, hope, and contentment should be maintained; however, he or she should be encouraged to recognize personal limitations so as not to overextend or overexert.

When the "honeymoon" period ends, the second stage of adaptation to hemodialysis, the period of disenchantment and discouragement begins. The stage of disenchantment and discouragement lasts approximately three to twelve months and is characterized by a distinct change in the individual's effective behavior. The onset of this period of adaptation may be very abrupt or gradual; however, it frequently occurs in relation to a specific stressful event. The specific stressful event may be the individual's planned or actual resumption of employment or household duties. Feelings of contentment, confidence, and hope markedly decrease and/or disappear and in their place are feelings of helplessness and sadness. The afflicted person has begun to recognize his or her loss of wellness.

During the stage of disenchantment and discouragement the afflicted person manifests an increase in dependent behavior. The individual may refuse to make decisions, be demanding of others, verbally abuse family and health team members, and demonstrate regressed emotional reactions. The major difficulty at this time lies in the individual's dependence upon the dialysis machine for survival and the required therapy's stringent restrictions. Diet and fluid intake are critically controlled, and free time is limited since dialysis therapy can consume as much as twenty to thirty hours a week. Thus, the afflicted person experiences a dependence/independence conflict. In addition to the dependence/independence conflict, depression can result during the stage of disenchantment and discouragement. The afflicted person questions the value of existence and the quality of life. When these feelings of depression are not transient, health team members must be aware of the potential existence of suicidal ideations. Surveys have indicated that the incidence of suicide in hemodialysis patients is more than 100 times that of the general population (Abram, Moore, and Westerfelt, 1971).

The nurse's role during the period of disenchantment and discouragement is to assist the afflicted person in coping with the dependence/independence conflict and with feelings of depression (Levy, 1981). To assist the dialysis patient in dealing with the dependence/independence conflict, it is helpful to point out that the reality of the illness requires dependence upon the dialysis machine and health team members and/or family to carry out the dialysis treatment. Reassurrance that dependence in these two forms are necessary and socially acceptable must be provided. On the other hand, regressive behavior, verbal abuse toward others, and demanding behavior are neither necessary nor socially acceptable forms of dependence. The overly dependent dialysis patient may need encouragement to look at his or her behavior when using these socially unacceptable forms of dependence. When the patient lashes out at family or health team members, he or she needs to be reminded that this behavior is inappropriate; however, reassurance that he or she is acceptable as a person needs to be expressed. For example, if a husband who is undergoing home dialysis therapy verbally strikes out at his wife, she may find it therapeutic to respond with, "Honey, I love you very much, but sometimes what you say to me is very upsetting!"

To foster independence, the dialysant should avoid the use of night clothes and the use of a bed during the dialysis treatment since the presence of these two items aid in placing the individual in the dependent role of illness. In addition, the individual should actively participate in health care therapies by planning and by carrying out diet and fluid restrictions. Positive feedback from others should be forthcoming when the individual demonstrates increased initiative in these activities. Involvement is especially important during dialysis therapy because all too often the individual may want to retreat into sleep during therapy. One of the few times that sleep during the entire process would be advisable is when the treatment is set up during sleeping hours for the sole purpose of allowing for sleep and therapy simultaneously. Such an arrangement may be necessary when attempts are being made to meet the time demands of a work schedule. However, many dialysis patients find it difficult to sleep through the entire therapy because they are anxious about the successful completion of the dialysis procedure.

To assist the dialysant in dealing with feelings of depression, the nurse should get him or her involved in activities with others since expressions of depression often are manifestations of anger about being dependent upon others and about the lack of physical freedom. Card playing, leather tooling, conversation, and watching television in a group are but a few possibilities. To allow the depressed hemodialysis patient to retreat into his or her own world only adds to feelings of anger and subsequent depression. Above all, the nurse must be aware of the possible presence of suicidal ideations so that appropriate therapeutic intervention can be taken. It may be necessary to make a contract with the individual about approaching a member of the health care team whenever feelings of self-harm occur or to place the patient on one-to-one observations. In addition, appropriate members of the health care team (e.g., psychiatric clinical nurse specialist and/or psychiatrist) should be notified so that more intense therapeutic intervention may be instituted.

The third and final stage of adaptation to hemodialysis, the period of long-term adaptation, is characterized by the afflicted person's manifestation of some degree of acceptance of the limitations, shortcomings, and complications of maintenance hemodialysis. Generally the transition between the stage of disenchantment and discouragement and the stage of adaptation is gradual. The stage of long-term adaptation is marked by fluctuations in the afflicted person's sense of psychological and physical well-being. In other words, the individual may experience periods of contentment alternating with periods of depression of varying duration. During both the stages of contentment and depression, the afflicted person's primary defense mechanism is denial. Denial used by these individuals tends to be more extensive than the denial used by patients with other physical illnesses since it appears to serve an effective adaptive function. During periods of depression, denial protects the individual from experiencing even more intense feelings of helplessness while during episodes of contentment it aids in preserving a sense of well-being.

During the stage of long-term adaptation anger may be manifested in the form of verbal expression or noncompliance to medical regimens (e.g., not following dietary restrictions or not taking proper care of the shunt site). However, despite the use of denial and the expression of anger, the hemodialysis patient in the stage of long-term adaptation generally is able to deal with his or her new way of life.

The nurse's role during the stage of adaptation is to assist the afflicted person in dealing with the behavioral manifestations of denial and anger. Since both denial and anger serve a purpose for the hemodialysis patient, the nurse should avoid attempting to remove either one of these protective behavioral mechanisms, but the individual's denial and anger should not be supported by the nurse, the family, or any member of the health care team. Rather, the afflicted individual requires assistance in looking at his or her behavior and rechannelling it to a more socially acceptable mode. For example, if the home dialysis patient feels angry, he or she should be encouraged to become involved in such activities as dusting, vacuuming, typing, or painting instead of verbally chastising others. In the hospital setting such activities as watching an active sports event or doing handicrafts can aid in releasing pent-up feelings of aggression. In addition, family members, the nurse, and other members of the health care team need to be available and willing to listen to the hemodialysis patient verbalize his or her feelings. Even though the afflicted individual may have reached the point of resolving the loss of wellness, he or she continues to require psychological support from others in the form of patience and understanding.

The individual undergoing hemodialysis is not the only person who suffers from the psychological impact of this demanding therapy. The family of the afflicted individual also must contend with the emotional assaults created by hemodialysis. One of the major family changes that occurs when an individual undergoes dialysis is alteration in family structure. When the afflicted person is being maintained on dialysis in the acute care setting, other family members may be required to assume some of the responsibilities that have been carried out in the past by the dialysis patient. If the dialysis patient is a married woman, her husband and children may have to assume more responsibility in keeping the home clean, shopping for groceries, and washing the family clothing. If the dialysis patient is a married man, his wife and children may find it necessary to do such jobs as mowing the lawn, taking the car in for repairs, and contacting a carpenter for necessary household repairs. The jobs assumed by family members, of course, will depend upon which tasks each family member assumed prior to the afflicted individual's illness.

If the afflicted person is maintained on hemodialysis in the home setting, family members will find it necessary to carry out the actual dialysis procedure in addition to assuming some of the family responsibilities previously carried out by the dialysis patient. Clinicians have noted that, in the case of the married dialysis patient, the spouse's role plays a major part in the success or failure of home dialysis therapy. Successful home dialysis tends to be at risk if the spouse is naturally dependent upon the patient-partner (Streltzer, Finkelstein, Feigenbaum, Kitsen, and Cohn, 1976). Although home dialysis offers advantages such as greater flexibility in scheduling time, increased mobility, and a sense of control over the illness, it also places additional demands upon the spouse or family member responsible for carrying out the therapy.

The nurse's role involves assisting the family members to deal with the alterations in family structure that occur as a result of dialysis therapy. Involving the family and the dialysis patient in group and/or family therapy proves beneficial to the patient and family members, encouraging them to share feelings about alterations in their family structure as a result of the illness. Group therapy sessions give the opportunity to explore, along with others having similar problems, ways to cope with family structure alterations. In the case of home dialysis, it is advisable for the nurse to involve as many family members as possible in assisting with the dialysis treatment. Young children can assist by running errands for the parent involved in carrying out the treatment, or by visiting, playing games, or watching T.V. with the parent on the dialysis machine. Older children can be taught the dialysis treatment so that the responsibilities and demands of the therapy are not placed solely upon one family member. The dialysis patient, however, should be informed of the reason for sharing responsibilities so that he or she does not interpret this action as rejection by the spouse or by any other family member. When involving family members in the therapy it must be remembered that guilt can be elicited if the family member feels responsible for the dialysant's progressive deterioration in health status. This is particularly significant in regard to children. Should guilt be elicited, it would be advisable for the nurse to assist the family member in examining his or her guilt feelings in regards to the focus of their guilt, the reality base for the guilt, and what might be done to alter the guilt feelings

Somatic Impact

The individual undergoing hemodialysis suffers several impacts to his or her body image. These somatic impacts include skin discoloration, hair loss, weight fluctuations, the presence of an arteriovenous shunt or an arteriovenous fistula, and the incorporation of the dialysis machine as part of one's self.

Individuals who undergo hemodialysis manifest a characteristic change in skin color as a result of kidney malfunction. The nailbeds and mucous membranes become pale due to anemia, which generally is present. The skin of white individuals takes on a sallow, yellow-brown cast and the skin of blacks becomes darker in color. Both of these alterations are caused by the combination of anemia and of melanin deposits. The color changes are most evident in the exposed areas of the face and hands since light tends to accentuate its presence.

To assist the afflicted person in dealing with the characteristic alterations in skin color, it is beneficial to point out that this somatic alteration is part of the disease process. The individual becomes aware that skin color changes are expected and occur in other individuals afflicted with the same alterations in kidney function. As the individual shares his or her concerns about skin color changes, the nurse can take this opportunity to point out how clothing of certain colors and hues accentuate skin color alterations. The afflicted person may want to experiment with wearing different colors of clothing and avoid those which are unflattering. The light-skinned individual may find that certain shades of yellow and green will accentuate the presence of a sallow, yellow-brown cast while the black-skinned individual may find that dark colors such as navy blue, brown, or black draw attention to the darkened color.

The amount and distribution of hair loss, another alteration in body image, will vary among individuals undergoing hemodialysis. Whether the hair loss is on the head or on the rest of the body, the afflicted individual requires reassurance that the hair will grow back. Some dialysis patients have been known to lose and regrow hair several times over a five-year period. If the hair loss occurs predominantly on the head, the nurse may find it beneficial to suggest a restyling of the hair in an attempt to cover areas of little or no growth. If the hair loss is extensive, the use of a wig or hair piece may be advisable. Should the hair loss occur predominantly on the arms, legs, and chest, the nurse's approach should be governed by the afflicted individual's response to such a loss. For example, the female actually may view hair loss on the legs as an advantage. The male, however, may view hair loss on the chest as a visible loss of masculinity and, as a result, be more comfortable wearing shirts that button up to the collar.

Fluctuation in weight, a third alteration in body image, often occurs as a result of the interplay between the afflicted person's disease process and the dialysis therapy. Between dialysis therapies fluid tends to accumulate in the body due to electrolyte and waste product retention. As the person undergoes hemodialysis, fluid is removed along with the excess electrolytes and waste products with the outcome of weight loss. It is not uncommon for dialysis patients to see their weight loss as a positive secondary gain and some dialysants are concerned only with how much weight they have lost as a result of the therapy.

The presence of an arteriovenous shunt or a subcutaneous arteriovenous (A-V) fistula (two means of access to the bloodstream for hemodialysis) imposes a potential fourth alteration in body image. The arteriovenous shunt is the method in which the arterial system and the venous system are connected by a cannula. The cannula is placed in the nondominant limb so that the cannulated limb can be favored by the individual. If the afflicted individual's work calls for the use of both arms, the nondominant leg is utilized. Should the hemodialysis patient use his or her legs extensively, an arm site may be preferred. The home dialysis patient generally has the shunt site in the leg so that both arms are free for carrying out the dialysis procedure. The presence of an arteriovenous shunt necessitates an external cannula and a bulky dressing. The shunt site requires daily cleansing and the application of a sterile dressing that must be kept on at all times since the most frequent complication resulting from the insertion of an external cannula is wound infection. However, the presence of the visible cannula and dressing can cause the afflicted person to be self-conscious about bodily appearance since it draws attention to the presence of the illness and to the existence of the therapy.

To deal with these feelings, the nurse will find it beneficial to encourage the afflicted person to wear loose-fitting clothing over the cannula site. Women with cannulas in the lower extremity may find it convenient to wear pantsuits while those with cannulas in the upper extremity may find wearing long puff-sleeved blouses or dresses quite appealing. Dealing with the manner of dress in relation to the presence of a cannula may not be as significant a problem for men as it is for women, since men are more accustomed to wearing long-legged trousers and long-sleeved shirts.

The subcutaneous arteriovenous fistula, another method of access to the bloodstream, is a surgically created connection between the arterial system and the venous system. An anastomosis of the cephalic vein and the radial or brachial artery is made to create an opening between a large vein and a large artery. The leakage of arterial blood into the venous system causes the veins to become engorged, thus making it a convenient site for needle insertion. The advantage of the A-V fistula is the lack of need for daily cleansing and bulky dressing since a cannula is not in place; however, venipunctures are necessary for each dialysis treatment.

The role of the nurse in dealing with the presence of the A-V fistula involves assisting the afflicted person to cope with discomfort each time a venipuncture is performed. Encouraging the use of diversional tactics to distract the individual during needle insertion may prove helpful. These diversionary tactics may include the use of self-induced hypnosis, deep-breathing exercises, or simply engaging the individual in conversation.

The incorporation of the dialysis machine as part of one's self is probably the greatest assault that hemodialysis has on the afflicted person's body image. Since the afflicted individual is dependent for life upon the machine, he or she may verbalize the existence of umbilical fantasies. The individual may describe personal dependence upon the machine in the context of a "fetal-placenta" relationship or may allude to the machine as making him or her into an "android" or a "zombie." Apart from feeling controlled by the machine, some dialysis patients may ascribe human qualities to the dialysis machine and actually speak to the machine as if it would respond. To deal with the hemodialysis patient's altered body image, as a result of the controlling and lifelike factors attributed to the dialysis machine, the dialysant needs to be encouraged to describe what meaning the dialysis machine holds for him or her. As the patient relays feelings about the machine, the nurse needs to point out that reactions toward the dialysis machine are not unusual. To cope with feelings related to the dialysis machine, the dialysis patient may find sharing feelings with other dialysants, in a group setting, very beneficial in providing reassurrance that his or her feelings are not unique. If the afflicted person is unable to contend appropriately with feelings about the dialysis machine, psychiatric intervention may be in order.

How the afflicted person copes with each of these somatic impacts is greatly affected by the developmental stage the person is experiencing at the time of dialysis. The hemodialysis patient who is between eighteen and forty-five years of age is in the stage of young adulthood. It is during this time that an individual begins to share oneself with others, both in friendship and in a mutually satisfying sexual relationship (Erikson, 1963). Because of dialysis therapy, the afflicted person may encounter difficulties merging his or her identity with others and, as a result, may develop a sense of isolation. The dialysant may feel unattractive because of hair loss and skin color changes and withdraw from the company of friends and relatives. The dialysant also may view the illness as a deterrent to achievement. Because of the extensive time required for dialysis therapy, the individual may feel incapable of demonstrating an acceptable image and believe that personal goals are unattainable. Unless the dialysant can be made to feel that he or she has something to offer others in friendship and in a mutually satisfying sexual relationship, intimacy will not be attained.

Between the ages of forty-five and sixty-five the individual enters the stage of adulthood. This stage spans the middle years of life. It is during this time that one focuses interest on establishing and guiding future generations (Erikson, 1963). The occurrence of renal alteration and resulting hemodialysis may lead the afflicted individual to feel incapable of guiding and directing future generations. Chronic defeatism and depression can result and the dialysant can retreat into isolation and self-pity. The individual subsequently views the ramifications of the affliction (e.g., skin color changes, hair loss, and time-consuming therapy) as premature old age. As a result, the individual can stagnate and retire to the rocking chair prematurely. Therefore, the dialysant in the stage of adulthood requires assistance in identifying how he or she can be generative.

The final stage of life, the stage of maturity, occurs from sixty-five years of age and over. During this period frequent thoughts of death occur and the individual's satisfaction in life comes from the acceptance of past triumphs and disappointments (Erikson, 1963). The adult's view of self is affected by how he or she feels perceived by others. With the occurrence of kidney malfunction and subsequent hemodialysis, the afflicted adult may question self-value. Thoughts of death often become more prevalent because of the presence of illness and the resulting therapy. Feelings of despair may become frequent. Therefore, the adult in the stage of maturity who is undergoing hemodialysis requires assistance in identifying self-worth.

Sexual Impact

Research has suggested that sexual activity is greatly affected in the individual undergoing hemodialysis. A survey conducted by Levy (1979) showed that hemodialysis patients of both sexes (but especially males) undergo substantial deterioration in sexual functioning. For males, the major sexual alterations are impotence and decreased libido (Jennrich, 1975). Male dialysants have reported as much as a 50 percent decrease in intercourse frequency between the onset of their disease process and the adjustment of maintenance hemodialysis (Bommer, Tschope, Ritz, and Andrassy, 1976). The male on hemodialysis often feels emasculated because of his total dependence on the dialysis machine. Since his wife often becomes the main source of economic support, additional losses in the male dialysant's self-esteem and masculinity occur. As a group, males maintained on hemodialysis tend to fail to resolve their sexual dysfunction problems. In fact, a large percentage of them experience a worsening of sexual functioning. It is likely that both physical and emotional factors play a major part in the cause of sexual dysfunction among male dialysants (Berkman, Katz, and Weissman, 1982; Levy, 1981).

Limited research has been conducted on the sexual dysfunction of the female dialysant. Amenorrhea and a decrease in the frequency of intercourse and orgasm, however, have been noted (Levy, 1973; Levy, 1979). Although some female dialysants have been known to experience an improvement in sexual function while being maintained on hemodialysis, the majority encountered a worsening in sexual functioning. Thus, both male and female dialysants sustain a severe impact to their sexuality as a result of alterations in kidney function and subsequent dialysis therapy.

The nurse's role in dealing with the sexual impact of hemodialysis is to assist the dialysant and sex partner in coping with sexual alterations. One of the most important nursing interventions for dealing with the sexual impact of hemodialysis is to inform the dialysant's sex partner about the possible alterations in sexual function that the dialysant may undergo. Nothing tends to be more devastating to the sexual life of a couple than the lack of information about sexual functioning on the part of one of the partners. In addition, the dialysant and sex partner should be informed about the factors that can contribute to the sexual alteration. For example, extreme tiredness as a result of therapy, the large blocks of time the therapy consumes, feelings of emasculation caused by the dependence upon both the dialysis machine and the spouse, fear of loss of sexual desirability because of hair loss and skin color changes, and fears of dislodgment of the arteriovenous shunt during coitus are but a few possible contributing factors.

To assist the couple in dealing with possible factors contributing to the dialysant's alteration in sexual functioning, the nurse needs to encourage the couple to identify and discuss ways in which they can facilitate the achievement of a mutually satisfying sexual relationship. If physical tiredness following therapy or the amount of time the therapy takes is a problem, the couple may find setting aside a specific time for sexual activity a helpful measure. Although spontaneity may be lost, complete or massive reduction in sexual activity can be prevented. If the male dialysant feels emasculated because of his dependence upon both the dialysis machine and his spouse, efforts should be made to reassure him of his masculinity. For example, encouraging the resumption of employment, maintaining joint decision making with the family structure, and avoiding the mechanical placement of the dialysant in the illness role (e.g., use of night clothes and a bed during dialysis treatment) are but a few possible suggestions. If the female dialysant encounters a decrease in feelings of sexual desirability because of hair loss and skin color changes, attempts should be made to reassure her of sexual desirability. Complimenting her on personal appearance or having her routinely visit a hairdresser are two possible interventions that can facilitate feelings of femininity. If fear of dislodging the arteriovenous shunt during coitus creates difficulties for the couple, the nurse should encourage the dialysant to check cannula connections and dressing secureness prior to engaging in sexual activity. It is advisable to explain how to avoid excessive use or pressure on the cannulated extremity. The dialysant also may find it helpful to avoid coital positions that place the cannulated extremity in a dependent position or that allow the sex partner to lie on the arm or leg.

Occupational Impact

Hemodialysis is an expensive health care regimen costing between $15,000 and $35,000 a year per patient (Levy, 1981). The treatment involves sophisticated equipment, the possible use of a uniquely designed setting, and the utilization of specially prepared personnel. The financial burden of the therapy formerly imposed upon the afflicted person and the family has been decreased significantly as a result of Public Law 92-603, Section 2991, which amended the Social Security Act in 1972. This amendment provides for Medicare coverage for eligible individuals requiring hemodialysis (U.S. Department of Health, Education, and Welfare, 1976). In 1979, congressional action extended further financial support to those persons treated in home dialysis programs. Nevertheless, an alteration in the standard of living may occur for the dialysant and the family as a result of the economic impact imposed by hemodialysis (Campbell and Campbell, 1978). If the dialysant is the breadwinner and is incapable of maintaining full-time employment, other members of the family may find it necessary to seek jobs to supplement the family income. Often jobs secured by other family members do not provide adequate salaries to meet the financial deficit created by the dialysant's decrease or loss of income; and a lowering of the family's standard of living results.

The occupational impact of hemodialysis is influenced by the afflicted person's adjustment to dialysis, the accessibility of home dialysis, and the dialysant's career endeavors. How successfully the individual has adjusted to the therapy is a primary factor affecting employability. The dialysant who has made an adjustment to the psychological and physical demands of the therapy is more likely to maintain employment than the dialysant who is poorly adjusted to the therapy. If activities are planned around the demands of treatment, there will be fewer difficulties in maintaining the dialysant's feelings of self-worth and in adaptation to long-term therapy (Farmer, Bewick, Parsons, and Snowden, 1979).

Another factor affecting the dialysant's employability is the accessibility of home hemodialysis. Since this form of dialysis is carried out in the privacy of one's home, there is conservation of time because the afflicted person does not have to go and come from the dialysis center for therapy. The dialysant can carry out any number of tasks and/or occupational pursuits while undergoing treatment in the privacy of the home. Thus individuals maintained on home hemodialysis have been noted to have higher rates of employment than those maintained on hemodialysis in nonhome settings.

The dialysant's career endeavor is a third factor affecting the occupational impact of hemodialysis. Employment rates tend to be higher for the dialysant in a professional career than for the dialysant engaged in manual labor. This can be attributed to the facts that manual labor often requires extensive use of the extremities and involves intense physical demands. Due to this extensive use of extremities by the manual laborer, the potential for traumatizing a cannulated extremity is great. In addition, because dialysis therapy causes temporary energy depletion, the manual laborer may be unable to meet required levels of productivity of a job with intense physical demands.

To aid the dialysant in contending with the occupational impact of the therapy, the nurse should assist him or her in dealing with the three major factors that affect employability: adjustment to dialysis; accessibility of home hemodialysis; and the dialysant's career endeavor. Since the dialysant's adjustment to the therapy plays a vital role in maintaining occupational pursuits, the nurse needs to assist the individual in working through his or her feelings about the therapy. The reader is advised to consult the sections on the psychological, somatic, and sexual impact of hemodialysis in this chapter for specific nursing interventions.

The accessibility of home hemodialysis, the second factor affecting the occupational impact of hemodialysis, may be a factor over which the nurse has little control. However, the professional nurse can play a major role in aiding both the dialysant and the family in adjusting to home hemodialysis. If the dialysant or the family encounters grave difficulties in dealing with this form of therapy, the dialysant may be forced to resume hemodialysis in the acute care setting. This move could decrease some of the possibilities for his or her maintenance of employment.

The nurse can assume an active part in aiding the dialysant to deal with the third factor affecting employability, the dialysant's career endeavor. The nurse's role involves assisting the dialysant in identifying and carrying out maneuvers that aid in maintaining employability. Since the presence of a cannula (for some dialysants) and excessive fatigue often create problems, the nurse may find it helpful to contact the occupational health nurse, the rehabilitation counselor, the social worker, and/or the occupational therapist for assistance. These specially prepared health team members can contact the dialysant's employer to see if necessary alterations in the work setting or in the dialysant's job responsibilities can be made. For example, jobs that lead to continual contamination of the cannula dressing (e.g., wet environments) often can be altered. Responsibilities that do not demand excessive use of the extremities (if the dialysant requires a cannula) or require excessive physical exertion might be arranged. In addition, the nurse will find it beneficial to discuss with the dialysis patient ways to prevent contamination of the cannula dressing and ways to conserve energy. Covering the cannula dressing with a piece of plastic that is sealed around the edges can aid in decreasing contamination in some settings. Arranging one's schedule and job responsibilities in order to avoid unnecessary trips to and from other locations within the work environment can be accomplished. By having the dialysant identify energy consuming work situations and ways of dealing with each of these situations, the likelihood of the individual's becoming unnecessarily fatigued will be decreased.

If the dialysant is unable to meet the demands of the job, even after initiating the above suggested maneuvers, a change in occupation may be required. Some dialysants have found working from their homes a feasible means of maintaining economic support. In this way rest and home hemodialysis are easily carried out. Jobs that might be performed in the home setting include repairing electronic equipment (i.e., television, radios, stereos), tailoring, maintaining professional office hours, or operating a small business attached to the house. In this case, the dialysant may find it necessary to engage family members in assisting with these forms of employment in order to avoid excessive strain and fatigue. When the means of employment is in the home, it often is easier to involve other family members than if the job were outside the home. Some dialysants, however, may have to undergo retraining in order to maintain a feasible means of employment while others may have to give up career endeavors completely.

Social Impact

One of the most devastating social impacts created by hemodialysis is the restriction placed upon oral intake. The dialysis patient continually is asked to restrict the consumption of certain foods and fluids and thus is unable to eat what he or she likes when desired. Social interactions that revolve around eating and drinking can pose problems for the dialysant unless necessary alterations are made in oral consumption. To assist the dialysis patient in dealing with dietary and fluid restrictions, the nurse needs to encourage the afflicted individual to find ways in which to deal with the imposed alteration in oral gratification. For example, some dialysants find that sucking on ice cubes, instead of drinking water, aids in decreasing the sensation of thirst and in decreasing the frustrations of fluid restriction. The dialysant, however, must account for the amount of water in the ice cubes when computing the total daily fluid intake. When dealing with food restriction, the dialysant should be encouraged to select favorite allowed foods while still consuming a balanced diet. Serving the food in an attractive way aids in palatability which, in turn, helps deal with the frustration resulting from required food restrictions. The nurse will find the dietician an invaluable colleague for providing guidance and assistance in selecting and preparing appropriate foods for the individual on dialysis.

If the dialysant plans to attend social functions involving food and drink, he or she can be instructed how to select from a menu or a hostess' table those items that are within diet restrictions. The dialysant should be advised to include the amount of fluid and type of food he or she wished to allot for the social function when planning and spacing the total twenty-four hour intake. Above all, the nurse and the family need to be understanding and supportive of the dialysant by providing positive reinforcement when attempts are made at maintaining food and fluid restrictions.

Travel often is restricted since the dialysant's mobility is greatly decreased because of the need to be close to a dialysis machine. Therefore, some patients have been known to travel in groups to other dialysis centers within and outside the United States. These trips are planned by organizations such as the National Association of Patients on Hemodialysis and Transplants. Medical problems and scheduling difficulties, however, often impede travel on the part of the dialysis patient since treatment units in the United States may be filled to capacity and unable to accept guest patients while overseas centers may be extremely expensive or closed to visitors. As a result, some dialysants have resorted to a compact travel hemodialysis system which can easily be transported by the patient to a hotel or motel room.

Although travel may be restricted for dialysis patients, these individuals need encouragement to continue interacting with family and friends. Research has shown that the dialysant often demonstrates a decrease in interest and in participation in both family and social activities (De-Nour, 1982). Lack of social contact often leads to feelings of frustration and depression which, in turn, impede the dialysant's adjustment to the necessary long-term therapy. The nurse needs to encourage the dialysant and the family to plan social and family activities that are not exhausting and that do not occur immediately after therapy since this is a time of extreme fatigue. The type of activities selected will vary among dialysants since each afflicted person's activity tolerance, personal motivation, and interest area differ.

SUMMARY

As a result of the malfunction of their kidneys, approximately 35,000 Americans are maintained on hemodialysis, 15 percent of whom are dialyzed in their homes. Dialysis is the passage of particles from an area of high concentration to an area of low concentration across a semipermeable membrane. The basic goals of hemodialysis are to remove end products of protein metabolism from the blood, to maintain a safe concentration of serum electrolytes, to correct acidosis and replenish the blood's bicarbonate system, and to remove excess fluid from the blood.

As a result of the afflicted person's dependence for life upon the dialysis machine, impacts are created upon his or her psychological well-being, somatic identity, sexuality, occupational identity, and social role. Thus, the nurse must assist the individual undergoing hemodialysis to deal, to the best of his or her ability, with each of these impacts.

Patient Situation   Dr. H. D., a thirty-seven-year-old white college professor, who is married and the mother of two children, ages fourteen years and ten years, has been undergoing hemodialysis for the past six months. The D.'s have decided that in the family's best interest it would be advisable for Dr. H. D. to be maintained on home hemodialysis. As a result, the D's are undergoing a home hemodialysis orientation program. During the orientation program the nurse in charge identified problems related to Dr. H. D.'s psychological well-being, somatic identity, sexuality, occupational identity, and social role.

Following are Dr. H. D.'s nursing care plan and patient care cardex dealing with each of these areas of concern.

NURSING CARE PLAN

Nursing Diagnoses	Objectives	Nursing Interventions	Principles/Rationale	Evaluations
Psychological Impact Unresolved dependence/independence conflict manifested by the expectation that husband and children should wait on her.	To assist Dr. H. D. in dealing with her dependence/independence conflict.	Point out to Dr. H. D. that the reality of her illness requires dependence upon the dialysis machine and family members for carrying out the dialysis therapy. Point out behaviors that are unacceptable manifestations of dependence (e.g., demanding behavior and verbal abuse).	Informing the dialysant of acceptable and unacceptable forms of dependence regarding dialysis therapy can aid in decreasing unacceptable demonstrations of dependence.	The nurse would observe for: Dr. H. D.'s decreased manifestation of unacceptable forms of dependence.
		Encourage Dr. H. D. to look at her behavior when she utilizes unacceptable manifestations of dependence (e.g., demanding behavior).	Having the dialysant examine personal behavior aids in the development of insight.	
	To foster independence in Dr. H. D.	Encourage Dr. H. D. to take an active part in her therapy (e.g., planning diet and fluid restrictions).	Active participation in one's own care aids in fostering independence.	Dr. H. D.'s increased demonstration of independence.
		Encourage Dr. H. D.'s family to provide positive feedback to Dr. H. D. each time she assumes more independence.	Positive feedback regarding improved behavior aids in building the dialysant's self-esteem.	

Somatic Impact		Nursing Intervention	Rationale	Evaluation
Somatic Impact Alteration in body image manifested by expressed concern about personal appearance because of her sallow, yellow-brown skin and the presence of a cannula in her leg.	To assist Dr. H. D. to cope with her altered body image.	Encourage Dr. H. D. to wear street clothes and to sit in a comfortable recliner when carrying out dialysis therapy. Encourage Dr. H. D. to become involved in activities during her dialysis therapy (e.g., reading, grading papers, preparing lectures). Point out to Dr. H. D. that her skin color changes are a part of the disease process.	Avoiding the use of night clothes and a bed during dialysis therapy aids in preventing the mechanical placement of the dialysant in the dependent role of illness. Activity during dialysis therapy aids in fostering independence. Realizing that certain alterations in body image are expected as a result of the disease process aids in decreasing anxiety related to their occurrence.	The nurse would observe for: Dr. H. D.'s verbalization about how she views herself and how she plans to deal with her altered bodily appearance.
	To enhance Dr. H. D.'s feelings of self-worth.	Encourage Dr. H. D. to select clothing colors that do not accentuate her skin color changes (e.g., avoid certain shades of yellow and green). Encourage Dr. H. D. to wear loose-fitting clothing over the cannula (e.g., pantsuits). Encourage Dr. H. D. to inspect routinely the shunt site and carry out daily dressing changes.	Feeling attractive to one's self and to others facilitates feelings of self-worth. Maintaining good care of the shunt site aids in preventing further alterations in body image caused by the breakdown of the shunt site.	Dr. H. D.'s verbalization of how she will alter her clothing style and colors to avoid accentuating her altered body image.

(cont.)

317

NURSING CARE PLAN (cont.)

Nursing Diagnoses	Objectives	Nursing Interventions	Principles/Rationale	Evaluations
Sexual Impact Sexual dysfunction manifested by expressed concern about decreased libido.	To facilitate a healthy and mutually satisfying sexual relationship between the D.'s.	Inform Mr. D. that a decrease in libido is not an uncommon occurrence for individuals maintained on hemodialysis.	Spouses aware of the possible existence of sexual alterations occurring in their partners are more likely to be understanding of their partner's problem and are likely to feel less frustrated with the situation.	The nurse would observe for: Dr. H. D.'s verbalization of an increased satisfaction in her sexual relationship with her husband.
		Inform the D.'s of the possible factors that can contribute to the sexual alteration (e.g., tiredness, time consumed by the dialysis therapy, and fears of loss of sexual desirability as a result of skin color changes and the presence of the arteriovenous shunt).	Being aware of factors that can contribute to a sexual alteration aids in assisting the couple in identifying possible ways of coping with the alteration.	
		Encourage the D.'s to discuss and identify ways in which they can facilitate the achievement of a mutually satisfying sexual relationship (e.g., setting aside a specific time for sexual activity, having Mr. D. reassure Dr. H. D. of her sexual desirability, and carrying out maneuvers that aid in preventing dislodgment or pressure on the cannula).	Couples who work together to identify ways to improve their sex life are more likely to achieve mutual satisfaction.	
Occupational Impact Potential job management deficit manifested by expressed concern about being unable to maintain	To decrease Dr. H. D.'s concern about being incapacitated as a result of her hemodialysis.	Point out to Dr. H. D. that dialysants on home hemodialysis tend to report a higher rate of employment than dialysants maintained on acute care setting dialysis.	Knowing the incidence of employability among dialysants aids in decreasing the afflicted individual's anxiety about job maintainence.	The nurse would observe for: Dr. H. D.'s verbalization about possible ways to alter her work situation so that she can maintain her teaching responsibilities.

318

Problem / Goal	Nursing Interventions	Rationale	Evaluation
	Encourage Dr. H. D. to plan job-related activities around her therapy and to carry out certain job responsibilities while on dialysis (e.g., reading, computing grades, and writing student evaluations). Consult with the occupational health nurse, the rehabilitation counselor, the social worker, and/or the occupational therapist.	Dialysants who learn to plan their life's activities around the demands of their therapy encounter fewer difficulties in maintaining employment. Health team members specially prepared to deal with the occupational impacts of dialysis are in a position to contact the dialysant's employer to see if necessary alterations in the work setting or in the dialysant's job responsibilities can be made.	Dr. H. D.'s verbalization that with alterations she feels she will be able to maintain her teaching activities.
Social Impact Potential social isolation manifested by expressed concern about being unable to entertain colleagues and business associates in her home. To decrease Dr. H. D.'s concern about being unable to socialize. To prevent Dr. H. D.'s withdrawal from social contacts.	Encourage Dr. H. D. to think of ways to incorporate her daily food and fluid restrictions into a home social function. Encourage Dr. H. D. to serve her food in an attractive way. Encourage Dr. H. D.'s family to be supportive of her as she attempts to carry out food and fluid restrictions when in a social setting.	Actually involving the dialysant in planning social activities aids in decreasing the chances of withdrawal from social contacts. Attractively prepared food aids in palatibility and, in turn, decreases frustration resulting from food restrictions. Positive reinforcement for a job well done in the social setting aids in increasing the dialysant's feelings of self-worth and aids in preventing the individual from withdrawing from social interactions.	The nurse would observe for: Dr. H. D.'s verbalization about how she plans to carry out social entertaining in her home and at the same time incorporate her food and fluid restrictions.

PATIENT CARE CARDEX

PATIENT'S NAME: ___Dr. H. D.___

AGE: ___37 years___

MARITAL STATUS: ___Married___

SIGNIFICANT OTHERS: ___Husband and two children___

___(14 years and 10 years)___

MEDICAL DIAGNOSIS: ___Chronic renal failure___

SEX: ___Female___

OCCUPATION: ___College professor___

Nursing Diagnoses

Psychological: Unresolved dependence/independence conflict manifested by the expectation that husband and children should wait on her.

Nursing Approaches

1. Point out that the reality of the illness requires dependence upon the dialysis machine and family members for carrying out the therapy.
2. Point out behavior that is an unacceptable manifestation of dependence (e.g., demanding behavior).
3. Encourage to look at behavior when utilizing unacceptable manifestations of dependence.
4. Encourage family members to provide positive feedback each time more independence is assumed.
5. Encourage to wear street clothes and to sit in a comfortable recliner when carrying out dialysis therapy.
6. Encourage to become involved in activities during dialysis therapy (e.g., reading, grading papers, preparing lectures).

Somatic: Alteration in body image manifested by expressed concern about personal appearance because of her sallow, yellow-brown skin and the presence of a cannula in her leg.

1. Point out that skin color changes are a part of the disease process.
2. Encourage to select clothing colors that do not accentuate skin color changes (e.g., avoid certain shades of yellow and green).
3. Encourage to wear loose-fitting clothing over the cannula.
4. Encourage to inspect routinely the shunt site and carry out daily dressing changes.

Sexual: Sexual dysfunction manifested by expressed concern about decreased libido.

1. Inform husband that decreased libido is not an uncommon occurrence for individuals maintained on hemodialysis.
2. Inform both partners of the possible factors that can contribute to sexual alterations (e.g., tiredness or fears of loss of sexual desirability).
3. Encourage both partners to discuss and identify with each other ways in which they can facilitate the achievement of a mutually satisfying sexual relationship (e.g., setting aside a specific time for sexual activity).

Occupational: Potential job management deficit manifested by expressed concern about being unable to maintain teaching responsibilities.

1. Point out that dialysants on home dialysis tend to maintain a higher rate of employment than dialysants maintained on acute care dialysis.
2. Encourage to plan job-related activities around therapy and to carry out job-related activities during therapy.
3. Consult with the occupational health nurse, the rehabilitation counselor, the social worker, and/or the occupational therapist.

Social: Potential social isolation manifested by expressed concern about being unable to entertain colleagues and business associates in her home.

1. Encourage to think of ways to incorporate daily food and fluid restrictions into the home social function.
2. Encourage to serve food in an attractive way.
3. Encourage family to be supportive during attempts to carry out fluid and food restrictions when in a social setting.

REFERENCES

ABEL, J., RAWNTREE, L., and TURNER, B. The removal of diffusible substances from the circulating blood by means of dialysis, *Transactions of the Association of American Physicians,* 1913, *28,* 51–54.

ABRAM, J., MOORE, G., and WESTERFELT, G. Suicidal behavior in chronic dialysis patients, *American Journal of Psychiatry,* 1971, *127* (9), 1199–1204.

BERKMAN, A., KATZ, L., and WEISSMAN, R. Sexuality and the life-style of home dialysis patients, *Archives and Physical Medicine and Rehabilitation,* 1982, *63* (6), 272–275.

BOMMER, J., TSCHOPE, W., RITZ, E., and ANDRASSY, K. Sexual behavior of hemodialyzed patients, *Clinical Nephrology,* 1976, *6* (1), 315–318.

CAMPBELL, J., and CAMPBELL, A. The social and economic cost of end-stage renal disease: A patient's perspective, *New England Journal of Medicine,* 1978, *299* (8), 386–392.

DE-NOUR, A. Social adjustment of chronic dialysis patients, *American Journal of Psychiatry,* 1982, *139* (1), 97–100.

ERIKSON, E. *Childhood and society.* New York: W.W. Norton and Co., Inc., 1963.

FARMER, C., BEWICK M., PARSONS, V., and SNOWDEN, A. Survival on home haemodialysis: its relationship with physical symptomatology, psychosocial background and psychiatric morbidity, *Psychological Medicine,* 1979, *9* (3), 515–523.

JENNRICH, J. Some aspects of the nursing care for patients on hemodialysis, *Heart and Lung,* 1975, *4* (6), 885–889.

LEVY, N. Psychological reactions to machine dependency: Hemodialysis, *Psychiatric Clinics of North America,* 1981, *4* (2), 351–363.

LEVY, N. Sexual adjustment to maintenance hemodialysis and renal transplantation: national survey by questionnaire: preliminary report, *Transactions of the American Society for Artificial Internal Organs,* 1973, *19,* 138–143.

LEVY, N. The sexual rehabilitation of the hemodialysis patient, *Sexuality and Disability,* 1979, *2,* 60–68.

MILLER, P. Problems of the urinary system. In W. Phipps, B. Long, and N. Woods (Eds.), *Medical-surgical nursing: concepts and clinical practice.* St. Louis: C.V. Mosby, 1983.

RAJAPAKSA, T. Maintenance hemodialysis: how to help patients cope, *Medical Times,* 1979, *107* (10), 86–88, 91–92.

REICHSMAN, F., and LEVY, N. Problems in adaptation to maintenance hemodialysis, *Archives of Internal Medicine,* 1972, *130* (12), 859–865.

STRELTZER, J., FINKELSTEIN, F., FEIGENBAUM, H., KITSEN, J., and COHN, G. The spouse's role in home hemodialysis, *Archives of General Psychiatry,* 1976, *33* (1), 55–58.

U.S. DEPARTMENT OF HEALTH, EDUCATION AND WELFARE. Living with end-stage renal disease. Washington, D.C.: Public Health Service. (Health Services Administration. Bureau of Quality Assurance.) U.S. Government Printing Office, 1976.

WINEMAN, R. End-stage renal disease, *Dialysis and Transplantation,* 1978, *7,* 1034–1047, 1064.

INDEX